Polycystic Ovary Syndrome

Polycystic Ovary Syndrome

Editor: Margaret Booth

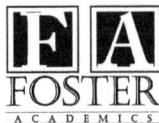

FOSTER
ACADEMICS

www.fosteracademics.com

www.fosteracademics.com

FA
FOSTER
ACADEMICS

Cataloging-in-Publication Data

Polycystic ovary syndrome / edited by Margaret Booth.
    p. cm.
Includes bibliographical references and index.
ISBN 978-1-63242-663-5
1. Polycystic ovary syndrome. 2. Ovaries--Cysts. 3. Ovaries--Diseases.
4. Syndromes. I. Booth, Margaret.
RG480.S7 P65 2019
618.1--dc23

Foster Academics,
118-35 Queens Blvd., Suite 400,
Forest Hills, NY 11375, USA

ISBN 978-1-63242-663-5 (Hardback)

Contents

Preface

The increase in androgens levels in women results in heavy periods or no menstrual periods, pelvic pain, excess facial and body hair, difficulty in getting pregnant, acne, etc. This set of symptoms may be termed as polycystic ovary syndrome (PCOS) and affects between 2-20% of women between the ages of 18 and 44. Some of the conditions associated with PCOS are obesity, Type 2 diabetes, obstructive sleep apnea, mood disorders, heart disease, etc. It occurs due to genetic and environmental factors. It is diagnosed through an ultrasound based on high androgen levels, presence of ovarian cysts and lack of ovulation. PCOS has no known cure, but can be treated with certain lifestyle changes such as exercise and weight loss. This book is compiled in such a manner, that it will provide in-depth knowledge about polycystic ovary syndrome. The topics covered in this extensive book deal with the core aspects of the causative factors and consequences of polycystic ovary syndrome as well as the interventions aimed at its management. It will help the readers in keeping pace with the rapid changes in this field.

The information shared in this book is based on empirical researches made by veterans in this field of study. The elaborative information provided in this book will help the readers further their scope of knowledge leading to advancements in this field.

Finally, I would like to thank my fellow researchers who gave constructive feedback and my family members who supported me at every step of my research.

Editor

Association between circulating adiponectin levels and polycystic ovarian syndrome

Saira Saeed Mirza[1], Kashif Shafique[2,3*], Abdul Rauf Shaikh[4], Naveed Ali Khan[5] and Masood Anwar Qureshi[6]

Abstract

Background: Low adiponectin levels in polycystic ovarian syndrome (PCOS) have been largely attributed to obesity which is common among these patients. In addition, evidence also suggests that low adiponectin in PCOS may be related to insulin resistance (IR) in these women. However, studies on the role of adiponectin in younger and lean patients are limited. Therefore, the aim of the present study was to examine the association of adiponectin levels in young and lean women with PCOS.

Methods: A case–control study was conducted at the Dow University of Health Sciences, Karachi, Pakistan. Cases were 75 patients of PCOS with Body Mass Index (BMI) <23 aged 16–35 years and 75 healthy age and BMI matched controls were selected from family and friends of the cases. Demographic details, family history and past medical history were obtained through interview by a physician. Anthropometric measurements included weight and height of the participants. Fasting glucose, total cholesterol, high-density lipoprotein (HDL), insulin, adiponectin, and androgen levels were determined. IR was calculated using homeostasis model assessment for insulin resistance (HOMA-IR). Logistic regression models were used to assess the association between adiponectin and PCOS after adjusting for co-variates.

Results: On multivariable analysis, PCOS cases were 3.2 times more likely to have low adiponectin level (OR = 3.2, 95% CI 1.49-6.90, p-value 0.003) compared to the controls after adjustment for age, BMI, family history, marital status, total cholesterol, HDL level and IR. Females with a family history of PCOS were significantly more likely to have lower adiponectin (OR = 3.32, 95% CI 1.27-8.67, p-value 0.014) compared to those who did not have a family history of PCOS. The associations of IR and family history with low adiponectin level also remained statistically significant after adjustments for covariates.

Conclusion: Serum adiponectin levels are independently associated with PCOS and are only partly explained by IR. Adiponectin level may serve as a potential independent biomarker for diagnosis of PCOS in young and lean women with fewer symptoms, or women with a family history of PCOS.

Introduction

The polycystic ovarian syndrome (PCOS) is the most common endocrine disorder affecting reproductive age women worldwide [1]. Clinical features of PCOS namely hirsutism, acne, and alopecia originate from high circulating levels of androgens, menstrual irregularities from anovulatory cycles [2], and obesity is thought to originate from both the underlying IR [1] and high androgen levels in these patients [3]. The alarming tribulations associated with the syndrome are past the reproductive axis and these women are at a greater risk of developing the metabolic syndrome at an early age because of IR and obesity [4-6] observed in 30-60% of PCOS patients [7].

In recent years, role of adipose tissue hormones, particularly adiponectin has been implicated in the pathogenesis of PCOS [8,9]. Adiponectin has antiatherogenic, anti-diabetic, anti-inflammatory and insulin sensitizing effects, and is negatively related to the degree of adiposity in healthy individuals [10]. Despite being an adipokine, low levels of adiponectin have been found more closely related to the degree of IR than adiposity itself [11]. Studies have also shown that both insulin action and circulating levels of adiponectin are lower in women with PCOS [12].

* Correspondence: Kashif.shafique@glasgow.ac.uk
[2]Institute of Health and Wellbeing, University of Glasgow, 1-Lilybank Gardens, G12 8RZ Glasgow, UK
[3]School of Public Health, Dow University of Health Sciences, Karachi, Pakistan
Full list of author information is available at the end of the article

There are some variations in age at presentation of PCOS between different countries. Furthermore, its typical features like a combination of obesity, hirsutism, acne, alopecia, and irregular menstruation [13] are absent in many women whereas patients manifest with PCOS at a younger age, and without any significant history of its symptoms. Also, obesity and symptoms of hyperandrogenism are also lower in those patients who are lean and presenting a younger age [13].

Although low adiponectin levels have been associated with PCOS which is mainly attributed to obesity among these patients, studies have also suggested that low adiponectin in PCOS may be related to IR in these women. However, the role of adiponectin in younger and lean patients has been examined only in few studies. In these women, it is not certain that to what extent, the IR determines the levels of adiponectin. If adiponectin levels in younger and lean women provide similar association with PCOS as in obese patients, the level of adiponectin may be a useful proxy measure of an ongoing ovarian disease in women with atypical presentation of PCOS. Therefore, we examined the association of adiponectin levels with PCOS in younger and lean women.

Methods
Selection of cases
We recruited 75 newly diagnosed PCOS patients aged between 16–35 years with desirable BMI, from the outpatient departments of Gynecology units of two public sector hospitals Civil hospital Karachiand Lady Dufferin hospital, Karachi, Pakistan. Desirable BMI was defined as BMI < 23 according to the Asian reference values for BMI [14]. PCOS was diagnosed using the Rotterdam Criteria [15] which states that PCOS is diagnosed if patient have any two of the following three features, 1) oligo/amenorrhea and/or anovulation, 2) hyperandrogenism and/or hyperandrogenemia, and 3) polycystic ovaries on ultrasound after exclusion of other etiologies. Oligomenorrhea was defined as infrequent menstruation or less than 9 menstrual periods per year. Amenorrhea was defined as absence or abnormal cessation of menses for three months or more [15]. For diagnostic purposes, since we recruited already diagnosed patients of PCOS, presence of either clinical hyperandrogenism or biochemical hyperandrogenemia was considered acceptable, whichever used by the diagnosing gynecologist. Hyperandrogenism was defined as a score of 7 or more on the Ferriman Gallaway index, or apparent severe hirsutism, acne and alopecia [2].

We did not include pregnant PCOS patients. In addition, patients with type 2 diabetes mellitus, chronic liver disease, thyroid dysfunction, and using medications such as steroids, contraceptives, hypoglycemic/antidiabetic drugs were not included in the study.

Selection of controls
Controls were 75 age-matched healthy females with regular menstrual cycle from family and friends of the cases. Controls also had BMI within desirable range. Females taking medication, including steroids and contraceptives were not included.

Demographic information, detailed menstrual and reproductive history, family history of menstrual or reproductive problems, past medical history, and anthropometric profile were recorded. Fasting blood samples were drawn from all participants for assessment of blood glucose, lipid profile, adiponectin, insulin and androgen levels. Fasting serum adiponectin was estimated using the Bio-Rad PR 3100 which uses Enzyme Linked ImmunoSorbent Assay (ELISA) technique of quantitative hormone estimation. Adiponectin was categorized using the median value of the sample, 13.0 μU/ml.

Written informed consent was obtained from all study participants. The study was approved by the Ethics Committee/Institutional Review Board (IRB), Dow University of Health Sciences.

Covariates
Age, marital status, family history of PCOS, BMI, IR, total blood cholesterol level and HDL were used as covariates. Age was categorized into 5-year age groups. For marital status, women were grouped into married and unmarried. Family history was inquired during the interview. Participants were asked questions about the presence/history of the following complaints in their first degree (mother and/or sisters), and/or second degree (aunts and/or cousins) relatives:

1. History of PCOS
2. History of any menstrual problems
3. Problems in conception
4. Excess facial hair, baldness, and/or acne resistant to treatment

From the last three questions, presence of any two, was also considered as a positive history of PCOS, and finally participants were categorized as having a negative or a positive family history of PCOS.

BMI was calculated using the standard formula. IR was calculated using HOMA-IR [16]. HOMA-IR calculates the IR by dividing the product of fasting blood glucose level (mg/dl) and serum insulin level (μU/ml) by a constant, i.e. 405. A HOMA-IR value of 2.5 or above were considered as insulin resistant [16]. Fasting blood glucose was estimated using the automatic biochemical analyzer (Hitachi 902) which uses the photometric technique of glucose estimation. Fasting serum insulin was estimated, using IMMULITE 1000 analyzer which is a solid-phase, two site chemiluminescentimmunometric assay. Lipid profile, (total serum cholesterol and HDL were the parameters of interest) was done by enzymatic calorimetric test. We measured free serum testosterone in fasting state; hyperandrogenemia was defined as free serum testosterone levels higher than 100 ng/ml [17].

Statistical analysis

Data were analyzed using the STATA Software Version 12 (StataCorp, College Station, TX, USA). Results are presented as means and standard deviations. Threshold for statistical significance was set at p < 0.05. Socio-demographic and other biochemical measures were compared between cases and control using the independent sample t-test and chi-squared test for continuous and categorical variables, respectively. To analyze the association between study variables, adiponectin was used as the dependent variable and age, marital status, family history of PCOS, BMI, total cholesterol, HDL and IR were used as independent variables in logistic regression models. To assess the association between adiponectin with PCOS, both univariable and multivariable models were used. Multivariable regression model included age, marital status, family history of PCOS, BMI, total cholesterol, HDL, and IR as co-variates.

Results

A total of 150 individuals participated in this study, of which 75 were diagnosed PCOS cases and 75 controls. The mean age of sample was 25.6 (SD 6.12), with no statistically significant difference between cases and controls (p-value 0.76). The majority of participants were married (n = 80, 53.3%), with no significant difference in distribution of married individuals between cases and controls (p-value 0.33). Furthermore, there was no significant difference in total cholesterol (p-value 0.72), HDL (p-value 0.19) and family history of PCOS among cases and controls (p-value 0.08). However, there were significant differences in BMI and adiponectin level between cases and controls. PCOS Cases had significantly higher BMI (mean difference 0.97, p-value .02) and lower adiponectin level (mean difference 5.73, p-value <0.001). The demographic and other characteristics of study sample are described in Table 1.

Univariable analysis to assess the association between PCOS and adiponectin level (adiponectin ≤13.0), revealed that cases were 2.7 times more likely (OR = 2.67, 95% CI 1.38-5.16, p-value 0.004) to have lower adiponectin compared to controls. Females with a family history of PCOS were significantly more likely to have to lower adiponectin (OR = 3.11, 95% CI 1.33-7.26, p-value 0.009) compared to those who did not have a family history of PCOS (Table 2). IR also showed a statistically significant negative association with low adiponectin (p-value 0.001). Other factors including age, BMI, marital status, total cholesterol level and HDL did not show statistically significant association with adiponectin (Table 2).

Table 1 Socio-demographic and biochemical characteristics of PCOS cases and controls

Characteristics	Cases		Controls		P-value
	n	(%)*	n	(%)*	
Total participants	75	(50.0)	75	(50.0)	
Age, mean(SD)	25.7	(6.0)	25.4	(6.3)	0.76
Age, categorical					
16-20	17	(22.7)	19	(25.3)	0.98
21-25	22	(29.3)	22	(29.3)	
26-30	12	(16.0)	11	(14.7)	
31-35	24	(32.0)	23	(30.7)	
Marital status					
Unmarried	38	(50.7)	32	(42.7)	0.33
Married	37	(49.3)	43	(57.3)	
Family history of PCOS					
No	63	(84.0)	54	(72.0)	0.08
Yes	12	(16.0)	21	(28.0)	
Body mass index, mean (SD)	19.3	(2.6)	18.3	(2.4)	0.02
Total cholesterol					
<6.2	68	(90.7)	69	(92.0)	0.72
≥6.2	7	(9.3)	6	(8.0)	
High density lipoprotein					
<1.29	35	(46.7)	43	(57.3)	0.19
≥1.29	40	(53.3)	32	(42.7)	
Insulin resistance	3.1	(2.1)	2.9	(2.7)	0.73
Adiponectin level, mean (SD)	12.4	(2.7)	18.2	(7.8)	<0.01
Adiponectin level, categorical					
≤13.0	27	(36.0)	45	(60.0)	<0.01
>13.0	48	(64.0)	30	(40.0)	

*n and percentages are mentioned until stated otherwise.

On multivariable analysis, the overall findings of univariable analysis remained consistent. PCOS cases were 3.2 times more likely to have low adiponectin level (OR = 3.2, 95% CI 1.49-6.90, p-value 0.003) compared to controls after adjustment for age, BMI, family history, marital status, total cholesterol level, HDL and IR. The associations of IR and family history with low adiponectin level also remained statistically significant after adjustments for covariates (Table 2).

A stratified analysis was also carried out based on age categories (≤25 years and >25 years) to assess the association of low adiponectin with PCOS. PCOS cases of age ≤25 years were 2.5 times more likely to have low adiponectin while cases of age >25 years were 2.9 times more likely to have low adiponectin, compared to their respective control groups (Figure 1). These associations changed slightly and remained statistically significant after adjustment for age, BMI, family history, marital status, total cholesterol level, HDL level and IR (Figure 1).

Table 2 The relationship of PCOS and other characteristics of low adiponectin level

Characteristics	Univariate analysis		P-value	Multivariate analysis		P-value
	Odds ratio	(95% CI)		Odds ratio	(95% CI)	
PCOS status						
Controls	1			1		
Cases	2.67	(1.38-5.16)	0.004	3.20	(1.49-6.90)	0.003
Age, categorical						
16-20	1			1		
21-25	0.54	(0.22-1.32)	0.179	0.53	(0.19-1.43)	0.207
26-30	1.34	(0.45-3.96)	0.597	0.92	(0.17-4.89)	0.924
31-35	0.68	0.29-1.64)	0.396	0.57	(0.12-2.71)	0.479
Marital status						
Unmarried	1			1		0.928
Married	0.94	(0.49-1.78)	0.844	1.06	(0.27-4.13)	
Family history of PCOS						
No	1			1		0.014
Yes	3.11	(1.33-7.26)	0.009	3.32	(1.27-8.67)	
Body mass index, mean (SD)	1.09	(0.96-1.24)	0.163	0.97	(0.84-1.13)	0.721
Total cholesterol						
<6.2	1			1		0.268
≥6.2	1.53	(0.47-4.92)	0.474	2.06	(0.57-7.40)	
High density lipoprotein						
<1.29	1			1		0.482
≥1.29	1.63	(0.86-3.12)	0.137	1.30	(0.63-2.69)	
Insulin resistance	1.29	(1.11-1.52)	0.001	1.23	(1.03-1.47)	0.023

Multivariate model include all covariates presented in this table.

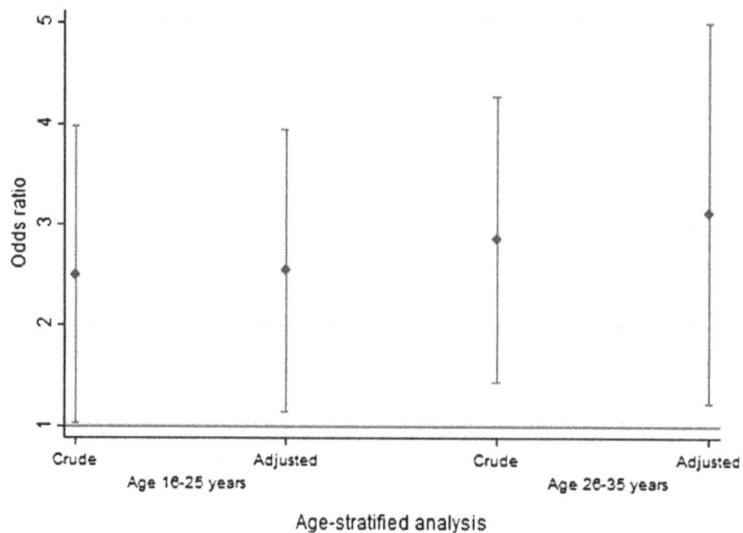

Figure 1 Age-specific relationship between PCOS and adiponectin level. Adjusted odds ratio are estimated after accounting for BMI, family history of PCOS, marital status, total cholesterol level, high density lipoprotein level and insulin resistance.

Discussion

Our findings suggest that PCOS women with a desirable BMI are significantly more likely to have low serum adiponectin levels. The association of PCOS with low adiponectin level remained consistent and statistically significant after adjustment for age, BMI, family history of PCOS, marital status, total cholesterol level, HDL and IR. This relationship between PCOS and low adiponectin also changed a little across different age groups. Furthermore, family histories of PCOS and IR were also significantly associated with lower adiponectin levels. We found low levels of adiponectin in lean young women with PCOS. Several studies have demonstrated reduced levels of serum adiponectin in women with PCOS [12,18-23]. Also, few of them have shown an association of low adiponectin levels in PCOS women irrespective of the weight and/or BMI of patients [12,18,20-22].

A systematic review and meta-analysis by Toulis et al., on a sub-analysis by using studies only with PCOS cases and controls matched on BMI, revealed that PCOS women had lower levels of adiponectin after controlling for the potential effects of obesity by BMI matching. This suggests that serum adiponectin levels are not independently determined by the degree of adiposity in women but underlying disease may also have some role. A possible explanation for this finding is that lower adiponectin levels in PCOS women might be a result of increasing IR in these patients [1] as supported by our study. As adiponectin is known to possess insulin-sensitizing, anti-diabetic properties and reduced circulating levels are also observed in type 2 diabetes mellitus [24], IR might possibly be a link between lower adiponectin level and development of polycystic ovarian syndrome; however, whether low adiponectin is a cause or a consequence of IR in PCOS remains debated. In addition, it has been observed in randomized controlled trials that treatment of PCOS patients with anti-diabetic medication as metformin [25,26], rosiglitazone [27], and pioglitazone [28], in addition to reductions in secretion of insulin and improvement in its action on glucose metabolism, also increases the adiponectin levels in circulation. However, in multivariable analysis, we observed lower adiponectin levels in women with PCOS, after adjusting for all possible confounders stated, including IR. Stratified analysis (data not shown) based on IR also showed a lower adiponectin level in PCOS women, suggesting that adiponectin levels in these women are regulated by certain unexplained factors other than IR. It could be possible that genetically predisposed women to PCOS might exhibit a lower secretion of adiponectin which may lead to other features/symptoms of PCOS with time.

We have also found an association of family history of PCOS and IR with lower adiponectin levels in PCOS women. Increasing evidence suggests that genetic factors play an important role in the pathogenesis of PCOS. Interestingly, prevalence of PCOS in South East Asians settled in United Kingdom was 52%, which is an 18% higher rate than the native population, suggestive of some genetic predisposition of PCOS among certain races [29]. In addition to familial clustering of PCOS in first degree relatives [30], it has been shown that the pre-pubertal daughters with normal BMI, of women with PCOS, manifest with disturbed metabolic profile including hypoadiponectenemia and hyperinsulinemia compared to daughters of healthy women [31]. In our study, controls were recruited from the family and friends of the cases. Cases and controls did not differ significantly regarding the history of PCOS. This might be argued that as history of PCOS is strongly related to the incidence of PCOS, however, it is not necessary that persons having PCOS always have a history of PCOS. This points towards the hypothesis that, although family history is an important risk factor, environmental triggers are also playing a role, e.g. diet, and exercise. In addition, PCOS is a syndrome and a polygenic causality cannot be ruled out. Dysfunctional changes in the metabolism of carbohydrates, insulin action, and steroid hormones have also been implicated. Therefore, a similar family history of PCOS can be explained as being one of the many contributory factors that cause PCOS, and a similarity of family history in cases and controls is not contradictory.

We found significantly lower levels of adiponectin in PCOS patients <25 years of age. It is possible that the younger age-group is the group with the involvement of a stronger genetic component in PCOS pathogenesis, which lead to an early manifestation of disease. This might indicate a more severe disease phenotype, which may worsen overtime, and become more resistant to treatment. Longitudinal studies can provide further insights, to better understand the course of disease in such patients. As we included lean women with PCOS, which is also a common presentation in clinics in Pakistan, our data suggest that lower adiponectin levels in women with PCOS are not only caused by the IR and obesity in these women. On the contrary, it might be interplay of family history of PCOS and IR, or these women have inherent low levels of adiponectin regardless of their BMI and degree of IR, which leads to development of the full-blown PCOS. Also, a positive family history of PCOS may evoke a disturbance in the insulin secretion in genetically predisposed individuals, giving rise to lower adiponectin levels and polycystic ovaries. Adiponectin thus may serve as a useful marker in detecting cases of PCOS with atypical presentation or in individuals with a family history of PCOS. Longitudinal studies are therefore warranted to understand the initiating point in development of PCOS in females having a family history of PCOS and IR.

Strengths and limitations

To our knowledge, this is the first study to investigate serum adiponectin levels in PCOS women in Pakistani population. However certain methodological considerations are worth-mentioning. Sample size was limited and the effect estimates may not be very precise, however, we found a statistically significant relationship between PCOS and adiponectin which remained significant even with this smaller sample. In addition, we calculated IR using HOMA-IR and not by the euglycemic/hyperglycemic clamp which is the gold standard to measure IR. However, HOMA-IR is a worldwide accepted surrogate marker for the calculation of IR. This may have potentially misclassified some individuals, however such misclassifications are likely to be non-differential and should lead to a null results. But in our study, we observed a statistically significant association both for IR and adiponectin with PCOS, which is unlikely due to a misclassification bias.

Conclusion

In conclusion, serum adiponectin levels in lean women with PCOS are only partly explained by IR. Adiponectin levels may serve as a potential independent biomarker for diagnosis of PCOS in lean women with fewer symptoms, or women with a family history of PCOS. Further research using prospective design may provide evidence on role of adiponectin in early diagnosis or detection of PCOS among young lean women.

Competing interests
All authors declare that they have no competing interests.

Authors' contributions
SSM, MAQ designed the study; KS, SSM and NAK carried out statistical analyses; all authors interpreted the results. SSM and NAK drafted the initial manuscript and all authors contributed to the final draft. MAQ supervised the research project. All authors read and approved the final manuscript.

Funding
Dow University of Health Sciences (DUHS) provided partial funding for biochemical tests of cases of PCOS. DUHS had no role in design, conduct and analysis of this study.

Author details
[1]Department of Epidemiology, University of Rotterdam, Rotterdam, The Netherlands. [2]Institute of Health and Wellbeing, University of Glasgow, 1-Lilybank Gardens, G12 8RZ Glasgow, UK. [3]School of Public Health, Dow University of Health Sciences, Karachi, Pakistan. [4]Department of Community Medicine, Dow University of Health Sciences, Karachi, Pakistan. [5]Department of Surgery, Dow University of Health Sciences, Karachi, Pakistan. [6]Institute of Basic Medical Sciences, Dow University of Health Sciences, Karachi, Pakistan.

References
1. Toulis KA, Goulis DG, Farmakiotis D, Georgopoulos NA, Katsikis I, Tarlatzis BC, et al: Adiponectin levels in women with polycystic ovary syndrome: a systematic review and a meta-analysis. Hum Reprod Update 2009, 15:297–307.
2. Ferriman D, Gallwey JD: Clinical assessment of body hair growth in women. J Clin Endocrinol 1961, 21:1440–1447.
3. Shroff R, Syrop CH, Davis W, Van Voorhis BJ, Dokras A: Risk of metabolic complications in the new PCOS phenotypes based on the Rotterdam criteria. Fertil Steril 2007, 88:1389–1395.
4. Cho LW, Randeva HS, Atkin SL: Cardiometabolic aspects of polycystic ovarian syndrome. Vasc Health Risk Manag 2007, 3:55–63.
5. Handelsman Y: Metabolic syndrome pathophysiology and clinical presentation. Toxicol Pathol 2009, 37:18–20.
6. Vuguin PM: Interventional studies for polycystic ovarian syndrome in children and adolescents. Ped Health 2010, 4:59–73.
7. Katulski K, Meczekalski B: Natural history of polycyclic ovary syndrome. Pol Merkur Lekarski 2010, 29:58–60.
8. Liu X, Zhang J, Li Y, Xu L, Wei D, Qiu D, et al: On the relationship between serum total adiponectin and insulin resistance in polycystic ovary syndrome. Sheng Wu Yi Xue Gong Cheng Xue Za Zhi 2010, 27:636–640.
9. Vrbikova J, Dvorakova K, Hill M, Vcelak J, Stanicka S, Vankova M, et al: Determinants of circulating adiponectin in women with polycystic ovary syndrome. Gynecol Obstet Invest 2005, 60:155–161.
10. Yamauchi T, Kamon J, Waki H, Terauchi Y, Kubota N, Hara K, et al: The fat-derived hormone adiponectin reverses insulin resistance associated with both lipoatrophy and obesity. Nat Med 2001, 7:941–946.
11. Weyer C, Funahashi T, Tanaka S, Hotta K, Matsuzawa Y, Pratley RE, et al: Hypoadiponectinemia in obesity and type 2 diabetes: close association with insulin resistance and hyperinsulinemia. J Clin Endocrinol Metab 2001, 86:1930–1935.
12. Aroda V, Ciaraldi TP, Chang SA, Dahan MH, Chang RJ, Henry RR: Circulating and cellular adiponectin in polycystic ovary syndrome: relationship to glucose tolerance and insulin action. Fertil Steril 2008, 89:1200–1208.
13. Azziz R: Controversy in clinical endocrinology: diagnosis of polycystic ovarian syndrome: the Rotterdam criteria are premature. J Clin Endocrinol Metab 2006, 91:781–785.
14. World Health Organization-International Obesity Task Force: The Asia-pacific perspective: redefining obesity and its treatment. Health communications Australia. 2000. http://www.wpro.who.int/nutrition/documents/docs/Redefiningobesity.pdf Accessed on 06-08-2013.
15. Rotterdam ESHRE/ASRM-Sponsored PCOS Consensus Workshop Group: Revised 2003 consensus on diagnostic criteria and long term health risks related to polycystic ovarian syndrome. Fertil Steril 2004, 81:19–25.
16. Matthews DR, Hosker JP, Rudenski AS, Naylor BA, Treacher DF, Turner RC: Homeostasis model assessment: insulin resistance and beta-cell function from fasting plasma glucose and insulin concentrations in man. Diabetologia 1985, 28:412–419.
17. Harrison S, Somani N, Bergfeld WF: Update on the management of hirsutism. Cleve Clin J Med 2010, 77:388–98.
18. Ardawi MS, Rouzi AA: Plasma adiponectin and insulin resistance in women with polycystic ovary syndrome. Fertil Steril 2005, 83:1708–1716.
19. Barber TM, Hazell M, Christodoulides C, Golding SJ, Alvey C, Burling K, et al: Serum levels of retinol-binding protein 4 and adiponectin in women with polycystic ovary syndrome: associations with visceral fat but no evidence for fat mass-independent effects on pathogenesis in this condition. J Clin Endocrinol Metab 2008, 93:2859–2865.
20. Carmina E, Orio F, Palomba S, Cascella T, Longo RA, Colao AM, et al: Evidence for altered adipocyte function in polycystic ovary syndrome. Eur J Endocrinol 2005, 152:389–394.
21. Escobar-Morreale HF, Villuendas G, Botella-Carretero JI, Alvarez-Blasco F, Sanchon R, Luque-Ramirez M, et al: Adiponectin and resistin in PCOS: a clinical, biochemical and molecular genetic study. Hum Reprod 2006, 21:2257–2265.
22. Sepilian V, Nagamani M: Adiponectin levels in women with polycystic ovary syndrome and severe insulin resistance. J Soc Gynecol Investig 2005, 12:129–134.
23. Wickham EP III, Cheang KI, Clore JN, Baillargeon JP, Nestler JE: Total and high-molecular weight adiponectin in women with the polycystic ovary syndrome. Metabolism 2011, 60:366–72.
24. Weyer C, Tataranni PA, Bogardus C, Pratley RE: Insulin resistance and insulin secretory dysfunction are independent predictors of worsening of glucose tolerance during each stage of type 2 diabetes development. Diabetes Care 2001, 24:89–94.
25. Agarwal N, Rice SP, Bolusani H, Luzio SD, Dunseath G, Ludgate M, et al: Metformin reduces arterial stiffness and improves endothelial function in young women with polycystic ovary syndrome: a randomized, placebo-controlled, crossover trial. J Clin Endocrinol Metab 2010, 95:722–730.

26. Elkind-Hirsch K, Marrioneaux O, Bhushan M, Vernor D, Bhushan R: **Comparison of single and combined treatment with exenatide and metformin on menstrual cyclicity in overweight women with polycystic ovary syndrome.** *J Clin Endocrinol Metab* 2008, **93:**2670–2678.

27. Majuri A, Santaniemi M, Rautio K, Kunnari A, Vartiainen J, Ruokonen A, *et al:* **Rosiglitazone treatment increases plasma levels of adiponectin and decreases levels of resistin in overweight women with PCOS: a randomized placebo-controlled study.** *Eur J Endocrinol* 2007, **156:**263–269.

28. Glintborg D, Frystyk J, Hojlund K, Andersen KK, Henriksen JE, Hermann AP, *et al:* **Total and high molecular weight (HMW) adiponectin levels and measures of glucose and lipid metabolism following pioglitazone treatment in a randomized placebo-controlled study in polycystic ovary syndrome.** *Clin Endocrinol (Oxf)* 2008, **68:**165–174.

29. Rodin DA, Bano G, Bland JM, Taylor K, Nussey SS: **Polycystic ovaries and associated metabolic abnormalities in Indian subcontinent Asian women.** *Clin Endocrinol (Oxf)* 1998, **49:**91–99.

30. Crosignani PG, Nicolosi AE: **Polycystic ovarian disease: heritability and heterogeneity.** *Hum Reprod Update* 2001, **7:**3–7.

31. Sir-Petermann T, Maliqueo M, Codner E, Echiburu B, Crisosto N, Perez V, *et al:* **Early metabolic derangements in daughters of women with polycystic ovary syndrome.** *J Clin Endocrinol Metab* 2007, **92:**4637–4642.

Effect of exercise intensity on weight changes and sexual hormones (androstenedione and free testosterone) in female rats with estradiol valerate-induced PCOS

Maryamosadat Miri[1], Hojatolah Karimi Jashni[2*] and Farzaneh Alipour[3]

Abstract

Introduction: Weight gain and fat accumulation are predisposing factors of PCOS. Life-style modification, including increasing physical activity, is the first line approach in managing PCOS. The objective of this study is to assess the effect of exercise intensity on weight changes, androstenedione and free testosterone level in female rats with estradiol valerate induced PCOS.

Method and materials: 40 female Wistar rats were selected (180 ± 20 g). They had every 2 to 3 consecutive estrous cycles during 12 to 14 days. The study was approved by ethical committee of Jahrom University of Medical Sciences. The first two groups were divided into control (n = 10) and polycystic (n = 30) that were induced PCOS by estradiol valerate injection after 60 days. The polycystic groups were divided into three groups of sham (n = 10), experiment group with low-intensity exercise (pco + l.exe) (n = 10) and experiment group with moderate intensity exercise (pco + m.exe) (n = 10). Exercises were performed during 6 sessions of 60 minutes per week for 8 weeks. (Moderate intensity: 28 m/min-70%–75%VO2Max. Low intensity (20 m/min-50%–55%VO2Max) running at 0 slope, 1 h/day, 6 days/week). ANOVA and LSD test were used for data analysis.

Results: In the present study, no significant differences were found in the decrease of total weights of rats. And also androstenedione level changes in experiment groups were higher compared to control group but no significant differences were found, also free testosterone level was significantly higher than the observer group.

Conclusion: According to weight changes and sexual hormones (Free testosterone and androstenedione) exercise training especially with low intensity may improve symptoms of polycystic ovary syndrome.

Keywords: Exercise intensity, Weight change, Androstenedione, Free testosterone

Introduction

It is certain that infertility is one of the main problems in today's medicine and its rate is increasing from 1955 and 10%–15% of the couples are suffering from that [1]. One of the causes of infertility is polycystic ovary syndrome (PCOS). PCOS is the most common endocrine abnormality in premenopausal women. It was first described by Stein and Leventhal in 1935, who found an association between amenorrhea, hirsutism, and obesity with polycystic ovaries. The authors reported on bilaterally enlarged ovaries, with a thick and whitened capsule [2]. This syndrome is characterized by hyperandrogenism, ovulatory dysfunction, irregular menstrual cycles, imbalance of sex hormones and polycystic ovarian morphology. Metabolic disturbances, such as insulin resistance and obesity are also associated with PCOS. It is thought to have a genetic etiology behind this syndrome, the severity and course of the disease is determined by lifestyle changes, especially body mass index [3].

On the other hand, the importance of exercise and mental health of individuals and society is obvious and is inseparable from the health of body and spirit. Attention

* Correspondence: Hojat_karimi@yahoo.co.in
[2]Department of Anatomy, Jahrom University of Medical Sciences, Jahrom, Iran
Full list of author information is available at the end of the article

Table 1 Comparison of means of all variables

	Moderate intensity	Low intensity	PCOS	Control
Free testosterone(ng/ml)	**0.494 ± 0.26 ***	0.319 ± 0.12	0.178 ± 0.08	0.343 ± 0.26
Androstenedione (ng/ml)	0.347 ± 0.172	0.273 ± 0.09	0.278 ± 0.16	0.261 ± 0.09
Weight total (gr)	28. 62 ± 17.70	34.55 ± 6.22	32.8 ± 19.27	28.66 ± 19.20
Final weight (gr)	204.11 ± 22.89	227.55 ± 16.14	210.6 ± 25.47	235.2 ± 49/82

* significant difference comparing PCOS ($p < 0.05$).

to women's exercise as much of their bodies' physiological needs is essential [4]. Physical activity and exercise cause levels of some hormones increase or decrease compared to resting level. Physical activity reduces estrogen and steroid hormone production [5]. Lifestyle intervention studies incorporating increased physical activity with reduced caloric intake show an improvement in ovulatory function, circulating androgen levels, inflammatory pattern, and insulin sensitivity in women with PCOS [6]. Furthermore, certain single-nucleotide polymorphisms associated with obesity contribute to elevated body mass index (BMI) in PCOS, supporting the concept that its phenotypes are a consequence of a polygenic mechanism [7].

Controversy exists about the effect of obesity on serum androgen production in PCOS. Some investigators have reported that testosterone and androstenedione levels are similar in obese and non obese PCOS patients [8,9]. However, it is well known that obesity generates a decrease in the sexual hormone-binding globulin, and therefore an increase in the levels of free androgens [10,11]. In contrast, dynamic studies have shown lower androstenedione levels in obese PCOS patients than in non obese PCOS patients [12,13]. Researchers believe that regular and light sports are a safe method. The effects of aerobic exercise on polycystic ovary syndrome was assessed in some papers, it is stated that, apart from the changes in body fat, level of sex hormones have been changed [6].

In the past, the effects of regular exercise with high intensity (80–85% maximal oxygen uptake), moderate intensity (70–75% maximal oxygen uptake) and low intensity (50–55% maximal oxygen uptake) were assessed. The result showed testosterone associated with high-intensity group was lower than inactive control group [14]. Since, the effect of exercise intensity in PCOS have not been assessed and regarding the importance of physical activity in rehabilitation of hormonal imbalances, we conducted this study to evaluate the effect of exercise intensity on weight changes, androstenedione and free testosterone levels in female rats with estradiol valerate-induced PCOS.

Method and materials

Animals
40 female Wistar rats were selected (180 ± 20 g). They had every 2 to 3 consecutive estrous cycles during 12 to 14 day. The rats were selected from Shiraz University of medical sciences and were kept in animal house of Jahrom University of medical sciences. Their cages were disinfected 3 times a week with alcohol 70% and enough water and also appropriate bottle was provided for them.

Approval
The study was approved by ethical committee of Jahrom University of Medical Sciences and morality was regarded.

Induction of PCOS
PCO phenotype is induced by of a variety of hormonal and non-hormonal methods, including testosterone, estradiol valerate, and dehydroepiandrosterone (DHT), adrenocorticotropic and long-term use of light. In this study, we used estradiol Valerate as an inducer. 30 rats were selected randomly from 40 ones. 4 mg estradiol validate which was dissolved in 0.2 mg Sesame oil was injected (IM) in their thigh.

Design
The first two groups were divided into control (n = 10) and polycystic (n = 30) that were induced PCOS by estradiol valerate injection after 60 days. The polycystic groups were divided into three groups of sham (n = 10), experiment groups (PCOS plus low-intensity exercise (n =10) and experiment group (PCOS plus moderate intensity exercise (n =10)). Exercises were performed during 6 sessions of 60 minutes per week which lasted 8 weeks. Moderate intensity: (28 m/min-70%–75%VO2Max. Low intensity (20 m/min-50%–55% VO2Max)running at 0 slope, 1 h/day, 6 days/week. The mice were anesthetized, then, of 5 ml of blood was obtained directly from the heart and was used for ELIZA. Exercise Programs.

Table 2 Variance analysis of final weights of rats (gr)

S.V	F.S	M.S	S.S	D.F
Group	1.964 ns	1990.76	5972/28	3
Error	-	1013.62	34463/11	34
Total	-	-	40435/39	37

ns (non-significant).

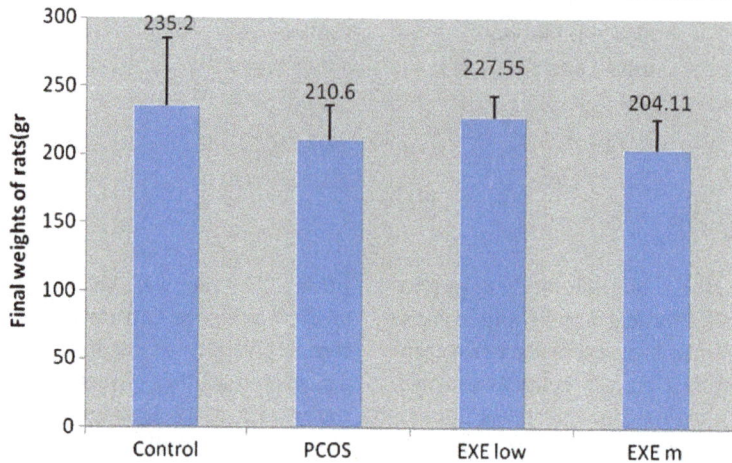

Figure 1 Changes of final weights of rats in experiment groups.

Exercise training protocol

The training group was exercised on a rodent motor-driven treadmill at a 0° slope for 60 min/day, 6 days/wk for 8 wk. During the 1st wk of training the rats ran at treadmill speed of 10 m/min for 15 min for adaptation. During the 2nd and 3rd wk of training the treadmill speed and exercise duration increased step by step until the animals ran for 60 min/day. The treadmill speed and exercise duration were then held constant for the remainder of the training period. We kept training frequency (6d/wk) and duration (60 min/d) constant. The exercise plan started with short-duration and light movements and gradually increased in intensity.

Vaginal smears and blood sampling

The estrus cycle stage was determined by microscopic analysis of the predominant cell types obtained via the vaginal smears taken daily (24) Vaginal smear test was taken within 60 days for reassurance of induction of PCOS in experiment groups. After vaginal smear test, we used animals having 2 or 3 regular estrous cycle within 12–14 days. Blood sampling directly from their heart was done through a 5 cc syringe after 32 hours following the last session. After isolation of blood serum, concentration of free testosterones, androstenedione was measured by ELIZA in Jahrom University of Medical Sciences.

Blood collection and tissue preparation

To derogate the effect of acute exercise, the rats were eventually anesthetized with diethyl ether and sodium pentobarbital (50 mg/kg, intraperitioneal injection) after a 12-h fast and 32 h after the last training session and their blood was gleaned from the abdominal aorta. Tubes containing plasma sample aliquots were kept frozen at –80°C until being analyzed.

Measurement

BioVendor kit was used for measurement of Free testosterone and androstenedione level in ELISA test.

Analyzing method

ANOVA test was used for comparison of mean and Standard deviation of hormones and tukey test for multi comparison of different groups was used in the studying groups $(p < 0.05)$ was considered as significant difference. ANOVA and LSD test for normal distributions was used.

Results

Results of final weights of rats

The results show that, no significant differences were found in the final weights of the rats compared to the control group. Final weights of rats in pco + exe.l and pco + exe.m did not have significant differences comparing the poly cystic group and also weight loss in pco + exe.l group was not significant comparing pco + exe.m group. Variance analysis of data was not significant. Also final weights of the rats have normal distribution. Regarding fissure value and data analysis, this factor does not have significant differences (Tables 1 and 2, Figure 1).

Table 3 Variance analysis of total weights of rats (gr)

S.V	F.S	M.S	S.S	D.F
Group	0.282 ns	68/49	205/48	3
Error	-	243/09	5834/23	24
Total	-	-	6039/71	27

ns (non-significant).

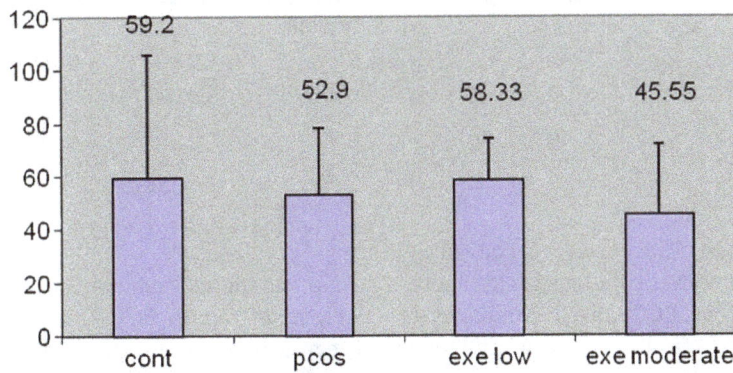

Figure 2 Changes of total weights of rats in experiment groups.

Results of total body weight of rats

Total weight means the difference of primary and final weights of rats. Although weight reduction is seen in our results, no significant difference was found in the total weights in the experiment groups comparing control group. And also data of the pco + exe.l group did not have significant differences comparing the polycystic group. No significant difference was found according to variance analysis (Table 3, Figure 2).

Results of body weight in 2 month protocol

Total body weight was measured within 2 month and recorded 18 times. Since most of weight changes were significant, data which were not significant are reported. Both experiment and polycystic groups did not have significant differences comparing the control group in this protocol. Weight changes are reported as below (Figure 3):

Weight of 6th time is not significant compared to the 5th and 4th ones. Also 10th compared to 9th and 15th compared to 12th, 13th and 14th ones furthermore, 18th compared to 16th were not significant.

Results of free testosterone changes in experiment group

The PCO + exe.m group showed a significant rise in free testosterone. No significant differences were found in the pco + exe.l group and polycystic group comparing the control group. Also pco + exe.l group did not have significant difference compared to polycystic group. The diagram shows that it has normal distribution. Also variance analysis was significant (Table 4, Figure 4).

Results of androstenedione changes in experiment group

Results showed that, androstenedione hormone changes in experiment group did not have significant difference

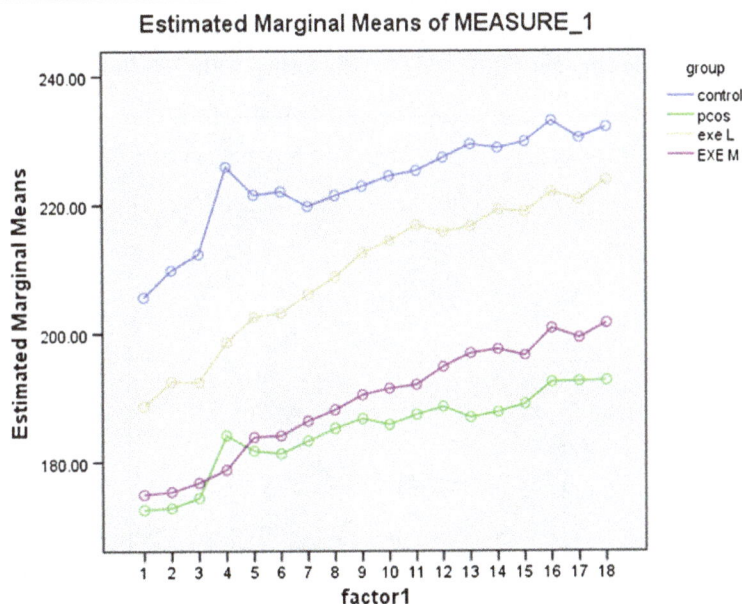

Figure 3 Weight changes during 2 month protocole.

Table 4 Variance analysis of free testosterone (ng)

S.V	F.S	M.S	S.S	D.F
Group	0. 015*	0.159	0.476	3
Error	-	0.040	1.353	34
Total	-	-	1.829	37

* (significant) p < 0.05.

Table 5 Variance analysis of androstenedione hormone (ng/ml)

S.V	F.S	M.S	S.S	D.F
Group	0. 720 ns	0.014	0.041	3
Error	-	0.019	0.649	34
Total	-	-	0.690	37

ns (non-significant).

compared to control group. There was no statistically significant difference between the decrease in androstenedione concentration in PCO + exe.l compared to Sham and there was no statistically significant difference between the increase in androstenedione concentration in pco + exe.m compared to sham and also the difference was not significant in PCO + exe.l group compared to PCO + exe.m. Androstenedione changes have normal distribution considering the diagram (Table 5, Figure 5).

Discussion

This study demonstrated that low intensity exercise may cause weight reduction and modify sexual hormones (androstenedione and Free testosterone) in polycystic ovary syndrome after 8 week. Polycystic ovary syndrome (PCOS) is related to the chronic anovulation, hyperandrogenemia, insulin resistance (IR)/hyperinsulinemia, and a high incidence of obesity.

It is emphasized that the most preferred and most effective method of treatment for PCOS is lifestyle modification. Researchers believe that PCOS is accompanied with androgen hormone rise and obesity. Although weight loss improves practically every parameter of PCOS, Wright et al. [15] concluded that differences in dietary intake and physical activity alone are not sufficient to explain differences in weight between women with and without PCOS. Our study confirms the findings by Wright et al. about lifestyle changes [9].

No significant differences were found in the final weights of rats in PCO + exe.l compared to the PCO + exe.m group and also the difference was not statistically significant between the total weights of rats in PCO + exe.m compared to PCO + exe.l group. Their weights were measured within 2 month and weight changes were reported daily. Weight changes were significant in 2nd up to 18th days comparing the first day. Some papers indicated that Physical activity has been found lower in PCOS patients than in control women [15]. The changes in lifestyle that incorporate an increase of physical activity and limited caloric intake have been beneficial in some studies. Regular physical activity is an important component to support the long-term reduction of overweight; however, the results are minimal with exercise alone [9]. An increase in physical activity is recommended for women with obesity and PCOS, as long as cardiovascular and orthopedic limitations are taken into consideration [16]. These are in consistent with our results.

Free testosterone rise in PCO + exe.m was significant comparing Sham. Free testosterone rise could be due to obesity and binding globulin reduction [17,18]. Effect of exercise intensity and its duration on menstruation have not been monitored. Another research showed that, significant rise of free testosterone was observed in women exercising with 75% intensity. They indicated that, rise

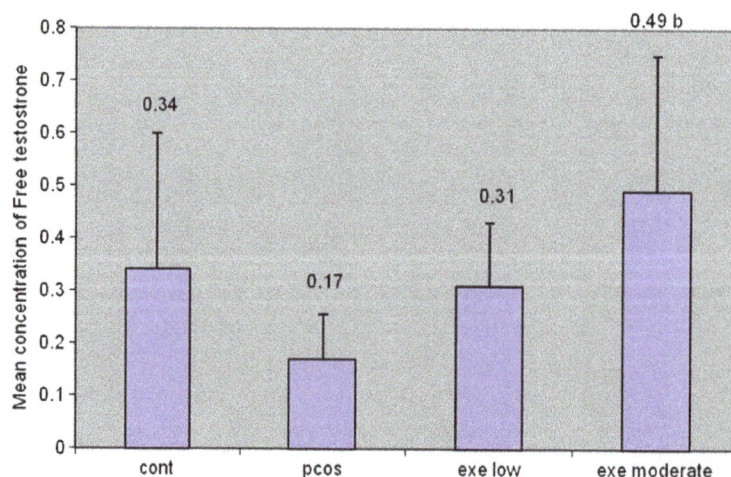

Figure 4 Changes of Free testosterone in experiment groups.

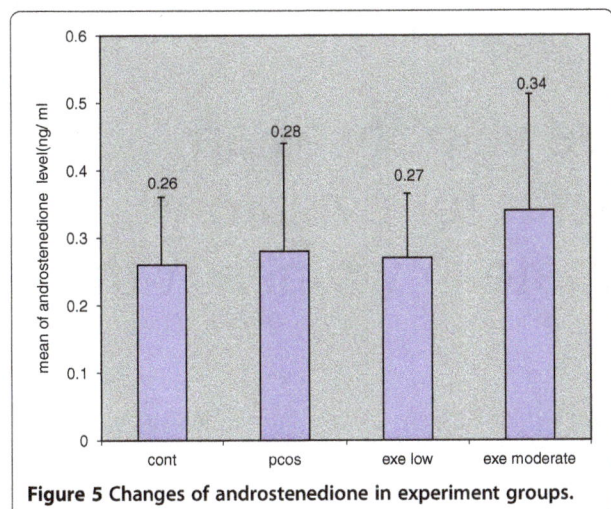

Figure 5 Changes of androstenedione in experiment groups.

Jahrom, Iran. [3]Student Research Committee, Jahrom University of Medical Sciences, Jahrom, Fars, Iran.

of hormone is because of decrease in clearance of testosterone due to hepatic blood serum flow reduction [19]. Other studies have found that obesity generates an increase of testosterone levels in PCOS patients [20-22]. But in our study, free testosterone changes in PCO + exe.l shows the sufficiency of low exercise intensity.

Although there are some researches over exercise effect on PCOS, there was not done over the exercise intensity effects on weight changes and sexual hormones (androstenedione and Free testosterone)in PCOS. Hence the present study demonstrated that low exercise intensity may modify weight changes and sexual hormones (androstenedione and Free testosterone) in polycystic ovary syndrome after 8 week better than moderate intensity.

Conclusion

Here we provided evidence that both low and moderate exercise intensity might enhance polycystic ovary syndrome and decrease its complications due to its effect on weight reduction and sex hormones (androstenedione and Free testosterone). Based on our results, low intensity exercise might be more effective and improve its symptoms.

Competing interests
The authors have no conflict of financial interests.

Authors' contributions
MM and HK evaluated the sexual hormone analysis.MM and FA performed the statistical analyses and drafted the manuscript. MM organized the exercise training and set the protocol, set the weight change and did the vaginal smear test.MM and FA performed ELISA test.HK helped draft the manuscript.MM and FA translated the manuscript and prepared it. All authors read and approved the final manuscript.

Acknowledgments
The authors thank Research Center of Jahrom University of Medical Sciences, Mr. Mohammad Momtaz and Michael Momtaz.

Author details
[1]Exercise Physiology, Jahrom University of Medical Sciences, Jahrom, Fars, Iran. [2]Department of Anatomy, Jahrom University of Medical Sciences,

References
1. Sarvari A, Naderi MM, Heidari M, Zarnani AH, Jeddi-Tehrani M, Sadeghi MR, Akhondi MM: Effect of environmental risk factor on human fertility. *J Reprod Infertil* 2010, **11**(4):341–355.
2. Marcondes JAM, Hayashida SY, Bachega TASS: Hirsutismo & Síndromes dos ovários policísticos. In *Endocrinologia*. Edited by Mendonça BB, Maciel RMB, Saad M. São Paulo, Brazil: Atheneu; 2007:635–682.
3. Forozanfard F: *Ovulation Step by Step*. Kashan: Printing, Publishing Morsel; 2010:81–105.
4. Hatami H, Razavi SM, Eftekhar AH, Majlesi F, Sayed Nozadi M, Parizadeh SMJ: *Text Book of Public Health*. 1st edition. Tehran: Arjmand Publications; 2006. P. 1656 2.
5. Hashemichashemi Z, Garavand N, Dehkordi KH, Ravasi A, Sardari M: Comparison of single bout of moderate intensity exercise on growth hormone active and inactive women. *Jundishapur J Med* 2011, **11**(2):147–156.
6. Christopher N, Tymchuk Sheva B, Tessler R, Bernard J: Changes in sex hormone-binding globulin, insulin, and serum lipids in postmenopausal women on a low-fat, high-fiber diet combined with exercise. *Nutr Cancer* 2000, **38**(2):158–162.
7. Franks S, Adams J, Mason H, Polson D: Ovulatory disorders in women with polycystic ovary syndrome. *Clin Obstet Gynaecol* 1985, **12**(3):605–632.
8. Singh KB, Mahajan DK, Wortsman J: Effect of obesity on the clinical and hormonal characteristics of the polycystic ovary syndrome. *J Reprod Med* 1994, **39**(10):805–808.
9. Hoeger M: Exercise therapy in polycystic ovary syndrome. *Semin Reprod Med* 2008, **26**(1):93–100.
10. Palomba S, Giallauria F, Falbo A, Russo T, Oppedisano R, Tolino A, Colao A, Vigorito C, Zullo F, Orio F: Structured exercise training programme versus hypocaloric hyperproteic diet in obese polycystic ovary syndrome patients with anovulatory infertility: a 24-week pilot study. *Hum Reprod* 2008, **23**:642–650.
11. Gilling-Smith C, Willis DS, Beard RW, Franks S: Hypersecretion of androstenedione by isolated thecal cells from polycystic ovaries. *J Clin Endocrinol Metab* 1994, **79**:1158–116512.
12. Dunaif A, Segal KR, Futterweit W, Dobrjansky A: Profound peripheral insulin resistance, independent of obesity, in polycystic ovary syndrome. *Diabetes* 1989, **38**(9):1165–1174.
13. dos Reis RM, Foss MC, de Moura MD, Ferriani RA, Silva de Sá MF: Insulin secretion in obese and non-obese women with polycystic ovary syndrome and its relationship with hyperandrogenism. *Gynecol Endocrinol* 1995, **9**(1):45–50.
14. Moran LJ, Harrison CL, Hutchison SK, Stepto N, Strauss BJ, Teede HJ: Exercise decreases anti-mullerian hormone in anovulatoryoverwight women with polycystic ovary syndrome-a pilot study. *Thieme eJournals* 2011:21989557. pubmed–as supplied by publisher.
15. Wright CE, Zborowski JV, Talbott EO, McHugh-Pemu K, Youk A: Dietary intake, physical activity, and obesity in women with polycystic ovary syndrome. *Int J Obes* 2004, **28**(8):1026–1032.
16. Moran LJ, Brinkworth G, Noakes M, Norman RJ: Effects of lifestyle modification in polycystic ovarian syndrome. *Reprod BioMed Online* 2006, **12**(5):569–578. Article no. 2166.
17. Pasquali R, Casimirri F, Balestra V, Flamia R, Melchionda N, Fabbri R, Barbara L: The relative contribution of androgens and insulin in determining abdominal fat distribution in 19 premenopausal women. *J Endocrinol Invest* 1991, **14**:839.
18. Peiris AN, Sothmann MS, Aiman EJ, Kissebah AH: The relationship of insulin to sex hormone binding globulin: role of adiposity. *Fertil Steril* 1989, **52**:69.
19. Consitt LA, Copeland JL, Tremblay MS: Hormone responses to resistance vs endurance exercise in premenopausal females. *Can J Appl Physiol* 2001, **26**(6):574–587.
20. Holte J, Bergh T, Berne C, Lithell H: Serum lipoprotein lipid profile in women with the polycystic ovary syndrome: relation to anthropometric, endocrine and metabolic variables. *Clin Endocrinol* 1994, **41**(4):463–471.

Brachial-to-ankle pulse wave velocity as an independent prognostic factor for ovulatory response to clomiphene citrate in women with polycystic ovary syndrome

Toshifumi Takahashi*, Hideki Igarashi, Shuichiro Hara, Mitsuyoshi Amita, Koki Matsuo, Ayumi Hasegawa and Hirohisa Kurachi

Abstract

Background: Polycystic ovary syndrome (PCOS) has a risk for cardiovascular disease. Increased arterial stiffness has been observed in women with PCOS. The purpose of the present study was to investigate whether the brachial-to-ankle pulse wave velocity (baPWV) is a prognostic factor for ovulatory response to clomiphene citrate (CC) in women with PCOS.

Methods: This study was a retrospective cohort study of 62 women with PCOS conducted from January 2009 to December 2012 at the university hospital, Yamagata, Japan. We analyzed 62 infertile PCOS patients who received CC. Ovulation was induced by 100 mg CC for 5 days. CC non-responder was defined as failure to ovulate for at least 2 consecutive CC-treatment cycles. The endocrine, metabolic, and cardiovascular parameters between CC responder (38 patients) and non-responder (24 patients) groups were analyzed.

Results: In univariate analysis, waist-to-hip ratio, level of free testosterone, percentages of patients with dyslipidemia, impaired glucose tolerance, and diabetes mellitus, blood glucose and insulin levels at 60 min and 120 min, the area under the curve of glucose and insulin after 75-g oral glucose intolerance test, and baPWV were significantly higher in CC non-responders compared with responders. In multivariate logistic regression analysis, both waist-to-hip ratio (odds ratio, 1.77; 95% confidence interval, 2.2–14.1; P = 0.04) and baPWV (odds ratio, 1.71; 95% confidence interval, 1.1–2.8; P = 0.03) were independent predictors of ovulation induction by CC in PCOS patients. The predictive values of waist-to-hip ratio and baPWV for the CC resistance in PCOS patients were determined by the receiver operating characteristic curves. The area under the curves for waist-to-hip ratio and baPWV were 0.76 and 0.77, respectively. Setting the threshold at 0.83 for waist-to-hip ratio offered the best compromise between specificity (0.65) and sensitivity (0.84), while the setting the threshold at 1,182 cm/s for baPWV offered the best compromise between specificity (0.80) and sensitivity (0.71).

Conclusions: Both metabolic and cardiovascular parameters were predictive for CC resistance in PCOS patients. The measurement of baPWV may be a useful tool to predict ovulation in PCOS patients who receive CC.

Keywords: Polycystic ovary syndrome, Clomiphene citrate, Brachial-to-ankle pulse wave velocity, Waist-to-hip ratio

* Correspondence: totakaha@med.id.yamagata-u.ac.jp
Department of Obstetrics and Gynecology, Yamagata University Faculty of Medicine, Yamagata 990-9585, Japan

Background

Polycystic ovary syndrome (PCOS) is a common ovulatory disorder in young women, which affects 5–10% of the population and results in infertility due to anovulation [1]. Clomiphene citrate (CC) is a first-line strategy to induce ovulation in women with PCOS. Although CC will induce ovulation in 60–80% of PCOS patients, the remainder are CC resistant [2,3]. CC-resistant women are recommended for other treatments, such as gonadotropin treatment or laparoscopic ovarian drilling to induce ovulation. Although gonadotropin therapy achieves higher ovulation and pregnancy rates, the treatment is associated with serious complications, such as ovarian hyperstimulation syndrome and multiple pregnancies [4,5]. Laparoscopic ovarian drilling is invasive and expensive [5,6].

Although the pathogenesis of PCOS is still unclear, the role of insulin resistance in the pathophysiology of PCOS has been established. Insulin resistance with compensatory hyperinsulinemia is common in women with PCOS [7]. Hyperinsulinemia directly contributes to an increase in androgen biosynthesis in the ovary [8] and a decrease in the level of hepatic sex hormone-binding globulin, resulting in an elevated free androgen level [9]. Hyperandrogenism within an ovary is believed to harm follicle development in PCOS. On the basis of these considerations, insulin-sensitizing drugs, such as metformin, pioglitazone, and rosiglitazone, have been used alone or in combination with CC in CC-resistant PCOS patients to induce ovulation [5].

The mechanisms of CC resistance in women with PCOS also remain unknown. Levels of testosterone [10] and blood glucose and blood glucose × immunoreactive insulin (IRI) at 120 min after oral glucose tolerance test have been reported as predictive markers in CC-resistant PCOS [11]. Because PCOS is associated with risk for developing type 2 diabetes mellitus [12], these reports support the idea that metabolic disorders could be involved in the mechanisms of CC-resistant PCOS.

Women with PCOS also are at risk for developing cardiovascular disease [13-16]. Increased arterial stiffness has been observed in women with PCOS compared to controls with normal menstrual cycles and normal androgen levels [17,18]. Brachial-to-ankle pulse wave velocity (baPWV) is a surrogate marker for arterial stiffness [19]. However, no reports concerning the association of cardiovascular parameters, such as baPWV, with ovulatory response to CC in women with PCOS have been published. The purpose of the present study was to investigate whether the baPWV is a prognostic factor for ovulatory response to CC in women with PCOS.

Methods

Subjects

This study was a retrospective cohort observational study. A total of 62 infertile patients diagnosed with PCOS from January 2009 to December 2012 in our hospital were recruited into the study. The ethics committee at Yamagata University Faculty of Medicine approved the study protocol. We previously reported that this cohort of seven women with PCOS who were CC-resistant successfully ovulated by co-treatment with bezafibrate and CC [20]. A written informed consent was obtained from all participants before entry into the study.

PCOS was diagnosed by the presence of oligomenorrhea or amenorrhea, polycystic ovaries on ultrasonography, and hyperandrogenemia or LH hypersecretion (elevated LH level and LH/FSH ratio) according to the 2007 criteria of the Japanese Society of Obstetrics and Gynecology (JSOG) [21]. Pelvic transvaginal ultrasound was performed using a 5 to 7.5-MHz probe in oligo-/amenorrheic women at random or days 3–5 after a spontaneous or a progestin-induced withdrawal bleeding. In the JSOG PCOS diagnostic criteria, a diagnosis of PCO was made if there were 10 or more follicles of 2–9 mm in diameter [21]. Because the prevalence of Japanese PCOS women with a sign of hyperandrogenism is very low [22], the clinical hyperandrogenism, such as hirsutism, is not included in the JSOG PCOS diagnostic criteria. Hyperandrogenemia was defined as an increase in the level of total testosterone, free testosterone or androstenedione concentration in the JSOG PCOS diagnostic criteria [21]. In the present study, we used the concentration of free testosterone over 1.0 pg/ml as hyperandrogenemia. The JSOG PCOS diagnostic criteria includes the Rotterdam 2003 criteria for PCOS [23]. Other etiologies such as congenital adrenal hyperplasia, androgen secreting tumor, or Cushing's syndrome were excluded [21,23]. Inclusion criteria included normal semen analysis according to World Health Organization criteria and normal hysterosalpingography within the preceding 6 months. Exclusion criteria included the presence of any infertility factors other than PCOS and the use of any medications, such as insulin sensitizers, lipid-lowering drugs, or anti-hypertensive drugs. Patients who were already diagnosed with impaired glucose tolerance or diabetes mellitus and smokers were also excluded from the study.

All patients were received CC (Shionogi Co. Ltd., Tokyo Japan) at 100 mg daily for 5 days from day 3–5 after a spontaneous or a progestin-induced withdrawal bleeding [20,24]. The patients were followed up with transvaginal ultrasound to record follicular growth from day 10–12 of the cycle. When a follicle of at least 18 mm was found, 5,000 IU of human chorionic gonadotropin (hCG, Mochida Co. Ltd., Tokyo Japan) was intramuscularly injected [25]. Artificial insemination with the husband's semen or natural intercourse was performed after the hCG injection. Serum progesterone was measured 7 days after hCG administration. Ovulation was determined as the vanishing of a follicle on transvaginal ultrasound, a rise in basal body temperature, and serum progesterone level >10 ng/ml at day 7 after hCG administration [20]. If no follicular growth was observed at day 21 of the menstrual cycle, we discontinued the measurement of follicle growth and recorded no ovarian response to CC. CC response was defined as confirmed ovulation in at least one cycle of CC administration [11]. CC non-response was defined as failure to demonstrate an ovarian response, and no ovulation for at least two consecutive cycles [20,26].

Hormonal assays

In the first cycle of CC treatment, all hormone measurements were performed on day 3–5 after a spontaneous or a progestin-induced withdrawal bleeding. Hormone concentrations were quantified using commercially available immunoassay kits. LH, FSH, PRL, and total testosterone were measured using an electrochemiluminescence immunoassay (ECLusys reagent LH, FSH, prolactin, testosterone II kit; Roche Diagnostics, Inc., Tokyo, Japan). Estradiol and progesterone levels were measured using a chemiluminescence immunoassay (Architect estradiol and progesterone kit; Abbott Japan, Inc., Tokyo, Japan). Free testosterone and dehydroepiandrosterone sulfate (DHEA-S) were measured by radioimmunoassay (DPC Free Testosterone Kit and DHEA-S kit; Mitsubishi Kagaku Iatron, Inc., Tokyo, Japan). Reliability criteria for total testosterone and free testosterone assays were established. The intra-assay coefficient of variation (CV) was 4.7–5.3% and the detection limit of the assay was 10 ng/dl for total testosterone, whereas the intra-assay CV was 5.7–7.4% and the detection limit of the assay was 0.24 pg/ml for free testosterone. All samples were assayed in duplicate.

Anthropometric measurements

In the first cycle of CC treatment, anthropometric measurements were performed on day 3–5 after a spontaneous or a progestin-induced withdrawal bleeding. Body height was measured to the nearest 0.5 cm using a stadiometer, and body weight (in light clothing without shoes) to the nearest 0.5 kg on a calibrated balance scale. Each patient's waist circumference was measured with a soft tape midway between the lowest rib and the iliac crest in the standing position. Hip circumference was measured at the widest part of the gluteal region, and the waist-to-hip ratio was calculated. Body mass index (BMI, kg/m^2) was calculated as weight in kilograms divided by the square of height in meters. Obesity was defined as BMI $\geq$ 30 kg/m^2.

Measurements of metabolic parameters

In the first cycle of CC treatment, a blood sample was collected by venipuncture on day 3–5 after a spontaneous or a progestin-induced withdrawal bleeding. Serum levels of triglycerides, low-density lipoprotein (LDL)

cholesterol, high-density lipoprotein (HDL) cholesterol, and total cholesterol were measured by an enzymatic assay. The diagnostic criteria for dyslipidemia were LDL cholesterol $\geq$ 140 mg/dl, HDL cholesterol < 40 mg/dl, or triglycerides $\geq$ 150 mg/dl according to the Japan Atherosclerosis Society's Guidelines for the Diagnosis and Prevention of Atherosclerotic Cardiovascular Diseases in Japanese [27].

Fasting plasma glucose (FPG) was measured by enzyme assay, and fasting IRI was measured by enzyme immunoassay. Glucose tolerance was determined by a 75-g oral glucose tolerance test (75-g OGTT). The diagnostic criteria for diabetes mellitus were in accordance with the Committee of the Japan Diabetes Society on the Diagnostic Criteria of Diabetes Mellitus [28]. Impaired glucose tolerance was defined as a 2-h postload plasma glucose level $\geq$ 140 mg/dl in subjects not meeting the criteria for diabetes mellitus [28]. The responses of glucose and insulin to 75-g OGTT were analyzed by calculating the area under the curve (AUC) for glucose and the AUC for insulin using a trapezoidal method. Insulin resistance was determined by homeostasis model assessment of insulin resistance (HOMA-IR) and quantitative insulin-sensitivity check index (QUICKI). The HOMA-IR was calculated using the formula FPG (mg/dl) × fasting IRI (μU/ml)/405, while the QUICKI was calculated as 1/(log fasting IRI [μU/ml] + log FPG [mg/dl]). Patients with HOMA-IR > 2.0 were considered insulin resistant. Fasting venous blood samples were taken on a random day, between 8:30 and 10:30 AM after a 12-h overnight fast, before initiation of ovulation induction with CC.

Measurements of cardiovascular parameters

In the first cycle of CC treatment, measurements of cardiovascular parameters were performed on day 3–5 after a spontaneous or a progestin-induced withdrawal bleeding. Blood pressure was measured in the supine position on the right arm after a 10-min rest; a standard sphygmomanometer of appropriate cuff size was used, and the first and fifth phases were recorded. Values used in the analysis are the average of 3 readings taken at 5-min intervals. The diagnostic criteria for hypertension were systolic blood pressure $\geq$ 140 mmHg or diastolic blood pressure $\geq$ 90 mmHg based on the Japanese Society of Hypertension Guidelines for the Management of Hypertension [29]. Mean blood pressure, which indicates overall peripheral resistance, was calculated as diastolic pressure plus one-third of the pulse pressure. baPWV, which indicates arterial stiffness, was measured using a volume-plethysmographic apparatus (form ABI; Omron Colin, Co., Ltd., Tokyo, Japan). The patient was examined in the supine position after resting for at least 5 min, with electrocardiogram electrodes placed on both wrists, a microphone to detect heart sounds placed on the left edge of the sternum, and cuffs wrapped on both the brachia and ankles. The intra- and interassay CV were < 8% for baPWV.

Statistical analysis

Because there were no studies in the literature on this subject, we were unable to estimate pretest power. Therefore, post hoc power analysis was performed by G*Power Software (version 3.1.9.2). Data were presented as mean ± SD if a normal distribution was expected; otherwise, median and range were used. In univariate analysis, differences in nominal variables between the groups were compared with the χ^2 test, unless the expected frequency was < 5, in which case, the Fisher's exact probability test was used. Differences in continuous variables were analyzed by nonparametric Mann-Whitney U test. The differences in continuous variables were compared between groups using the Student's t test. Multivariate logistic regression analysis was applied to evaluate the predictors for ovulatory response to CC in PCOS patients. $P > 0.10$ was used as a cutoff level to eliminate non-significant predictors from the prognostic model. The area under the receiver operating characteristic curve was used to assess the discriminative ability of the logistic models. Statistical analysis was performed with R software (The R Foundation for Statistical Computing, version 2.13.0). Significance was defined as $P < 0.05$.

Results

Thirty-eight PCOS patients (61%) were CC responders, and 24 (39%) were non-responders. Table 1 summarizes the clinical characteristics and endocrine parameters of the CC responder and non-responder groups. Age, BMI, the percentages of overweight ($25 \leq BMI < 30$) and obese (BMI ≥ 30) patients did not significantly differ between the groups. Waist-to-hip ratio was significantly higher among CC non-responders than CC responders. Although testosterone concentration did not differ between the groups, the level of free testosterone in CC non-responders was significantly higher than that in CC responders.

Table 2 summarizes the metabolic parameters in both groups. The percentage of CC non-responders with dyslipidemia was significantly higher than that of CC responders. The lipid parameters of triglycerides, LDL cholesterol, HDL cholesterol, and total cholesterol did not significantly differ between the groups. The percentage of patients with impaired glucose tolerance or diabetes mellitus was significantly higher among CC non-responders than CC responders. In assessing the glycemic and insulinemic response to 75-g OGTT, the levels of fasting glucose and IRI did not differ between groups, while the blood glucose and IRI levels at 60 min and 120 min and the

Table 1 Clinical characteristics and endocrine parameters of CC responsive and non-responsive patients with polycystic ovary syndrome

	CC responders (n = 38)	CC non-responders (n = 24)	P value
Age (y)	30.5 ± 4.7	31.5 ± 3.7	0.38
BMI (kg/m²)	23.7 ± 5.6	25.7 ± 6.4	0.21
No. of patients with < 18.5 BMI (%)	4 (11)	3 (13)	0.83
No. of patients with 18.5 ≤ BMI < 25 (%)	22 (58)	9 (38)	0.19
No. of patients with 25 ≤ BMI < 30 (%)	6 (16)	7 (29)	0.22
No. of patients with ≥ 30 BMI (%)	6 (16)	5 (21)	0.74
Gravida*	0 (0–3)	1 (0–4)	0.26
Parity*	0 (0–1)	0 (0–1)	0.82
Waist (cm)	78.2 ± 12.4	84.0 ± 12.3	0.11
Hip (cm)	95.82 ± 9.1	96.9 ± 8.8	0.67
Waist-to-hip ratio	0.81 ± 0.06	0.88 ± 0.07	0.001
LH (mIU/ml)	10.7 ± 3.8	12.3 ± 7.3	0.25
FSH (mIU/ml)	7.0 ± 1.7	6.6 ± 1.1	0.32
LH/FSH	1.6 ± 0.6	1.8 ± 0.9	0.23
PRL (ng/ml)	12.1 ± 5.8	12.3 ± 7.3	0.92
E2 (pg/ml)	46.93 ± 20.6	50.2 ± 18.2	0.54
Testosterone (ng/ml)	78.5 ± 25.8	99.6 ± 33.9	0.11
Free testosterone (pg/ml)	0.80 ± 0.34	1.17 ± 0.69	0.006
DHEA-S (µg/dl)	2095 ± 683	2284 ± 814	0.50

CC: clomiphene citrate, BMI: body mass index, DHEA-S: dehydroepiandrosterone sulfate.
*Median (range).

AUC of glucose and IRI were significantly higher among CC non-responders than in CC responders. The values of HOMA-IR and QUICKI, indicators for insulin resistance, did not significantly differ between the groups.

Table 3 summarizes the cardiovascular parameters in both groups. The levels of systolic, diastolic, and mean blood pressure did not significantly differ, while baPWV was significantly higher in the CC non-responder group than in CC responders.

In multivariate logistic regression analysis, both waist-to-hip ratio and baPWV were independent predictors for ovulatory response to CC in the PCOS patients (Table 4). Therefore, we validated the efficacy of measurement of waist-to-hip ratio and baPWV for the prediction of CC resistance in PCOS patients. Figure 1 shows the receiver operating characteristic curves of waist-to-hip ratio and baPWV for the prediction of CC resistance. The AUCs for waist-to-hip ratio and baPWV were 0.76 and 0.77, respectively. Setting the threshold at 0.83 for waist-to-hip ratio offered the best compromise between

Table 2 Metabolic parameters in CC responsive and non-responsive patients with polycystic ovary syndrome

	CC responders (n = 38)	CC non-responders (n = 24)	P value
No. of patients with dyslipidemia (%)	6 (16)	11 (38)	0.02
Triglycerides (mg/dl)	90.4 ± 44.9	117.1 ± 67.6	0.08
LDL cholesterol (mg/dl)	112.2 ± 44.6	116.0 ± 32.9	0.73
HDL cholesterol (mg/dl)	65.3 ± 13.5	60.1 ± 15.6	0.18
Total cholesterol (mg/dl)	192.0 ± 42.0	197.9 ± 31.6	0.57
No. of patients with IGT or DM (%)	4 (11)	11 (46)	0.004
75-g OGTT			
Plasma glucose (mg/dl)			
Fasting	88.9 ± 8.4	89.6 ± 7.5	0.76
60 min	129.0 ± 36.3	159.9 ± 48.4	0.01
120 min	112.1 ± 21.6	129.7 ± 41.9	0.04
AUC glucose (mg × h/dl)	936.9 ± 192.6	1080.9 ± 267.3	0.03
IRI (μU/ml)			
Fasting	9.6 ± 7.3	13.7 ± 9.7	0.09
60 min	67.1 ± 34.7	117.6 ± 90.0	0.007
120 min	61.2 ± 36.5	110.7 ± 107.5	0.02
AUC IRI (μU × h/ml)	473.3 ± 225.9	799.1 ± 609.1	0.009
HbA1c (%)	5.4 ± 0.4	5.6 ± 0.4	0.12
HOMA-IR	2.3 ± 1.9	3.4 ± 2.9	0.09
QUICKI	0.36 ± 0.04	0.34 ± 0.05	0.16

CC: clomiphene citrate, IGT: impaired glucose tolerance, DM: diabetes mellitus, AUC: area under the curve, IRI: immunoreactive insulin, HbA1c: hemoglobin A1c, HOMA-IR: homeostasis model assessment of insulin resistance, QUICKI: quantitative insulin-sensitivity check index.

specificity (0.65) and sensitivity (0.84), while the setting the threshold at 1,182 cm/s for baPWV offered the best compromise between specificity (0.80) and sensitivity (0.71). For patients with waist-to-hip ratio ≥ 0.83, the positive and negative predictive values were 0.72 and 0.79, respectively. For patients with baPWV ≥ 1,182 cm/s, the positive and negative predictive values were 0.69 and 0.81, respectively.

Table 3 Cardiovascular parameters in CC responsive and non-responsive patients with polycystic ovary syndrome

	CC responders (n = 38)	CC non-responders (n = 24)	P value
No. of patients with hypertension (%)	6 (16)	3 (13)	1.0
Systolic BP (mmHg)	118.5 ± 15.5	121.2 ± 16.1	0.54
Diastolic BP (mmHg)	69.3 ± 14.4	71.0 ± 11.8	0.64
Mean BP (mmHg)	85.7 ± 13.8	87.8 ± 12.9	0.58
baPWV (cm/s)	1113.9 ± 129.9	1249.2 ± 173.4	0.002

CC: clomiphene citrate, baPWV: brachial-to-ankle pulse wave velocity.

Table 4 Independent predictors for ovulatory response to CC in patients with polycystic ovary syndrome

Independent variables	Odds ratio (95% confidence interval)	P value
Waist-to-hip ratio	1.77 (2.2–14.1)	0.04
baPWV	1.71 (1.1–2.8)	0.03

CC: clomiphene citrate, baPWV: brachial-to-ankle pulse wave velocity.

Discussion

In the present study, we found that both metabolic and cardiovascular parameters were predictive for CC resistance in patients with PCOS. The measurement of waist-to-hip ratio and baPWV may be useful tools to predict the possibility for ovulation in PCOS patients who receive CC.

In the present study, waist-to-hip ratio was an independent predictor for ovulatory response to CC in PCOS patients. The waist-to-hip ratio correlates with visceral adiposity in obese and non-obese women with PCOS [30]. Douchi et al. reported that the ratio of trunk fat to leg fat, which indicates visceral adiposity, is a good predictor for CC resistance in women with PCOS [31], which is consistent with our findings. In their study, the trunk-to-leg fat ratio was measured by dual-energy X-ray absorptiometry. The measurement of waist-to-hip ratio is an easy and more convenient method to predict CC resistance in PCOS. Lord et al. reported that visceral adiposity, but not body weight, BMI, or subcutaneous adiposity, was strongly correlated with insulin resistance in women with PCOS [30]. The increased visceral adiposity

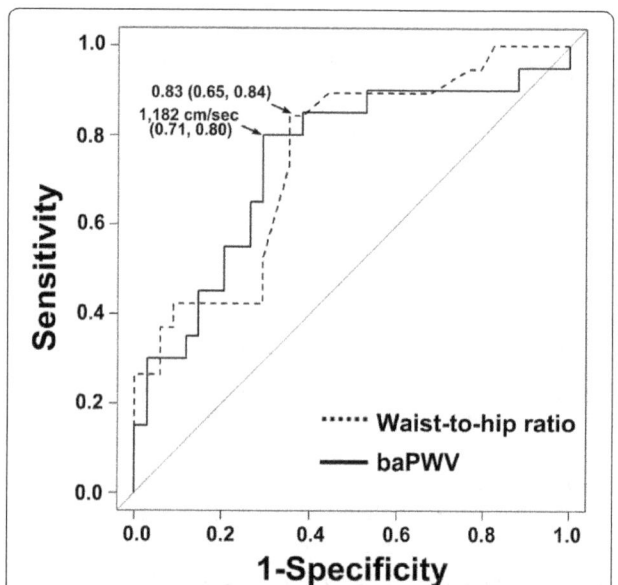

Figure 1 Receiver operating characteristic curve of waist-to-hip ratio and brachial-to-ankle pulse wave velocity (baPWV) to predict clomiphene citrate resistance in patients with polycystic ovary syndrome.

induces a decrease in adiponectin, which has an anti-inflammatory action, and an increase in inflammatory cytokines, such as tumor necrosis factor-α, interleukin-6, and free fatty acids, which raise insulin resistance [32]. The insulin resistance of peripheral tissues is thought to be an important etiological factor in PCOS [7]. These results support the hypothesis that increased visceral adiposity may be associated with CC resistance in PCOS women. Furthermore, waist-to-hip ratio is a well-known predictor for cardiovascular disease [33,34].

In the present study, baPWV was also an independent predictor for ovulatory response to CC in patients with PCOS. The baPWV is a surrogate marker for arterial stiffness [19] and a strong independent predictor of cardiovascular mortality in the patients with hypertension, end-stage renal disease, and diabetes [35-37]. An association between PCOS and arterial stiffness has been suggested [17,38-40]. Kelly et al. first reported that the brachial artery, but not aortic artery, PWV is significantly higher in reproductive-aged women with PCOS than in control women with regular menstrual cycles and normal androgen levels [17]. Meyer et al. also reported that central PWV in reproductive-aged women with PCOS is significantly higher than that in control women with regular menstrual cycles and normal androgen levels [39]. Moreover, Sasaki et al. reported that baPWV in reproductive-aged women with PCOS is significantly higher than that in control women with regular menstrual cycles and morphologically normal ovaries [18].

PWV is known to increase with age and hypertension in the general population [41]. Furthermore, several studies have reported that PWV increases in diabetic, dyslipidemia, and metabolic syndrome patients with insulin resistance [42,43]. Both total cholesterol and HOMA-IR, an indicator for insulin resistance, have been reported to correlate with PWV in women with PCOS [39]. Dyslipidemia is a well-known primary risk factor for the development of atherosclerosis and is very common in women with PCOS [44]. Therefore, dyslipidemia observed in reproductive-aged women with PCOS may influence early alteration of arterial structure, which leads to arterial stiffness.

No evidence of an association between PWV and CC resistance in women with PCOS has been previously reported. The precise mechanism for the increase in baPWV among CC non-responders compared to CC responders remains unclear. In the present study, although surrogate markers for insulin resistance, HOMA-IR and QUICKI, did not significantly differ between CC responders and non-responders, the percentage of patients with dyslipidemia and impaired glucose tolerance or diabetes mellitus in the CC non-responder group was higher compared to CC responders. Because PWV increases in patients with dyslipidemia and diabetes mellitus [43,45], these factors

may be one of the causes for the increase in baPWV among CC non-responders.

In the present study, free, but not total, testosterone level was also significantly higher in the CC non-responder group compared to CC responders. The free androgen index (FAI), which is obtained as the quotient 100 × total testosterone/SHBG, has been reported as higher in CC-resistant PCOS patients than in CC responders [46]. Moreover, Imani et al. reported that BMI, FAI, menstrual cycle history, and ovarian volume are useful predictors for CC resistance in infertile patients with World Health Organization group-II ovulatory disorders including PCOS [47]. These results indicate that hyperandrogenism, which may impair ovarian follicle development, may be involved in CC resistance in PCOS patients. In reproductive-aged women without PCOS, SHBG levels, but not total or free testosterone levels, were inversely associated with subclinical cardiovascular disease assessed by coronary artery calcified plaques and carotid artery intima-media thickness [48]. Creatsa et al. recently reported that higher serum testosterone and FAI are associated with subclinical atherosclerosis, while serum DHEA-S exhibits a negative association with arterial stiffness in healthy recently menopausal women [49]. These reports suggest that hyperandrogenism may be a link to the increased arterial stiffness observed in CC non-responsive PCOS patients.

In the present study, we could not explore the possible mechanisms involved in the increase in baPWV in CC-resistant PCOS patients. Further investigations are needed to demonstrate to link to the increase in arterial stiffness in CC-resistant PCOS. Because women with PCOS have multiple risk factors for cardiovascular disease (CVD) [14-16], such as impaired glucose tolerance, dyslipidemia, insulin resistance, and metabolic syndrome, the Androgen Excess and Polycystic Ovary Syndrome (AE-PCOS) Society published a consensus statement regarding assessment of CVD risk and CVD in women with PCOS [13].

Our study has certain limitations that should be noted. First, as PCOS was diagnosed according to the 2007 criteria of the JSOG [21], whose criteria matched the Rotterdam 2003 criteria [23], our findings might differ from other PCOS cohorts diagnosed by different criteria, such as National Institutes of Health 1990 and AE-PCOS. Because the prevalence of Japanese PCOS women with a sign of hyperandrogenism is very low compared to Caucasian women [22], the results of this study may not be extrapolated to other populations. Second, definitions vary the dose required to define CC-resistance ranging from 100 mg to 250 mg of CC [20,26,46,50,51]. In the present study, we defined CC non-responder as failure to ovulate with 100 mg of CC for at least 2 consecutive CC-treatment cycles. The CC non-responder in our study may ovulate in response to 150 mg of CC administration. However, the doses in excess of 100 mg per day are not approved by the Ministry of Health, Labour and Welfare of Japan as well as Food and Drug Administration of United States. Therefore, we could not prescribe more than 100 mg per day of CC in this study. Lastly, because of small sample size and retrospective study design, our findings should be interpreted with caution and confirmed by prospective study.

We performed a post hoc power analysis for the waist-to-hip ratio, baPWV, blood glucose and IRI levels at 60 min, and AUC of glucose and IRI with a two-sided level of significance of 0.05 and found a power of 0.98, 0.91, 0.84, 0.79, 0.64, and 0.76, respectively. After eliminating confounding factors, the both waist-to-hip ratio and baPWV were independent prognostic factors for ovulatory response to CC in patients with PCOS in multivariate analysis. Moreover, the measurement of waist-to-hip ratio and baPWV is quick and non-invasive to perform in comparison with blood sampling. Based on these results, both waist-to-hip ratio and baPWV might be candidates for prognostic factor for CC-resistant PCOS women.

In summary, the present study demonstrated that both metabolic and cardiovascular parameters were predictive for CC resistance in PCOS patients. The measurement of waist-to-hip ratio and baPWV may be useful tools to predict the possibility for ovulation in PCOS patients who receive CC. This study provides the first evidence of an association between arterial stiffness and CC resistance in patients with PCOS. A prospective study should be performed in order to access the clinical impact of measurement of baPWV for predicting CC-resistant PCOS women.

Abbreviations
PCOS: Polycystic ovary syndrome; CC: Clomiphene citrate; baPWV: Brachial-to-ankle pulse wave velocity; hCG: Human chorionic gonadotropin; DHEA-S: Dehydroepiandrosterone sulfate; CV: Coefficient of variation; BMI: Body mass index; LDL: Low-density lipoprotein; HDL: High-density lipoprotein; FPG: Fasting plasma glucose; IRI: Immunoreactive insulin; OGTT: Oral glucose tolerance test; AUC: Area under the curve; HOMA-IR: Homeostasis model assessment of insulin resistance; QUICKI: Quantitative insulin-sensitivity check index; CVD: Cardiovascular disease; FAI: Free androgen index; AE-PCOS: Androgen Excess and Polycystic Ovary Syndrome.

Competing interests
The authors declare that they have no competing interest.

Authors' contributions
TT contributed to study conception and design, acquisition, analysis and interpretation of data and drafting of the manuscript. HI, SH, MA, KM and AH contributed to acquisition and analysis of data. HK contributed to drafting of the manuscript and critical discussion. All the authors approved the manuscript.

Acknowledgement
This study was supported by a Grant-in-aid for General Science Research No. 22591815 to Toshifumi Takahashi, 22390308 and 24659723 to Hirohisa Kurachi, and the Global COE Program for Medical Sciences from the Japan Society for the Promotion of Science.

References
1. Asuncion M, Calvo RM, San Millan JL, Sancho J, Avila S, Escobar-Morreale HF: A prospective study of the prevalence of the polycystic ovary syndrome in unselected Caucasian women from Spain. *J Clin Endocrinol Metab* 2000, **85:**2434–2438.
2. Kousta E, White DM, Franks S: Modern use of clomiphene citrate in induction of ovulation. *Hum Reprod Update* 1997, **3:**359–365.
3. Pritts EA: Treatment of the infertile patient with polycystic ovarian syndrome. *Obstet Gynecol Surv* 2002, **57:**587–597.
4. Eijkemans MJC, Imani B, Mulders AGMGJ, Habbema JDF, Fauser BCJM: High singleton live birth rate following classical ovulation induction in normogonadotrophic anovulatory infertility (WHO 2). *Hum Reprod* 2003, **18:**2357–2362.
5. Thessaloniki EA-SPCWG: Consensus on infertility treatment related to polycystic ovary syndrome. *Fertil Steril* 2008, **89:**505–522.
6. Fernandez H, Morin-Surruca M, Torre A, Faivre E, Deffieux X, Gervaise A: Ovarian drilling for surgical treatment of polycystic ovarian syndrome: a comprehensive review. *Reprod Biomed Online* 2011, **22:**556–568.
7. Dunaif A: Insulin resistance and the polycystic ovary syndrome: mechanism and implications for pathogenesis. *Endocr Rev* 1997, **18:**774–800.
8. Adashi EY, Resnick CE, D'Ercole AJ, Svoboda ME, Van Wyk JJ: Insulin-like growth factors as intraovarian regulators of granulosa cell growth and function. *Endocr Rev* 1985, **6:**400–420.
9. Nestler JE, Powers LP, Matt DW, Steingold KA, Plymate SR, Rittmaster RS, Clore JN, Blackard WG: A direct effect of hyperinsulinemia on serum sex hormone-binding globulin levels in obese women with the polycystic ovary syndrome. *J Clin Endocrinol Metab* 1991, **72:**83–89.
10. Murakawa H, Hasegawa I, Kurabayashi T, Tanaka K: Polycystic ovary syndrome. Insulin resistance and ovulatory responses to clomiphene citrate. *J Reprod Med* 1999, **44:**23–27.
11. Kurabayashi T, Suzuki M, Fujita K, Murakawa H, Hasegawa I, Tanaka K: Prognostic factors for ovulatory response with clomiphene citrate in polycystic ovary syndrome. *Eur J Obstet Gynecol Reprod Biol* 2006, **126:**201–205.
12. Legro RS, Kunselman AR, Dodson WC, Dunaif A: Prevalence and predictors of risk for type 2 diabetes mellitus and impaired glucose tolerance in polycystic ovary syndrome: a prospective, controlled study in 254 affected women. *J Clin Endocrinol Metab* 1999, **84:**165–169.
13. Wild RA, Carmina E, Diamanti-Kandarakis E, Dokras A, Escobar-Morreale HF, Futterweit W, Lobo R, Norman RJ, Talbott E, Dumesic DA: Assessment of cardiovascular risk and prevention of cardiovascular disease in women with the polycystic ovary syndrome: a consensus statement by the Androgen Excess and Polycystic Ovary Syndrome (AE-PCOS) Society. *J Clin Endocrinol Metab* 2010, **95:**2038–2049.
14. Giallauria F, Orio F, Palomba S, Lombardi G, Colao A, Vigorito C: Cardiovascular risk in women with polycystic ovary syndrome. *J Cardiovasc Med (Hagerstown)* 2008, **9:**987–992.
15. Orio F, Vuolo L, Palomba S, Lombardi G, Colao A: Metabolic and cardiovascular consequences of polycystic ovary syndrome. *Minerva Ginecol* 2008, **60:**39–51.
16. Giallauria F, Orio F, Lombardi G, Colao A, Vigorito C, Tafuri MG, Palomba S: Relationship between heart rate recovery and inflammatory markers in patients with polycystic ovary syndrome: a cross-sectional study. *J Ovarian Res* 2009, **2:**3.
17. Kelly CJ, Speirs A, Gould GW, Petrie JR, Lyall H, Connell JM: Altered vascular function in young women with polycystic ovary syndrome. *J Clin Endocrinol Metab* 2002, **87:**742–746.
18. Sasaki A, Emi Y, Matsuda M, Sharula, Kamada Y, Chekir C, Hiramatsu Y, Nakatsuka M: Increased arterial stiffness in mildly-hypertensive women with polycystic ovary syndrome. *J Obstet Gynaecol Res* 2011, **37:**402–411.
19. Newman AB, Siscovick DS, Manolio TA, Polak J, Fried LP, Borhani NO, Wolfson SK: Ankle-arm index as a marker of atherosclerosis in the Cardiovascular Health Study. Cardiovascular Heart Study (CHS) Collaborative Research Group. *Circulation* 1993, **88:**837–845.
20. Hara S, Takahashi T, Amita M, Igarashi H, Kurachi H: Usefulness of bezafibrate for ovulation induction in clomiphene citrate-resistant polycystic ovary syndrome patients with dyslipidemia: a prospective pilot study of seven cases. *Gynecol Obstet Invest* 2010, **70:**166–172.

21. Mizunuma H, Irahara M: The Committee for Reproductive and Endocrine in Japan Society of Obstetrics and Gynecology. Annual report fro the determination of diagnostic criteria for polycystic ovary syndrome. *Acta Obstet Gynaecol Jpn* 2007, 59:1142–1147.

22. Carmina E, Koyama T, Chang L, Stanczyk FZ, Lobo RA: Does ethnicity influence the prevalence of adrenal hyperandrogenism and insulin resistance in polycystic ovary syndrome? *Am J Obstet Gynecol* 1992, 167:1807–1812.

23. Rotterdam ESHRE/ASRM-Sponsored PCOS Consensus Workshop G: Revised 2003 consensus on diagnostic criteria and long-term health risks related to polycystic ovary syndrome. *Fertil Steril* 2004, 81:19–25.

24. Homburg R: Clomiphene citrate–end of an era? a mini-review. *Hum Reprod* 2005, 2043–2051.

25. Padova G, Briguglia G, Tita P, Arpi ML, Munguira ME, Cafiso F, Cianci A, Ettore G, Pezzino V: Ovulation monitored by serum 17 beta-estradiol and ultrasound: differential ovarian response to human gonadotropins in various anovulatory states. *Acta Eur Fertil* 1988, 19:283–286.

26. Badawy A, Mosbah A, Tharwat A, Eid M: Extended letrozole therapy for ovulation induction in clomiphene-resistant women with polycystic ovary syndrome: a novel protocol. *Fertil Steril* 2009, 92:236–239.

27. Teramoto T, Sasaki J, Ueshima H, Egusa G, Kinoshita M, Shimamoto K, Daida H, Biro S, Hirobe K, Funahashi T, Yokote K, Yokode M: Diagnostic criteria for dyslipidemia. Executive summary of Japan Atherosclerosis Society (JAS) guideline for diagnosis and prevention of atherosclerotic cardiovascular diseases for Japanese. *J Atheroscler Thromb* 2007, 14:155–158.

28. Seino Y, Nanjo K, Tajima N, Kadowaki T, Kashiwagi A, Araki E, Ito C, Inagaki N, Iwamoto Y, Kasuga M, Hanafusa T, Haneda M, Ueki K: Report of the Committee on the Classification and Diagnostic Criteria of Diabetes Mellitus. *J Diabetes Invest* 2010, 1:212–228.

29. Ogihara T, Kikuchi K, Matsuoka H, Fujita T, Higaki J, Horiuchi M, Imai Y, Imaizumi T, Ito S, Iwao H, Kario K, Kawano Y, Kim-Mitsuyama S, Kimura G, Matsubara H, Matsuura H, Naruse M, Saito I, Shimada K, Shimamoto K, Suzuki H, Takishita S, Tanahashi N, Tsuchihashi T, Uchiyama M, Ueda S, Ueshima H, Umemura S, Ishimitsu T, Rakugi H: The Japanese Society of Hypertension Guidelines for the Management of Hypertension (JSH 2009). *Hypertens Res* 2009, 32:3–107.

30. Lord J, Thomas R, Fox B, Acharya U, Wilkin T: The central issue? Visceral fat mass is a good marker of insulin resistance and metabolic disturbance in women with polycystic ovary syndrome. *BJOG* 2006, 113:1203–1209.

31. Douchi T, Oki T, Yamasaki H, Nakae M, Imabayashi A, Nagata Y: Body fat patterning in polycystic ovary syndrome women as a predictor of the response to clomiphene. *Acta Obstet Gynecol Scand* 2004, 83:838–841.

32. Matsuzawa Y: Adiponectin: a key player in obesity related disorders. *Curr Pharm Des* 2010, 16:1896–1901.

33. de Koning L, Merchant AT, Pogue J, Anand SS: Waist circumference and waist-to-hip ratio as predictors of cardiovascular events: meta-regression analysis of prospective studies. *Eur Heart J* 2007, 28:850–856.

34. Wang Z, Hoy W: Waist circumference, body mass index, hip circumference and waist-to-hip ratio as predictors of cardiovascular disease in Aboriginal people. *Eur J Clin Nutr* 2004, 58:888–893.

35. Yokoyama H, Shoji T, Kimoto E, Shinohara K, Tanaka S, Koyama H, Emoto M, Nishizawa Y: Pulse wave velocity in lower-limb arteries among diabetic patients with peripheral arterial disease. *J Atheroscler Thromb* 2003, 10:253–258.

36. Laurent S, Boutouyrie P, Asmar R, Gautier I, Laloux B, Guize L, Ducimetiere P, Benetos A: Aortic stiffness is an independent predictor of all-cause and cardiovascular mortality in hypertensive patients. *Hypertension* 2001, 37:1236–1241.

37. Blacher J, Guerin AP, Pannier B, Marchais SJ, Safar ME, London GM: Impact of aortic stiffness on survival in end-stage renal disease. *Circulation* 1999, 99:2434–2439.

38. Lakhani K, Seifalian AM, Hardiman P: Impaired carotid viscoelastic properties in women with polycystic ovaries. *Circulation* 2002, 106:81–85.

39. Meyer C, McGrath BP, Teede HJ: Overweight women with polycystic ovary syndrome have evidence of subclinical cardiovascular disease. *J Clin Endocrinol Metab* 2005, 90:5711–5716.

40. Soares GM, Vieira CS, Martins WP, Franceschini SA, dos Reis RM, de Sa MF S, Ferriani RA: Increased arterial stiffness in nonobese women with polycystic ovary syndrome (PCOS) without comorbidities: one more characteristic inherent to the syndrome? *Clin Endocrinol (Oxf)* 2009, 71:406–411.

41. Hasegawa M, Nagao K, Kinoshita Y, Rodbard D, Asahina A: Increased pulse wave velocity and shortened pulse wave transmission time in hypertension and aging. *Cardiology* 1997, 88:147–151.

42. Tsubakimoto A, Saito I, Mannami T, Naito Y, Nakamura S, Dohi Y, Yonemasu K: Impact of metabolic syndrome on brachial-ankle pulse wave velocity in Japanese. *Hypertens Res* 2006, 29:29–37.

43. Cruickshank K, Riste L, Anderson SG, Wright JS, Dunn G, Gosling RG: Aortic pulse-wave velocity and its relationship to mortality in diabetes and glucose intolerance: an integrated index of vascular function? *Circulation* 2002, 106:2085–2090.

44. Legro RS, Kunselman AR, Dunaif A: Prevalence and predictors of dyslipidemia in women with polycystic ovary syndrome. *Am J Med* 2001, 111:607–613.

45. Yokoyama H, Kawasaki M, Ito Y, Minatoguchi S, Fujiwara H: Effects of fluvastatin on the carotid arterial media as assessed by integrated backscatter ultrasound compared with pulse-wave velocity. *J Am Coll Cardiol* 2005, 46:2031–2037.

46. Verit FF, Erel O, Kocyigit A: Association of increased total antioxidant capacity and anovulation in nonobese infertile patients with clomiphene citrate-resistant polycystic ovary syndrome. *Fertil Steril* 2007, 88:418–424.

47. Imani B, Eijkemans MJC, te Velde ER, Habbema JDF, Fauser BCJM: Predictors of Patients Remaining Anovulatory during Clomiphene Citrate Induction of Ovulation in Normogonadotropic Oligomenorrheic Infertility. *J Clin Endocrinol Metab* 1998, 83:2361–2365.

48. Calderon-Margalit R, Schwartz SM, Wellons MF, Lewis CE, Daviglus ML, Schreiner PJ, Williams OD, Sternfeld B, Carr JJ, O'Leary DH, Sidney S, Friedlander Y, Siscovick DS: Prospective association of serum androgens and sex hormone-binding globulin with subclinical cardiovascular disease in young adult women: the "Coronary Artery Risk Development in Young Adults" women's study. *J Clin Endocrinol Metab* 2010, 95:4424–4431.

49. Creatsa M, Armeni E, Stamatelopoulos K, Rizos D, Georgiopoulos G, Kazani M, Alexandrou A, Dendrinos S, Augoulea A, Papamichael C, Lambrinoudaki I: Circulating androgen levels are associated with subclinical atherosclerosis and arterial stiffness in healthy recently menopausal women. *Metabolism* 2012, 61:193–201.

50. Yarali H, Yildiz BO, Demirol A, Zeyneloglu HB, Yigit N, Bukulmez O, Koray Z: Co-administration of metformin during rFSH treatment in patients with clomiphene citrate-resistant polycystic ovarian syndrome: a prospective randomized trial. *Hum Reprod* 2002, 17:289–294.

51. Ahmed MI, Duleba AJ, El Shahat O, Ibrahim ME, Salem A: Naltrexone treatment in clomiphene resistant women with polycystic ovary syndrome. *Hum Reprod* 2008, 23:2564–2569.

Association of Gly972Arg variant of insulin receptor subtrate-1 and Gly1057Asp variant of insulin receptor subtrate-2 with polycystic ovary syndrome in the Chinese population

Ming-Wei Lin[1], Mei-Feng Huang[2,3] and Meng-Hsing Wu[2,3]*

Abstract

Objective: Polycystic ovary syndrome (PCOS) is a common endocrinologic disease in women. In the present study, we examined the relationship of the *IRS-1* Gly972Arg and *IRS-2* Gly1057Asp polymorphisms to PCOS and phenotypic features of PCOS in a Chinese population from Taiwan.

Materials and methods: A total of three hundred and forty genetically unrelated women with age from 18 to 45 years, including two hundred and forty-eight *PCOS* patients and ninety-two control subjects, were recruited. The hormone and biochemical measurements were evaluated for each woman. Genotyping of the *IRS-1* gene Gly972Arg variant and *IRS-2* gene Gly1057Asp variant were performed by using direct sequencing.

Results: We found significant difference in the genotypic distribution of *IRS-2* gene Gly1057Asp between the PCOS group and the control group (p = 0.004). The carriers of homozygous *IRS-2* Asp had an increased risk of PCOS compared with the carriers of Gly/Gly (OR 4.08, 95% C.I. 1.60-10.41, p = 0.003). No significant difference in genotype frequencies of *IRS-1* Gly972Arg was observed between two groups. We further investigated the effect of interaction of *IRS-1* Gly972Arg and *IRS-2* Gly1057Asp on the risk of PCOS and found that women carried *IRS-1* Gly/Arg or *IRS-2* Asp/Asp or carried both *IRS-1* Gly/Arg and *IRS-2* Asp/Asp had a much higher risk of PCOS compared with their counterpart, respectively (OR 2.49, 95% C.I. 1.16-5.37, p = 0.019; OR 11.87, 95% C.I. 1.21-116.84, p = 0.034). We further found, the non-obese PCOS patients carried significantly higher frequency of *IRS-2* Asp/Asp as compared with the control group (p = 0.004). A significant effect of interaction of carrying both *IRS-1* Gly/Arg and *IRS-2* Asp/Asp was also observed in the non-obese PCOS patients (p = 0.003), but not in the obese PCOS patients.

Conclusions: In this study, we found significant association of the variant of *IRS-2* gene as well as the interaction of *IRS-1* and *IRS-2* genes with PCOS, especially in non-obese women. Women with *IRS-2* homozygous Asp variant may be considered as a risk factor for PCOS that needs early detection to prevent further complication in the Chinese population from Taiwan.

Keyword: Polycystic ovary syndrome, Polymorphism, *Insulin receptor substrate −1*, *Insulin receptor substrate-2*

* Correspondence: mhwu68@mail.ncku.edu.tw
[2]Departments of Physiology, National Cheng Kung University College of Medicine, Tainan, Taiwan
[3]Departments of Obstetrics and Gynecology, National Cheng Kung University College of Medicine and Hospital, 138 Sheng-Li Road, 70428 Tainan, Taiwan
Full list of author information is available at the end of the article

Introduction

Polycystic ovary syndrome (PCOS) is a highly prevalent syndrome of ovarian dysfunction affecting approximately 5-10% of reproductive-aged women [1]. The PCOS is characterized by chronic anovulation, hyperandrogenism, and/ or the presence of polycystic ovary morphology. The syndrome demonstrates a significant reproductive and metabolic impact, and is associated with increased risk of type 2 diabetes, dyslipidemia, cardiovascular disease, endometrial carcinoma, and also leads to infertility [2-6]. In general, PCOS can be viewed as a heterogeneous androgen excess disorder with various degrees of gonadotropic and metabolic abnormalities determined by the interaction of multiple genetic and environmental factors. Insulin resistance, particularly in skeletal muscle and adipose tissue with sensitivity in ovarian tissue, affects up to 70% of women with PCOS and is a risk factor in PCOS women for developing type 2 diabetes [7,8]; however, the mechanisms for defects in insulin signaling in the disorder are complex [9] and have not been fully elucidated.

The insulin receptor is a heterotetramer consist of two α, β-dimers. The α-subunit contains the ligand-binding site, while the β-subunit contains a ligand-activated tyrosine kinase. Once tyrosine is phosphorylated, the insulin receptor phosphorylates two intracellular substrates, insulin receptor substrate-1 (IRS-1) and insulin receptor substrate-2 (IRS-2). The IRS-1 serves as a docking molecule for signaling and will activate the enzyme phosphatidylinositol 3-kinase (PI3K), a necessary step for the initiation of several effects of insulin such as glucose transport. When the IRS-1 is dysfunctional, the IRS-2 is the main docking protein for the intracellular propagation of the insulin signal [10]. However, the IRS-2 requires a higher insulin concentration for activation, the hallmark of insulin resistance.

The *IRS-1* gene is located on chromosome 2q36 and encodes a 1,242-amino acid protein with a molecular weight of 131.6 kDa. The most common variant, Gly972Arg (rs1801278), was reported to be associated with insulin resistance, type 2 diabetes and PCOS [11-14]. The *IRS-2* gene is located on chromosome 13q34 and encodes a protein of 1,354 amino acids. Moreover, the most common variant Gly1057Asp (rs1805097) in the *IRS-2* gene has also been reported to influence the susceptibility to insulin resistance and type 2 diabetes in PCOS women [15-17]. Two recent meta-analysis of PCOS studies reported that the *IRS-1* Gly972Arg polymorphism concerning the Gly/Arg *vs.* Gly/Gly genotype is significantly associated with the risk of developing PCOS and that this association is primarily mediated by increasing the levels of fasting insulin [18,19]. However, another meta-analysis of five studies with 519 cases and 883 controls failed to

demonstrate significant association between *IRS-2* Gly1057Asp polymorphism and PCOS [19].

Although the meta-analysis reported positive associations of the *IRS-1* Gly972Arg with PCOS and no association between the *IRS-2* Gly1057Asp polymorphism and PCOS, the results from different studies were controversial and were lack of data from Chinese ethnic origin. The aim of the study was to investigate if *IRS-1* Gly972Arg and *IRS-2* Gly1057Asp influence insulin resistance and are associated with risk of PCOS in the Chinese PCOS patients and controls from Taiwan.

Materials and methods
Subjects

A total of three hundred and forty genetically unrelated women with age from 18 to 45 years, including two hundred and forty-eight PCOS patients and ninety-two control subjects, were recruited from the Obstetrics and Gynecology clinics of the National Cheng Kung University Hospital (Tainan, Taiwan). This study was approved by the Institution Review Board of the hospital. Written informed consent was obtained from all participants. The study was in compliance with the Helsinki Declaration. All the participants are Han Chinese from the same geographical region in Taiwan.

The diagnosis of PCOS was assigned according to the 2003 Rotterdam criteria (The Rotterdam ESHRE/ASRM-sponsored PCOS consensus workshop group, 2004). The criteria are as follows: (i) oligo- and/or anovulation that is defined as the absence of menstruation for more than 35 days; (ii) clinical and/or biochemical signs of hyperandrogenism: the former is defined as and modified Ferriman-Gallwey score of 6 or greater with/without acne or androgenic alopecia, and the latter as total testosterone level of more than 0.95 ng/ml; and (iii) polycystic ovarian morphology identified by ultrasound scan. Women fulfilled any two of above three criteria were diagnosed as PCOS. The exclusion criteria included non-classic congenital adrenal hyperplasia, hyperprolactinemia, and androgen-secreting tumors. All the patients did not take any medication having effect on insulin levels or hormonal medications, including contraceptive pills, at least two months before their participating in the study. The control patients were enrolled from infertility clinic prior to entering an *in vitro* fertilization program due to tubal and/or male factors with free of menstrual cycle irregularities, clinical or biochemical hyperandrogenism, polycystic ovaries on ultrasound examination, or history of systemic/endocrine disease.

Hormone and biochemical measurement

The blood samples were obtained in the early follicular phase of menstrual cycle, but the random blood samples were obtained when amenorrheic. Biochemical assessment consisted of complete hormonal, including serum follicle stimulating hormone (FSH) luteinizing hormone (LH), thyroid-stimulating hormone (TSH), prolactin (PRL), estradiol (E_2), 17-OH-progesterone (17-OHP), total testosterone, and sex-hormone binding globulin (SHBG), and metabolic evaluation, including evaluation of lipid, glucose and insulin levels. All subjects received a 75-g glucose monohydrate in 350-ml water after a 10-h overnight fasting. A total of 5 ml blood sample was drawn before glucose loading and another 5 ml blood samples was drawn at 120 minutes after the glucose loading. Plasma glucose and insulin concentrations were determined by a glucose oxidase method in a glucose analyzer (model 2300, YSI, Yellow Springs, OH, USA) and by an automated chemiluminescence system (ADVIA Centaur Immunoassay System, Siemens Healthcare Diagnostics, Deerfield, IL, USA), respectively. Insulin resistance was evaluated using the homeostasis model analysis (HOMA) [fasting glucose (mg/dL) × fasting insulin (μU/mL)/405], quantitative insulin-sensitivity check index (QUICKI) [1/[log(fasting insulin) + log(fasting glucose)]], and the fasting glucose-to-insulin ratio (A/I).

Genotyping by re-sequencing

A total of 10 mL whole blood sample was taken from each subject for genotyping. Genomic deoxyribonucleic acid (DNA) was extracted from whole blood using the GeneMark extraction Kit (GeneMark Technology Co., Ltd., Tainan, Taiwan, ROC) according to the manufacturer's instruction. Genotypings of the *IRS-1* gene Gly972Arg variant (rs 1801278) and the *IRS-2* gene Gly1057Asp (rs1805097) variant were performed by using direct sequencing. The primer sequences for the *IRS-1* Gly972Arg polymorphism were 5'-GGGTCGAG ATGGGCAGACT-3' and 5'-GGGACAACTCATCTGC ATGGT-3'; while for the *IRS-2* Gly1057Asp polymorphism were 5'-GGAGCTGTACCGCCTGCC-3' and 5'-AC CAAAAGCCATCTCGGTGT-3', respectively. Twenty to fifty nanograms of total genomic DNA was amplified in a total volume of twenty-five microliter containing 900 nM primers, and 12.5 ul of Taq-Man universal PCR master mix (Perkin-Elmer, Applied Biosystems Division) by using the standard polymerase chain reaction (PCR) techniques. The PCR amplification was performed with the following conditions: 95°C, 10 min; followed by 40 cycles of 95°C 1 min, 53°C 30 secs., and 72°C 30 secs. The final step was 72°C for 10 minutes. The PCR reactions were performed in 96-well microtiter plates and the sequencing reactions were performed using the ABI BigDye Terminator reagents (Applied Biosystems, Foster City, CA). The PCR products were sent to the Nucleic Acid Sequencing Center of National Cheng-Kung University

for sequencing by using the ABI 3100 DNA sequencer (Applied Biosystems, Foster City, CA). The sequence data were analyzed by using the PolyPhred software (v5.04) [20]. The genotypes were assigned to the subjects independently by two individuals blinded to the subject information.

Statistical analysis

Data were expressed as mean ± SD or number (%). Two-sample *t* test was applied to compare the mean differences between groups. Differences in genotypic frequencies and categorical data between groups were compared by using

Table 1 Descriptive characteristics of the study participants

	PCOS group	Control group	p^a
Subjects (n)	248	92	
Age (years)	28.2 ± 5.4	32.4 ± 5.5	< 0.001
Body weight (kg)	62.7 ± 14.8	56.9 ± 10.3	< 0.001
Body height (cm)	159.4 ± 5.3	159.7 ± 5.3	0.681
BMI (kg/m²)	24.7 ± 5.5	22.3 ± 4.0	< 0.001
Waist circumference (cm)	83.9 ± 13.5	82.7 ± 12.2	0.705
Systolic BP (mmHg)	117 ± 15	115 ± 14	0.178
Diastolic BP (mmHg)	70 ± 11	70 ± 11	0.852
Total cholesterol (mg/dL)	181.9 ± 43.0	189.9 ± 35.5	0.285
Triglycerides (mg/dL)	104.3 ± 67.5	91.6 ± 46.0	0.258
HDL-C (mg/dL)	53.8 ± 12.8	58.6 ± 17.4	0.063
LDL-C (mg/dL)	114.4 ± 43.8	115.3 ± 32.2	0.914
Fasting insulin	9.9 ± 10.5	9.3 ± 15.5	0.733
2 hr insulin	54.8 ± 52.0	32.5 ± 26.5	< 0.001
HbA1C (%)	5.5 ± 0.5	5.3 ± 0.3	0.037
AC (mg/dL)	89.4 ± 12.0	87.6 ± 5.3	0.086
PC (mg/dL)	110.4 ± 36.2	99.0 ± 25.9	0.036
HOMA index (mg/L)	2.3 ± 2.6	2.0 ± 3.4	0.542
A/I (AC/ Fasting Insulin)	16.7 ± 11.7	17.9 ± 11.4	0.489
QUICKI index (mg/L)	3.4 ± 0.8	3.5 ± 0.7	0.674
SHBG (nmol/L)	37.8 ± 29.7	59.6 ± 53.8	0.007
17-OHP (ng/mL)	1.8 ± 1.4	2.0 ± 1.3	0.529
Hirsutism score	5.6 ± 3.8	3.2 ± 2.9	0.016
TSH (μU/mL)	2.1 ± 1.3	2 .0 ± 1.0	0.618
LH (mIU/mL)	8.0 ± 5.3	4.3 ± 2.5	< 0.001
FSH (mIU/mL)	5.6 ± 2.0	6.0 ± 2.4	0.212
E2 (pg/mL)	45.8 ± 22.9	43.1 ± 27.5	0.484
Testosterone (ng/mL)	0.55 ± 0.31	0.35 ± 0.19	< 0.001
Free androgen index	5.98 ± 4.61	4.04 ± 4.02	0.043
PRL (ng/mL)	12.5 ± 6.4	13.5 ± 6.3	0.248

[a]Compared by t test.

Pearson's chi-squared tests. Hardy-Weinberg equilibrium at each SNP was tested using Pearson's chi-squared tests. Logistic regression analyses were performed to examine the differences in genotypic frequencies and interaction of two SNPs between the PCOS and control groups. Odds ratios and 95% confidence interval (ORs ± 95% CI) from the logistic regression model after controlling for other covariates were used to estimate the magnitude of the association between genotype and PCOS. The statistical analyses were performed using the SPSS program (Version 17.0, SPSS Inc., Chicago, IL, USA). A p value less than 0.05 was considered as statistically significant.

Results
Clinical and biochemical characteristics of the study population
The clinical and biochemical characteristics of the PCOS and control groups were summarized in Table 1. The PCOS subjects were significant younger and had higher body weight and body mass index as compared with the control subjects. As we could expect, the levels of LH, testosterone, free androgen index, SHBG and Hirsutism score were significantly higher in the PCOS group than in the control group. Moreover, the PCOS patients also had significantly elevated levels of glucose, insulin at 2 hour during the oral glucose tolerance test, and HbA1C (glucose: 110.4 ± 36.2 mg/dL; insulin: 54.8 ± 52.0 mg/dL; HbA1C: 5.5 ± 0.5 (%)) compared with the control subjects (glucose: 99.0 ± 25.9 mg/dL; insulin: 32.5 ± 26.5 mg/dL; HbA1C: 5.3 ± 0.3 (%)). The results remained significant after adjusting the age effect between the PCOS and control groups.

IRS-1 and IRS-2 genotypes and gene-gene interaction
There was significant difference in IRS-2 gene Gly1057Asp genotypic distribution between the PCOS group and the control group (chi-squared test p = 0.004). The carriers of homozygous IRS-2 Asp had an increased risk of PCOS compared with the carriers of Gly/Gly after adjusting for age and BMI (OR =4.08, 95% C.I. 1.60-10.41, p = 0.003) (Table 2). However, no significant difference in genotype frequencies of IRS-1 Gly972Arg was observed between two groups (Table 2). The IRS-1 Gly972Arg variant was in Hardy-Weinberg equilibrium, but the IRS-2 Gly1057Asp variant was not in Hardy-Weinberg equilibrium in both PCOS and control groups.

When we further investigated the effect of interaction of IRS-1 Gly972Arg and IRS-2 Gly1057Asp on the risk of PCOS, we found that women carried IRS-1 Gly/Arg or IRS-2 Asp/Asp had an increased risk of PCOS (OR = 2.49, 95% C.I. 1.16-5.37, p = 0.019). Moreover, carriers of both IRS-1 Gly/Arg and IRS-2 Asp/Asp had a much higher risk of PCOS compared with their counterpart (OR = 11.87, 95% C.I. 1.21-116.84, p = 0.034) (Table 2).

IRS-2 genotype and clinical phenotypes
We then evaluated the association between IRS-2 Gly1057Asp genotype and clinical phenotypes in all subjects of both PCOS (n = 95) and control (n = 74) groups and found the levels of fasting insulin, and

Table 2 Genotypic distribution of polymorphisms in the _IRS1_ and _IRS2_ genes between the PCOS group and control group

	PCOS group	Control group	p^a	OR (95% C.I.)	p^b
IRS-1 Gly972Arg	(n = 248)	(n = 92)			
GG	220 (88.7%)	84 (91.3%)	0.622	1	
GA	28 (11.3%)	8 (8.7%)		1.03 (0.42-2.53)	0.942
IRS-2 Gly1057Asp	(n = 95)	(n = 74)			
GG	12 (12.6%)	25 (33.8%)		1	
GA	18 (18.9%)	13 (17.6%)	0.004	2.77 (0.87-8.81)	0.084
AA	65 (68.4%)	36 (48.6%)		4.08 (1.60-10.41)	0.003
GG + GA	30 (31.6%)	38 (51.4%)	0.015	1	
AA	65 (68.4%)	36 (48.6%)		2.52 (1.21-5.26)	0.014
IRS-1 and _IRS-2_	(n = 95)	(n = 74)			
GG/GG + GA	26 (27.4%)	35 (47.3%)		1	
GA/AA	58 (61.1%)	38 (51.4%)	0.003	2.49 (1.16-5.37)	0.019
GA and AA	11 (11.6%)	1 (1.4%)		11.87 (1.21-116.84)	0.034

[a]Compared by chi-square test.
[b]Compared by logistic regression after adjusting for age and BMI.

HOMA index were significantly higher in women carrying the homozygous Asp/Asp genotype than their counterparts (Gly/Gly and Gly/Asp) (Table 3). However, when we focused on the PCOS group, the association between *IRS-2* genotype and clinical phenotypes became statistically insignificant (data not shown).

IRS-1 and *IRS-2* genotypes and obesity

When the study subjects were classified into obese (obese: BMI ≥ 27 kg/m^2) (PCOS n = 72; Control n = 9) and non-obese groups (BMI < 27 kg/m^2) (PCOS n = 176; Control n = 83), the non-obese PCOS patients carried significantly

Table 3 Relationship between clinical phenotypes and genotypes of the *IRS-2 Gly1057Asp* polymorphism

	GG + GA	AA	p^a
Subjects (n)	68	101	
Age (years)	30.0 ± 6.2	29.7 ± 6.0	0.688
Body weight (kg)	58.7 ± 13.4	61.3 ± 13.3	0.208
Body height (cm)	159.8 ± 5.3	160.1 ± 5.6	0.779
BMI (kg/m^2)	23.0 ± 5.0	23.9 ± 4.8	0.219
Waist circumference (cm)	80.8 ± 12.1	86.2 ± 11.6	0.058
Systolic BP (mmHg)	113 ± 12	117 ± 15	0.055
Diastolic BP (mmHg)	69 ± 10	71 ± 11	0.209
Total cholesterol (mg/dL)	181.7 ± 48.3	180.6 ± 45.5	0.908
Triglycerides (mg/dL)	91.3 ± 59.5	110.8 ± 68.3	0.152
HDL-C (mg/dL)	55.6 ± 12.0	54.3 ± 13.6	0.653
LDL-C (mg/dL)	111.2 ± 33.4	114.7 ± 28.3	0.598
Fasting insulin	6.7 ± 6.1	11.0 ± 15.3	0.025
2 hr insulin	38.3 ± 31.6	54.2 ± 56.7	0.087
HbA1C (%)	5.4 ± 0.3	5.5 ± 0.5	0.544
AC (mg/dL)	87.6 ± 5.8	90.4 ± 16.8	0.164
PC (mg/dL)	105.4 ± 29.9	109.3 ± 40.2	0.557
HOMA index (mg/L)	1.5 ± 1.6	2.6 ± 3.8	0.022
A/I (AC/ Fasting Insulin)	19.1 ± 11.3	17.4 ± 12.3	0.427
QUICKI index (mg/L)	3.6 ± 0.8	3.5 ± 0.8	0.454
SHBG (nmol/L)	48.5 ± 41.9	40.2 ± 42.5	0.337
17-OHP (ng/mL)	1.8 ± 1.3	2.0 ± 1.4	0.400
Hirsutism score	4.6 ± 3.3	5.8 ± 3.9	0.289
TSH (µU/mL)	2.4 ± 1.5	2.0 ± 0.9	0.044
LH (mIU/mL)	6.8 ± 4.5	7.6 ± 5.5	0.367
FSH (mIU/mL)	5.6 ± 2.3	6.0 ± 2.3	0.445
E2 (pg/mL)	42.5 ± 23.4	48.2 ± 25.5	0.217
Testosterone (ng/mL)	0.4 ± 0.3	0.5 ± 0.3	0.289
Free androgen index	4.60 ± 3.61	6.01 ± 4.61	0.217
PRL (ng/mL)	12.8 ± 6.5	12.3 ± 6.1	0.692

^{a}Compared by t test.

higher frequency of *IRS-2* Asp/Asp as compared with the control group (p = 0.004) (Table 4). A significant effect of interaction of carrying both *IRS-1* Gly/Arg and *IRS-2* Asp/Asp was also observed in the non-obese PCOS patients (p = 0.003), but not in the obese PCOS patients (p = 0.834).

Discussion

PCOS is a highly prevalent syndrome of ovarian dysfunction and affects up to 10% of reproductive age women, nearly half of whom will develop impaired glucose tolerance or type 2 diabetes [8]. This predisposition to type 2 diabetes is a consequence of defects in both insulin action [9] and insulin secretion [15]. Recently, several polymorphisms in *IRS-1* and *IRS-2* have been implicated in PCOS [16,21]. However, the results in PCOS patients were in considerable disagreement and, therefore, the role of these variants in the pathogenesis of insulin resistance and PCOS remains debatable. In the present study, we found significant association of the variants of *IRS-2* gene as well as the interaction of *IRS-1* and *IRS-2* genes with PCOS, especially in non-obese women. We also found significantly increased levels of fasting insulin, and elevated HOMA index in women carrying the homozygous Asp/Asp genotype than their counterpart (Gly/Asp and Gly/Gly).

In our study, we found women with homozygous *IRS-2* Asp genotypes had a significantly increased risk of PCOS compared with the carriers of homozygous *IRS-2* Gly (OR = 4.08, 95% CI: 1.60-10.41). We also observed women with the *IRS-2* Asp/Asp genotype had significantly higher fasting insulin and HOMA index compared with those with Gly/Asp and Gly/Gly genotypes. However, Ehrmann et al. reported that the *IRS-2* Gly/Gly genotype carriers of their nondiabetic subjects had significantly higher 2-h oral glucose tolerance test glucose levels compared with those with Gly/Asp and Asp/Asp genotypes in whites or Gly/Asp genotype in African-Americans [15]. The susceptibility allele of *IRS-2* Gly1057Asp reported in our population is completely opposite from those reported in other populations. When we further examined the minor allele frequency of *IRS-2* Gly1057Asp in different populations, we observed that the Gly is the minor allele in our population, while it is Asp in Caucasians and African Americans [19]. The increased homozygous *IRS-2* Asp polymorphism in the population from Taiwan might be due to different evolutionary force, such as genetic drift, or selection pressure. It may be also due to different techniques used for genotyping of allelic variants. Our study used PCR following by re-sequencing to conduct our genotyping which will produce more reliable genotypes.

We did not find significant difference in genotype frequencies of *IRS-1* Gly972Arg between the PCOS and

Table 4 Genotypic distribution of polymorphisms in the *IRS1* and *IRS2* genes between the control group and the PCO group stratified by BMI

	Non-obese group (BMI <27)			Obese group (BMI ≥ 27)		
	PCOS group (n = 176)	Control group (n = 83)	p^a	PCOS group (n = 72)	Control group (n = 9)	p^b
IRS-1 Gly972Arg						
GG	156 (88.6%)	77 (92.8%)	0.792	64 (88.9%)	7 (77.8%)	0.307
GA	20 (11.4%)	6 (7.2%)		8 (11.1%)	2 (22.2%)	
IRS-2 Gly1057Asp	(n = 70)	(n = 68)		(n = 25)	(n = 6)	
GG	8 (11.4%)	24 (35.3%)	0.004	4 (16.0%)	1 (16.7%)	1.000
GA	15 (21.4%)	12 (17.6%)		3 (12.0%)	1 (16.7%)	
AA	47 (67.1%)	32 (47.1%)		18 (72.0%)	4 (66.7%)	
GG + GA	23 (32.9%)	36 (52.9%)	0.027	7 (28.0%)	2 (33.3%)	1,000
AA	47 (67.1%)	32 (47.1%)		18 (72.0%)	4 (66.7%)	
IRS-1 and *IRS-2*	(n = 70)	(n = 68)		(n = 25)	(n = 6)	
GG / GG + GA	20 (28.6%)	33 (48.5%)	0.003	6 (24.0%)	2 (3.3%)	0.834
GA / AA	43 (61.4%)	35 (51.5%)		15 (60.0%)	3 (50.0%)	
GA and AA	7 (10.0%)	0 (0.0%)		4 (16.0%)	1 (16.7%)	

[a,b]Comparison between the PCOS group and the control group by chi-square test.

control groups. Our finding is contradictory to the results from meta-analysis [19]. This inconclusive results in our population deserved further investigations with larger independent sample in the Chinese population from Taiwan.

We found the *IRS-1* Gly972Arg variant was in Hardy-Weinberg equilibrium, but the *IRS-2* Gly1057Asp variant was not in Hardy-Weinberg equilibrium in both PCOS and control groups. The possible reasons why the *IRS-1* SNP in the control group is in equilibrium while it is not for the *IRS-2* marker may be due to different selection pressure for *IRS-1* and *IRS-2* variants or the *IRS-2* Gly1057Arg variant is a recent mutation.

Our study found significant association of the variants of *IRS-2* gene as well as the interaction of *IRS-1* and *IRS-2* genes with PCOS. The magnitudes of associations were more profound in non-obese women group (Table 4). A couple of studies reported that the association of the Asp1057 allele in *IRS-2* with type 2 diabetes may be mediated by interaction of the polymorphism with obesity on several diabetes-related traits [20,22]. The exact molecular mechanism of *IRS-2* Gly1057Asp polymorphism on insulin action is not clear, but it is speculated that this variant introduces an exchange of a charged amino acid (Asp) with a neutral one (Gly) in the domain of IRS-2 molecule located in between two putative tyrosine phosphorylation sites (at positions 1042 & 1072) of the protein. This could produce alterations in downstream signaling through IRS-2 [22].

In this study, despite the PCOS subjects were significant younger, with higher risk of morphologic change,

glucose intolerance, and endocrine dysfunction than the control subjects (Table 1), we only found increased levels of fasting insulin, and elevated HOMA index in women carrying the homozygous Asp/Asp genotype than their counterpart (Gly/Gly and Gly/Asp) (Table 3). It may be probable that women with *IRS-2* homozygous Asp variant are more likely to show early signs of metabolic risks rather than to be associated with the development of PCOS.

In our previous study, the level of interleukin-6, which is considered as an early low-grade chronic inflammatory marker, was increased in PCOS women. But the elevated interleukin-6 level was reduced significantly after metformin treatment, especially among PCOS women with *IRS-2* homozygous Asp variant [23]. In this study, we did not have the information of metformin treatment, thus we are unable to evaluate the effect of metformin treatment.

There are several limitations in the study. Firstly, our control subjects were recruited from outpatient department of the hospital, so they might not be well-presented as in the general population. We were also aware that the inclusion and exclusion criteria of control subjects we applied in the study might result in over-estimation of the odds ratio of the *IRS-2* gene on PCOS [24]. The control subjects of the study were enrolled from infertility clinic prior to entering an in vitro fertilization program due to tubal and/or male factors with free of menstrual cycle irregularities, clinical or biochemical hyperandrogenism, polycystic ovaries on ultrasound examination, or history of systemic/endocrine disease. General speaking, they were normal in endocrine function, but were recruited due to infertility problem. Therefore, they could be viewed as normal in male factor but mechanical reason in tubal factor. The issue of over-estimation of odds ratio might not be as severe as we suspect. Secondly, despite we found that the levels of 2-hour insulin, glucose, and HbA1C in the PCOS group significantly higher than the control group, however, we could not find significant differences in HOMA index, A/I, and QUICK index between two groups. The possible reason is that our PCOS group is significantly younger than the control group. For younger PCOS women, the insulin sensitivity/resistance may be normal or only mild hyperinsulinemia. Thirdly, in the oral glucose tolerance test, we only measured the glucose and insulin levels at the fasting and 2-hour time points, thus may limit us to capture the entire picture of insulin sensitivity/resistance during the time course. Lastly, although significant association of the variant of *IRS-2* gene and its interaction effect with *IRS-1* gene related to PCOS was found, the sample size of our study is relatively small. In order to confirm our findings, further larger well-designed studies, especially in different ethnic populations are warranted.

In summary, we found significant association of the variants of *IRS-2* gene as well as the interaction of *IRS-1* and *IRS-2* genes with PCOS, especially in non-obese women. Women with *IRS-2* homozygous Asp variant may be considered as a risk factor for PCOS that needs early detection to prevent further complications in the Chinese population of Taiwan.

Competing interests
The authors declare that they have no competing interests.

Authors' contributions
M-F H carried out the molecular genetic studies, participated in the sequence alignment. M-W L participated in the design of the study, performed the statistical analysis and wrote the manuscript. M-H W designed the study, performed the clinical diagnosis, processed the samples, supervised the project, and wrote the manuscript. All authors read and approved the final manuscript.

Acknowledgments
This work was supported by research grants DOH94-TD-D-113-037 and DOH95-TD-D-113-033 (to M-H Wu) from Department of Health, Executive Yuan, Taiwan, R.O.C. and in part by the Ministry of Education, Taiwan, Aim for the Top University Plan of National Yang-Ming University and by the UST-UCSD International Center of Excellence in Advanced Bioengineering sponsored by the Taiwan Ministry of Science and Technology I-RiCE Program under Grant Number: NSC102-2911-I-009-101 (to M-W Lin).

Author details
[1]Institute of Public Health, National Yang-Ming University, Taipei, Taiwan. [2]Departments of Physiology, National Cheng Kung University College of Medicine, Tainan, Taiwan. [3]Departments of Obstetrics and Gynecology, National Cheng Kung University College of Medicine and Hospital, 138 Sheng-Li Road, 70428 Tainan, Taiwan.

References
1. Azziz R, Woods KS, Reyna R, Key TJ, Knochenhauer ES, Yildiz BO: **The prevalence and features of the polycystic ovary syndrome in an unselected population.** *J Clin Endocrinol Metab* 2004, 89:2745–2749.
2. Hardiman P, Pillay OC, Atiomo W: **Polycystic ovary syndrome and endometrial carcinoma.** *Lancet* 2003, 361:1810–1812.
3. Legro RS: **Polycystic ovary syndrome and cardiovascular disease: a premature association?** *Endocr Rev* 2003, 24:302–312.
4. Ovalle F, Azziz R: **Insulin resistance, polycystic ovary syndrome, and type 2 diabetes mellitus.** *Fertil Steril* 2002, 77:1095–1105.
5. Legro RS, Arslanian SA, Ehrmann DA, Hoeger KM, Murad MH, Pasquali R, Welt CK: **Diagnosis and treatment of polycystic ovary syndrome: an endocrine society clinical practice guideline.** *J Clin Endocrinol Metab* 2013, 98:4565–4592.
6. Orio F, Palomba S: **Reproductive endocrinology: new guidelines for the diagnosis and treatment of PCOS.** *Nat Rev Endocrinol* 2014, 10:130–132.
7. Dunaif A: **Insulin resistance and the polycystic ovary syndrome: mechanism and implications for pathogenesis.** *Endocr Rev* 1997, 18:774–800.
8. Ehrmann DA, Barnes RB, Rosenfield RL, Cavaghan MK, Imperial J: **Prevalence of impaired glucose tolerance and diabetes in women with polycystic ovary syndrome.** *Diabetes Care* 1999, 22:141–146.
9. Dunaif A, Wu X, Lee A, Diamanti-Kandarakis E: **Defects in insulin receptor signaling in vivo in the polycystic ovary syndrome (PCOS).** *Am J Physiol Endocrinol Metab* 2001, 281:E392–E399.
10. Ogihara T, Isobe T, Ichimura T, Taoka M, Funaki M, Sakoda H, Onishi Y, Inukai K, Anai M, Fukushima Y, Kikuchi M, Yazaki Y, Oka Y, Asano T: **14-3-3 protein binds to insulin receptor substrate-1, one of the binding sites of which is in the phosphotyrosine binding domain.** *J Biol Chem* 1997, 272:25267–25274.
11. Baba T, Endo T, Sata F, Honnma H, Kitajima Y, Hayashi T, Manase K, Kanaya M, Yamada H, Minakami H, Kishi R, Saito T: **Polycystic ovary syndrome is associated with genetic polymorphism in the insulin signaling gene IRS-1 but not ENPP1 in a Japanese population.** *Life Sci* 2007, 81:850–854.
12. Dilek S, Ertunc D, Tok EC, Erdal EM, Aktas A: **Association of Gly972Arg variant of insulin receptor substrate-1 with metabolic features in women with polycystic ovary syndrome.** *Fertil Steril* 2005, 84:407–412.
13. Pappalardo MA, Russo GT, Pedone A, Pizzo A, Borrielli I, Stabile G, Artenisio AC, Amato A, Calvani M, Cucinotta D, Trimarchi F, Benvenga S: **Very high frequency of the polymorphism for the insulin receptor substrate 1 (IRS-1) at codon 972 (glycine972arginine) in Southern Italian women with polycystic ovary syndrome.** *Horm Metab Res* 2010, 42:575–584.
14. Sir-Petermann T, Angel B, Maliqueo M, Santos JL, Riesco MV, Toloza H, Perez-Bravo F: **Insulin secretion in women who have polycystic ovary syndrome and carry the Gly972Arg variant of insulin receptor substrate-1 in response to a high-glycemic or low-glycemic carbohydrate load.** *Nutrition* 2004, 20:905–910.
15. Ehrmann DA, Tang X, Yoshiuchi I, Cox NJ, Bell GI: **Relationship of insulin receptor substrate-1 and –2 genotypes to phenotypic features of polycystic ovary syndrome.** *J Clin Endocrinol Metab* 2002, 87:4297–4300.
16. El Mkadem SA, Lautier C, Macari F, Molinari N, Lefebvre P, Renard E, Gris JC, Cros G, Daures JP, Bringer J, White MF, Grigorescu F: **Role of allelic variants Gly972Arg of IRS-1 and Gly1057Asp of IRS-2 in moderate-to-severe insulin resistance of women with polycystic ovary syndrome.** *Diabetes* 2001, 50:2164–2168.
17. Villuendas G, Botella-Carretero JI, Roldan B, Sancho J, Escobar-Morreale HF, San Millan JL: **Polymorphisms in the insulin receptor substrate-1 (IRS-1) gene and the insulin receptor substrate-2 (IRS-2) gene influence glucose homeostasis and body mass index in women with polycystic ovary syndrome and non-hyperandrogenic controls.** *Hum Reprod* 2005, 20:3184–3191.
18. Ioannidis A, Ikonomi E, Dimou NL, Douma L, Bagos PG: **Polymorphisms of the insulin receptor and the insulin receptor substrates genes in polycystic ovary syndrome: a Mendelian randomization meta-analysis.** *Mol Genet Metab* 2010, 99:174–183.
19. Ruan Y, Ma J, Xie X: **Association of IRS-1 and IRS-2 genes polymorphisms with polycystic ovary syndrome: a meta-analysis.** *Endocr J* 2012, 59:601–609.
20. Stephens M, Sloan JS, Robertson PD, Scheet P, Nickerson DA: **Automating sequence-based detection and genotyping of SNPs from diploid samples.** *Nat Genet* 2006, 38:375–381.
21. Sir-Petermann T, Perez-Bravo F, Angel B, Maliqueo M, Calvillan M, Palomino A: **G972R polymorphism of IRS-1 in women with polycystic ovary syndrome.** *Diabetologia* 2001, 44:1200–1201.

22. Mammarella S, Romano F, Di Valerio A, Creati B, Esposito Diana L, Palmirotta R, Capani F, Vitullo P, Volpe G, Battista P, Della Loggia F, Mariani-Costantini R, Cama A: **Interaction between the G1057D variant of IRS-2 and overweight in the pathogenesis of type 2 diabetes.** *Hum Mol Genet* 2000, **9:**2517–2521.
23. Lin YS, Tsai SJ, Lin MW, Yang CT, Huang MF, Wu MH: **Interleukin-6 as an early chronic inflammatory marker in polycystic ovary syndrome with insulin receptor substrate-2 polymorphism.** *Am J Reprod Immunol* 2011, **66:**527–533.
24. Bloom MS, Schisterman EF, Hediger ML: **Selecting controls is not selecting "normals": design and analysis issues for studying the etiology of polycystic ovary syndrome.** *Fertil Steril* 2006, **86:**1–12.

5

The transcriptome of corona radiata cells from individual MII oocytes that after ICSI developed to embryos selected for transfer: PCOS women compared to healthy women

5

Marie Louise Wissing[1*], Si Brask Sonne[2], David Westergaard[3], Kho do Nguyen[4], Kirstine Belling[3], Thomas Høst[1] and Anne Lis Mikkelsen[1]

Abstract

Background: Corona radiata cells (CRCs) refer to the fraction of cumulus cells just adjacent to the oocyte. The CRCs are closely connected to the oocyte throughout maturation and their gene expression profiles might reflect oocyte quality. Polycystic ovary syndrome (PCOS) is a common cause of infertility. It is controversial whether PCOS associate with diminished oocyte quality. The purpose of this study was to compare individual human CRC samples between PCOS patients and controls.

Methods: All patients were stimulated by the long gonadotropin-releasing hormone (GnRH) agonist protocol. The CRC samples originated from individual oocytes developing into embryos selected for transfer. CRCs were isolated in a two-step denudation procedure, separating outer cumulus cells from the inner CRCs. Extracted RNA was amplified and transcriptome profiling was performed with Human Agilent® arrays.

Results: The transcriptomes of CRCs showed no individual genes with significant differential expression between PCOS and controls, but gene set enrichment analysis identified several cell cycle- and DNA replication pathways overexpressed in PCOS CRCs (FDR < 0.05). Five of the genes contributing to the up-regulated cell cycle pathways in the PCOS CRCs were selected for qRT-PCR validation in ten PCOS and ten control CRC samples. qRT-PCR confirmed significant up-regulation in PCOS CRCs of cell cycle progression genes *HIST1H4C* (FC = 2.7), *UBE2C* (FC = 2.6) and cell cycle related transcription factor *E2F4* (FC = 2.5).

Conclusion: The overexpression of cell cycle-related genes and cell cycle pathways in PCOS CRCs could indicate a disturbed or delayed final maturation and differentiation of the CRCs in response to the human chorionic gonadotropin (hCG) surge. However, this had no effect on the *in vitro* development of the corresponding embryos. Future studies are needed to clarify whether the up-regulated cell cycle pathways in PCOS CRCs have any clinical implications.

Keywords: Corona radiata cells, Transcriptome, Gene expression, PCOS, Oocyte quality

* Correspondence: mlwi@regionsjaelland.dk
[1]Department of Gynecology-Obstetrics, Holbaek Fertility Clinic, Holbaek Hospital, Smedelundsgade 60, 4300 Holbaek, Denmark
Full list of author information is available at the end of the article

Background

Polycystic Ovary Syndrome (PCOS) is the most prevalent endocrine disorder of women in the reproductive age and represents a combination of polycystic ovaries, oligo/anovulation and hyperandrogenism [1]. The follicular microenvironment previously found to be altered in PCOS women might influence oocyte maturation and oocyte developmental competence [2,3]. Previous studies of PCOS women compared to healthy women revealed gene expression differences in metaphase II (MII) oocytes [4], in cumulus cells of individual MII oocytes with unknown developmental potential [5] and pooled, cultured cumulus cells [6]. Ribosomal RNA content was increased in cumulus cells of PCOS women [7], which could indicate a higher rate of proliferation; also granulosa cells from PCOS women have been shown to be hyperproliferative [3]. These alterations may suggest an altered oocyte quality in PCOS patients compared to controls. However, they do not necessarily extrapolate to the clinical situation, where only oocytes developing into top quality embryos are used for transfer. A meta-analysis showed that PCOS women had a similar number of top quality embryos and similar rates of pregnancy and live births compared to healthy women undergoing in vitro fertilization (IVF), but PCOS patients had more oocytes retrieved and a significantly lower fertilization rate [8].

Corona radiata cells (CRCs) refer to the innermost layer of the cumulus cells, which is in direct contact with the zona pellucida of the oocyte. Throughout folliculogenesis and until the luteinizing hormone (LH) surge for final oocyte maturation, transzonal projections exist between the oocyte and the CRCs, allowing exchange of substances between the oocyte and the CRCs [9]. We hypothesize that transcriptomic analysis of CRCs would serve as a non-invasive method of gaining deeper understanding of the microenvironment of the oocyte. Since PCOS and non-PCOS women undergoing IVF had the same clinical outcome [8], we wanted to find out whether the transcriptomic profile of CRCs would differ between PCOS and controls in clinically relevant samples of CRCs from embryos chosen for transfer.

Materials and methods

This study was approved by The Danish Ethical Science Committee (SJ-156) and conducted in accordance with the Helsinki Declaration and all participants gave informed consent before inclusion in the study.

Study population

Ten women with PCOS and ten healthy, regularly cycling women without known disease (controls) were included. Exclusion criteria were diabetes type 1 or 2, impaired thyroid, renal or hepatic function, congenital adrenal hyperplasia, endometriosis, premature ovarian failure, hypothalamic amenorrhea or age >35 years.

Diagnosis of PCOS was made according to the Rotterdam Consensus Criteria [1]. For all control women, indication for intracytoplasmic sperm injection (ICSI) was a partner with infertility (defined as <5 million progressively moving spermatozoa/ml). For the PCOS women, half (5/10) of the couples were referred to ICSI because of male infertility and the rest after 4–6 failed attempts of intra-uterine insemination (IUI).

Baseline examination

Participants were included in the study based on a focused gynecological history and objective examination including transvaginal ultrasound of the ovaries and uterus. Blood samples were drawn after an overnight fast at 08.30-09.00 a.m. on cycle day (cd) 3–5 for regularly cycling women and on a random day for amenorrhoeic women. All androgen analyses were done at the same laboratory (Statens Serum Institut, SSI, Copenhagen, Denmark) in order to minimize variability. Total testosterone was measured by the CHS™ MSMS Steroids Kit (PerkinElmers®, Waltham, Massachusetts, USA) with intra-assay variation of 9.6% and inter-assay variation of 10.6%. Sex hormone-binding globulin (SHBG) was measured by Architect i2000 analyzer (Abbott®, Abbott Park, Illinois, USA) with an intra-assay variation of 2.8% and an inter-assay variation of 5.8%. Free testosterone was calculated from total testosterone and SHBG [10]. LH and follicle-stimulating hormone (FSH) were measured by immunoassay (LH: ref 11732234, FSH: ref 11775863, Roche Diagnostics, Mannheim, Germany).

Ovarian stimulation

Ovarian stimulation was achieved by the long gonadotropin-releasing hormone (GnRH) agonist protocol. Pituitary desensitization with buserelin 0.5 mg (Suprefact®, Sanofi-Aventis, Paris, France) was started on cd 21 in regularly menstruating women and at cd 15 for oligo/amenorrhoeic women starting with ethinylestradiol 30 mg/desogestrel 150 mg daily from the 1st day of bleeding (Marvelon®, Organon/Microgyn®, Bayer Pharma, Leverkusen, Germany) and until cd 21. Controlled ovarian stimulation with recombinant FSH (rFSH) (Puregon®, Organon, Oss, Netherlands) was started after at least 14 days of desensitization. Follicle growth was monitored by transvaginal ultrasound. Recombinant human chorionic gonadotropin (rhCG) 6500 IU (Ovitrelle®, Modugno, Italy) was administered when at least three follicles reached the size of 17 mm. Oocyte Pick-up (OPU) was performed 36 hours later under transvaginal ultrasound guidance. Luteal phase support (Lutinus®, Ferring©, Copenhagen, Denmark) was given from the day of transfer and until the pregnancy test. We adhered to the Danish National Criteria of elective single transfer for all patients <37 years of age. Transvaginal ultrasound was performed three weeks after a positive hCG blood test to confirm intrauterine clinical pregnancy.

Isolation of corona radiata cells, fertilization and time lapse incubation of embryos

Following OPU, cumulus-oocyte complexes were washed several times in Fertilization medium (Cook, Eight Mile Plains, Queensland, Australia) to remove cell debris, and incubated for two hours in Fertilization medium (Cook, Eight Mile Plains, Queensland, Australia). Then the oocytes were transferred to a droplet of Cleavage medium (Cook, Eight Mile Plains, Queensland, Australia) and denudated in a two-step procedure: First, the cumulus cells were removed by gentle pipetting in 20 µl Cumulase® (Origio, Måløv, Denmark) with a 1–10 µl Eppendorf Pipette using a Dual filter PCR clean 20 µl tip (Eppendorf, Hamburg, Germany). Then the oocyte with the remaining CRCs was transferred to 10 µl Cumulase® (Origio, Måløv, Denmark) and the CRCs were removed by gentle pipetting with a Denudation pipette 0.134-0.145 mm (Vitrolife, Göteborg, Sweden). Immediately after oocyte denudation, individual droplets containing the CRCs were transferred to DNA Lobind Eppendorf tubes (Eppendorf, Hamburg, Germany), snap frozen in liquid nitrogen and stored at −80°C until RNA extraction. MII oocytes were fertilized by ICSI within ten minutes after denudation, and incubated in individual wells in an Embryoscope® (Unisense Fertilitech, Aarhus, Denmark), which gave the opportunity to track the development of all fertilized oocytes until transfer (day 2), or, for the untransferred embryos, until vitrification as top quality blastocyst or disposal at day 5/6. Analysis of the images was done with the EmbryoViewer® Software (Unisense FertiliTech Aarhus, Denmark). The time from ICSI to the following events were annotated: Pronuclei breakdown (defined as the first picture frame where the pronuclei disappeared), 1st cleavage (defined as the first picture frame where the zygote turned into two cells) and cleavage to four cells (defined as the first picture frame where four cells were observed the first time).

Selection of CRC samples used in the study

The CRC samples used in this study came from oocytes developing into top quality embryos: All transferred embryos were top quality embryos according to the ALPHA/ESHRE consensus [11] scoring points in short: Four cells at day 2, low fragmentation (cut-off 25% fragmentation), cell cycle specific cell size, no multinucleation. Vitrified top quality blastocysts day 5/6 had score 3–6 AA/AB according to the blastocyst classification proposed by Gardner and Schoolcraft [12]. The fate of the ten oocytes corresponding to the CRC samples used were as follows: In the PCOS group, ten transferred embryos gave three clinical pregnancies, resulting in two live births and one

missed abortion in gestational week 7 and seven negative hCG tests 14 days after oocyte retrieval; In the control group, three top quality blastocysts were vitrified for later use, and seven transferred embryos gave three clinical pregnancies with two live births and one missed abortion in gestational week 7.

RNA extraction and amplification

Total RNA was extracted by the RNAequeous® micro-kit from Ambion (Life Technologies, Paisley, UK) according to manufacturer's instructions. The samples were analyzed for total RNA concentration by Qubit® (Life Technologies, Paisley, UK) and total RNA quality and level of degradation using an Agilent 2100 Bioanalyzer and RNA 6000 Pico LabChip according to the manufacturer's instructions (Agilent Technologies, Waldbronn, Germany). All of the RNA samples showed two distinct peaks representing 18S and 28S rRNA, which indicated good quality RNA and presented RNA Integrity Number (RIN) from 6–9.4. Total RNA of 50 ng was amplified and converted into cDNA using the Ovation Pico WTA System V2 RNA Amplification System from NuGEN® Inc. (NuGEN®, San Carlos, California, USA).

Microarray experiment

cDNA was coupled to a Cyanine 3-dUTP fluorescent dye (Cy3) using the Oligonucleotide Array-Based CGH for Genomic DNA Analysis, Enzymatic Labeling for Blood, Cells or Tissues (protocol version 6.2, Agilent Technologies, Santa Clara, California, USA). Cy3-labeled cDNA was hybridized to Agilent Human Gene Expression Microarrays 4 × 44k v2 (G4845A) using the One-Color Microarray-Based Gene Expression Analysis, Quick Amp Labeling (version 5.7 protocol, Agilent Technologies, Santa Clara, California, USA) and scanned using an Agilent DNA Microarray scanner (Agilent Technologies, Santa Clara, California, USA). For microarray analysis, we used six CRC samples from PCOS women, and six from healthy controls (12 arrays in total).

Quantitative reverse-transcriptase PCR

The following TaqMan® Gene Expression Assays (predesigned) (Applied Biosystems, Life Technologies Europe, Nærum, Denmark) were used (Assay ID-No: Hs00168719_m1 (Cyclophillin B/PPIB), Hs00171034_m1 (Cyclin T2, CCNT2), Hs00543883_s1 (histone cluster 1, H4c/HIST1H4C), Hs00608098_m1 (E2F transcription factor 4, p107/p130-binding/E2F4), and Hs00964100_g1 (ubiquitin-conjugating enzyme E2C/UBE2C)). Sample triplicates were prepared according to the manufacturer's instructions. A total reaction volume of 20 µL was prepared on ice containing 10 µL TaqMan® Gene Expression Master Mix (2X), 1 µL TaqMan® Gene Expression Assay Mix (20X), 4 µL cDNA

5 ng/µl, and 5 µL RNase-free water. The samples were then centrifuged at 1,100 × g at 4°C for 5 minutes.

Gene expression was quantified using the MX3005 qPCR system (Agilent Technologies Denmark, Hørsholm, Denmark) under the following thermal cycling conditions: 95°C for 10 minutes, 40 cycles of 95°C for 15 seconds and 60°C for 1 minute. The data was normalized to *cyclophillin* (PPIB) [13], and relative quantification calculated according to the Comparative CT Method (ABI user bulletin # 2, 2001). qRT-PCR was performed on ten PCOS CRC samples and ten control CRC samples.

Gene expression microarray processing and analysis
Array quality was assessed with the arrayQualityMetrics R package [14], which used a variety of statistical tests combined with data visualization to mark outliers. Evaluation was done manually on a per array basis. Pre-processing of microarray data was done with the LIMMA software [15,16] available from the Bioconductor project [17]. Normalization between arrays was done by quantile normalization [18]. For genes with multiple probes, the intensity was defined as the median of all probes mapping to that gene.

Statistically significant differences between PCOS and control CRC samples in expression of individual transcripts were assessed by the LIMMA moderated t-test [16] using the Benjamin-Hochberg method of correction of P-values for multiple testing.

Statistical significance of biological themes was investigated for the entire dataset with the Gene Set Enrichment Analysis (GSEA) software version 2.0.12 (http://www.broadinstitute.org/gsea/index.jsp) [19,20]. In short, the GSEA algorithm ranked genes according to their expression level. By default, genes were ranked using the Signal-2-Noise metric, a more robust measure than both mean and median values, and very robust against outliers:

$$Signal2Noise = \frac{\mu_{pcos} - \mu_{control}}{sd_{pcos} + sd_{control}}$$

The enrichment of a pathway was assessed by walking through the list of ranked genes, incrementing a running sum score when encountering a gene found in the pathway, and decreasing it when encountering a gene not in the pathway. According to the authors, this corresponded to a weighted Kolmogorov-Smirnov-like statistic. Statistical significance was assessed by permutating the ranked list of genes a thousand times. Genes which were either poorly expressed, had high intra-variation in the group or had low variance between the PCOS and control group populated the middle of the ranked list, and thus did not contribute to the running sum score. We specifically investigated the pathways contained in the databases KEGG

[21] and REACTOME [22]. Normalized enrichment score (NES) is defined as:

$$NES = \frac{\text{actual ES}}{mean \text{ (ESs against all permutations of the dataset)}}$$

NES was reported together with the false discovery rate (FDR). We reported pathways with FDR ≤0.05.

All samples were MIAME compliant and were handled according to SOP in the microarray Center. The 12 arrays were submitted to ArrayExpress (http://www.ebi.ac.uk/arrayexpress/) at EMBL using MIAMExpress. The experiment accession number is E-MEXP-3985.

Statistics
Differences in baseline parameters between groups were tested by Mann–Whitney test (Graphpad Prism v. 6, San Diego, California, USA). Differences between groups in developmental timing of the embryos corresponding to the selected CRC samples were evaluated by Students t-test (Graphpad Prism v. 6, San Diego, California, USA). Differences between PCOS and control CRC samples in gene expression of selected genes in the qRT-PCR experiment were evaluated by Bayesian parameter estimation [23]. A comparison was considered significant if the 95% HDI (Highest Density Interval) did not contain the value 0.

Results
Baseline parameters of study groups
The PCOS and control group differed according to PCOS status. The PCOS group exhibited oligomenorrhea, polycystic ovaries and hyperandrogenaemia (Table 1). Age, BMI and basal FSH were similar across groups (Table 1). Embryo kinetic timings of the embryos corresponding to the selected CRC samples did not differ between groups (Table 1).

Quality of the arrays
There were no apparent outliers based on the arrayQualityMetrics reports.

Differentially expressed genes
After correction for multiple testing, no individual genes in the microarray experiment showed significant differential expression between PCOS CRC samples and control CRC samples (Additional file 1).

Gene set enrichment analysis
GSEA showed upregulation of 24 pathways with FDR < 0.05 in PCOS CRCs compared to control CRCs (Table 2). Especially pathways involved in cell cycle and DNA replication were up-regulated in PCOS CRCs (Table 2). Additional file 2 shows the full pathway list with the

Table 1 Baseline descriptive parameters of the study participants and the average developmental timings of the embryos corresponding to the CRC samples used in the study

	PCOS	Controls	p-value
Age	27,3±3,4	27,8±4	ns
BMI	24±4,8	22,4±3,5	ns
No of antral follicles/ one plane	15,8±5,4	8,2±1,7	<0,0001
No of menstrual bleedings/year	1,8±3,2	12±0	<0,0001
Total testosterone	2,8±1,1	1,2±0,3	0,0003
Free testosterone	0,03931±0,02532	0,014±0,0042	0,0029
SHBG	78±26	79±21	ns
LH/FSH	1,6±0,8	0,8±0,3	0,03
Time of 2PN breakdown (h)	23.2±3.8	21.8±2.4	ns
Time of 1st Cleavage (h)	26±4.1	24.3±2.5	ns
Time of cleavage to 4 cells (h)	38.3±5	36.4±4.2	ns

p-value <0,05 considered significant. Not significant = ns.

Table 2 Gene set enrichment analysis of the transcriptome of CRCs of individual oocytes developing into embryos selected for transfer

Pathway	No of genes enriched/total number of genes in the pathway	FDR	NES
Reactome Cell Cycle	127/421	0.001	0.42
Reactome G2 M Checkpoints	17/45	0.001	0.61
KEGG DNA Replication	20/36	0.001	0.65
Reactome Meiotic Recombination	35/86	0.001	0.59
Reactome Packaging of Telomere Ends	25/48	0.001	0.63
Reactome Activation of the Pre Replicative Complex	14/31	0.001	0.60
Reactome RNA POL I RNA POL III and Mitochondrial Transcription	45/122	0.001	0.53
Reactome RNA POL I Transcription	35/89	0.001	0.55
Reactome RNA POL I Promotor Opening	32/62	0.001	0.64
Reactome Activation of ATR in Response to Replication Stress	15/38	0.001	0.63
Reactome Deposition of new CENPA containing Nucleosomes at the Centromere	34/64	0.001	0.60
Reactome DNA strand Elongation	20/30	0.001	0.69
Reactome Telomere Maintenance	39/75	0.001	0.61
Reactome Cell Cycle Mitotic	94/325	0.01	0.41
Reactome Meiosis	45/116	0.01	0.49
Reactome Amyloids	34/83	0.01	0.51
Reactome lagging strand synthesis	12/19	0.01	0.69
Reactome Mitotic M M G1 Phases	55/137	0.03	0.42
Reactome Mitotic Prometaphase	32/87	0.03	0.47
Reactome DNA replication	56/192	0.03	0.42
Reactome Meiotic Synapsis	34/73	0.03	0.50
Reactome Chromosome Maintenance	55/122	0.03	0.42
Reactome Extension of Telomeres	13/27	0.03	0.59
Reactome Transcription	61/210	0.04	0.41

PCOS women compared controls (n = 6 PCOS arrays vs n = 6 control arrays). Enriched pathways with FDR <0.05 were listed. NES = normalized enrichment score. All enriched pathways were upregulated in PCOS CRC samples.

genes contributing to the up-regulation of these pathways in PCOS CRC samples.

Quantitative reverse transcriptase PCR

Five of the genes contributing to the up-regulated cell cycle pathways in the PCOS CRCs were selected for qRT-PCR validation. We selected genes with different functions in the cell cycle. Gene expression by qRT-PCR were in accordance with the microarray data for three out of five genes tested (Figure 1). According to the qRT-PCR results, PCOS CRC samples showed significant up-regulation of *HIST1H4C* (FC = 2.7, 95% HDI 0.436-4.49), *UBE2C* (FC (Fold Change) = 2.6, 95% HDI 0.00438-3.21) and *E2F4* (FC = 2.5, 95% HDI 0.571-5.33). *CCND2* and *CCNT2* showed equal expression between groups in the qRT-PCR experiment while the microarray data showed a 1.4 higher expression in the PCOS CRC samples (Figure 1).

Discussion

In this study, we present for the first time a transcriptomic analysis of individual human CRC samples from oocytes used for transfer or blastocyst vitrification in PCOS and controls. We did not find any significantly differentially expressed individual genes after correction for multiple testing in the present microarray study of PCOS CRCs and control CRCs from MII oocytes developing into top quality embryos. This is in contrast to the study by Haouzi *et al.* [5] who found 3,700 significantly differentially expressed genes between PCOS and control cumulus cells from MII oocytes of unspecified developmental potential with the same number of arrays per group as in the present study (six PCOS vs. six control arrays). However, the apparent inconsistency between the present study and the study by Haouzi *et al.* [5] could be explained by the different study designs and experimental approaches: Firstly, we used enzymatically isolated CRCs, which

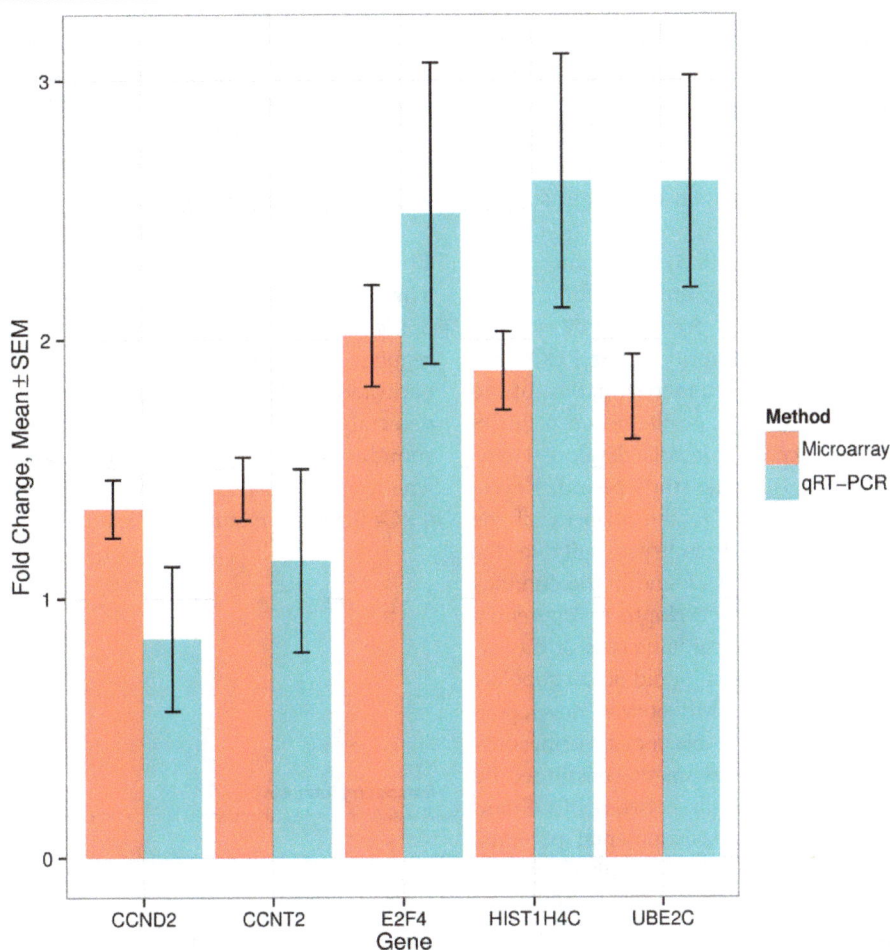

Figure 1 Comparison between microarray and qRT-PCR results for 5 selected genes in PCOS and control CRC samples. Fold change (PCOS/controls) ± Standard Error of the Mean (SEM). Red bars represented microarray results and blue bars represented qRT-PCR results. Microarray experiment: 6 PCOS CRC arrays vs. 6 control CRC arrays. qRT-PCR experiment: 10 PCOS CRC samples vs. 10 control CRC samples. The up-regulation of *UBE2C, HIST1H4C* and *E2F4* in PCOS CRCs found in the microarray experiment was in line with the qRT-PCR results, whereas the 1.4 fold up-regulation of *CCND2* and *CCNT2* in PCOS CRCs found in the microarray experiment could not be confirmed by qRT-PCR.

constitute the innermost cells closest to the oocyte, whereas Haouzi *et al.* [5] used mechanically cut cumulus cells. Several previous studies have successfully used enzymatically isolated cumulus cells [24-29] and CRCs [30,31] to investigate gene expression differences according to e.g. oocyte quality. Cumulase® used for denudation is a pure, recombinant and specific hyaluronidase and we would not expect the short exposure to mask gene expression differences. To the best of our knowledge, no studies have investigated gene expression differences according to isolation procedure of cumulus cells. Secondly, we used CRC samples from MII oocytes capable of developing into top quality embryos, whereas in former studies on gene expression in cumulus cells from PCOS patients [5,6], the developmental potential of the oocytes was not tracked. The strict use of CRCs from MII oocytes developing into top quality embryos in the present microarray study might explain why there were no individual genes with significant differential expression between PCOS and controls. Previous studies have shown that the transcriptome of cumulus cells from MII oocytes of poor developmental competence differed from cumulus cells of MII oocytes with high developmental competence [24,26,29,31-36]. These previous findings underlined the importance of oocyte selection, when comparing cumulus cells or CRCs in relation to a certain condition, such as PCOS.

During the study period, 10% (5/51) of women diagnosed with PCOS did not develop embryos for transfer or blastocyst vitrification. In the present study, we did not examine CRCs from this minority of the PCOS patients. This might have led to an underestimation of the differences in CRC transcriptomic profile between PCOS patients and controls since all controls developed embryos useful for transfer during the study period. Nevertheless, our data were applicable to the majority of the PCOS patients who developed embryos suitable for transfer: Transcriptomic aberrations found in the cumulus cells of MII oocytes of unknown developmental potential from PCOS women [5] or in the cumulus cells of the entire oocyte pool from PCOS women [6] did not extrapolate to the transcriptome of CRCs of MII oocytes developing into embryos used for transfer or blastocyst vitrification. This indicated that the microenvironment constituted by the CRCs did not differ substantially between PCOS and controls for oocytes with good developmental potential and it is in line with previous findings of similar implantation and pregnancy rates in PCOS patients and non-PCOS patients undergoing IVF [8].

The minority of PCOS patients with no embryos suitable for transfer constituted a clinically interesting subgroup with clearly impaired oocyte quality, and future studies on oocyte quality in PCOS should focus on this subgroup as a distinct entity within the PCOS population.

The GSEA showed up-regulation of pathways involved in cell cycle and DNA replication in PCOS CRCs. This is in line with previous studies showing hyperproliferative cumulus [7] and granulosa [3] cells in PCOS. The LH/hCG surge for final oocyte maturation dramatically down-regulate cell cycle genes in human granulosa cells [37] as well as in rodent cumulus-oocyte-complexes [38]. In agreement with this, cell cycle pathways were up-regulated in human cumulus cells of MI oocytes compared to cumulus cells of MII oocytes [39]. We speculate that the up-regulation of cell cycle pathways in PCOS CRCs could be an indicator of disturbed or delayed final maturation of the cumulus cells/CRCs in response to the LH/hCG trigger.

The three cell cycle-related genes which showed significant up-regulation in PCOS CRCs represented different aspects of cell cycle: HIST1H4C is a replication-dependent histone exclusively transcribed during the S-phase of the cell cycle [40,41], UBE2C is required for destruction of mitotic cyclins and cell cycle progression [42], and E2F4 is a transcription factor and exerted a range of functions, mainly in cell cycle, DNA repair, ubiquitination and stress response pathways [43]. In light of the multitude of regulatory functions exerted by E2F4, the significant 2.5 fold up-regulation in PCOS CRCs according to the qRT-PCR experiment might have interesting biological implications, which should be explored in future studies.

Conclusion

The transcriptomic analysis of CRCs from oocytes developing into embryos selected for transfer showed up-regulation of cell cycle pathways and DNA replication pathways in PCOS CRC samples, however, this had no detectable effect on *in vitro* development of the corresponding embryos. Future studies are needed to clarify whether the up-regulated cell cycle pathways in PCOS CRCs have any clinical implications.

Competing interests
The authors declare that they have no competing interests.

Authors' contributions
MLWI planned the study, recruited patients, collected materials, extracted RNA, performed qRT-PCR and wrote the manuscript. SBS extracted RNA and revised the manuscript. DW and KB performed the bio-informatical analyses and revised the manuscript. KDN performed the microarray experiment. THT planned the study and helped with collecting materials. ALM planned the study and revised the manuscript. All authors have read and approved the final version of the manuscript.

Acknowledgements
We thank the staff in the IVF lab of Holbæk Fertility Clinic for their assistance in isolating corona cell samples. The study was supported by a grant from Nordic InfuCare.

Author details
[1]Department of Gynecology-Obstetrics, Holbaek Fertility Clinic, Holbaek Hospital, Smedelundsgade 60, 4300 Holbaek, Denmark. [2]Institute of Biology, University of Copenhagen, 2100 Copenhagen, Denmark. [3]Department of Systems Biology, Center for Biological Sequence Analysis, Technical University of Denmark, Kemitorvet building 208, 2800 Lyngby, Denmark. [4]DTU Multi Assay Core, Technical University of Denmark DTU, 2800 Lyngby, Denmark.

References

1. Rotterdam ESHRE/ASRM-Sponsored PCOS Consensus Workshop Group: **Revised 2003 consensus on diagnostic criteria and long-term health risks related to polycystic ovary syndrome.** *Fertil Steril* 2004, **81:**19–25.
2. Desforges-Bullet V, Gallo C, Lefebvre C, Pigny P, Dewailly D, Catteau-Jonard S: **Increased anti-Müllerian hormone and decreased FSH levels in follicular fluid obtained in women with polycystic ovaries at the time of follicle puncture for in vitro fertilization.** *Fertil Steril* 2010, **94:**198–204.
3. Stubbs SA, Stark J, Dilworth SM, Franks S, Hardy K: **Abnormal preantral folliculogenesis in polycystic ovaries is associated with increased granulosa cell division.** *J Clin Endocrinol Metab* 2007, **92:**4418–4426.
4. Wood JR, Dumesic DA, Abbott DH, Strauss JF: **Molecular abnormalities in oocytes from women with polycystic ovary syndrome revealed by microarray analysis.** *J Clin Endocrinol Metab* 2007, **92:**705–713.
5. Haouzi D, Assou S, Monzo C, Vincens C, Dechaud H, Hamamah S: **Altered gene expression profile in cumulus cells of mature MII oocytes from patients with polycystic ovary syndrome.** *Hum Reprod* 2012, **27:**3523–3530.
6. Kenigsberg S, Bentov Y, Chalifa-Caspi V, Potashnik G, Ofir R, Birk OS: **Gene expression microarray profiles of cumulus cells in lean and overweight-obese polycystic ovary syndrome patients.** *Mol Hum Reprod* 2009, **15:**89–103.
7. Polzikov M, Yakovenko S, Voznesenskaya J, Troshina M, Zatsepina O: **Overexpression of ribosomal RNA in cumulus cells of patients with polycystic ovary syndrome.** *J Assist Reprod Genet* 2012, **29:**1141–1145.
8. Heijnen EMEW, Eijkemans MJC, Hughes EG, Laven JSE, Macklon NS, Fauser BCJM: **A meta-analysis of outcomes of conventional IVF in women with polycystic ovary syndrome.** *Hum Reprod Update* 2006, **12:**13–21.
9. Albertini DF, Combelles CM, Benecchi E, Carabatsos MJ: **Cellular basis for paracrine regulation of ovarian follicle development.** *Reproduction (Cambridge, England)* 2001, **121:**647–653.
10. Vermeulen A, Verdonck L, Kaufman JM: **A critical evaluation of simple methods for the estimation of free testosterone in serum.** *J Clin Endocrinol Metab* 1999, **84:**3666–3672.
11. Alpha Scientists in Reproductive Medicine and ESHRE Special Interest Group of Embryology: **The Istanbul consensus workshop on embryo assessment: proceedings of an expert meeting.** *Hum Reprod* 2011, **26:**1270–1283.
12. Gardner DK, Schoolcraft WB: **Culture and transfer of human blastocysts.** *Curr Opin Obstet Gynecol* 1999, **11:**307–311.
13. Teixeira Filho FL, Baracat EC, Lee TH, Suh CS, Matsui M, Chang RJ, Shimasaki S, Erickson GF: **Aberrant expression of growth differentiation factor-9 in oocytes of women with polycystic ovary syndrome.** *J Clin Endocrinol Metab* 2002, **87:**1337–1344.
14. Kauffmann A, Gentleman R, Huber W: **ArrayQualityMetrics–a bioconductor package for quality assessment of microarray data.** *Bioinformatics (Oxford, England)* 2009, **25:**415–416.
15. Bolstad BM, Irizarry RA, Astrand M, Speed TP: **A comparison of normalization methods for high density oligonucleotide array data based on variance and bias.** *Bioinformatics (Oxford, England)* 2003, **19:**185–193.
16. Smyth GK: **Linear models and empirical bayes methods for assessing differential expression in microarray experiments.** *Stat Appl Genet Mol Biol* 2004, **3:**Article3.
17. Gentleman RC, Carey VJ, Bates DM, Bolstad B, Dettling M, Dudoit S, Ellis B, Gautier L, Ge Y, Gentry J, Hornik K, Hothorn T, Huber W, Iacus S, Irizarry R, Leisch F, Li C, Maechler M, Rossini AJ, Sawitzki G, Smith C, Smyth G, Tierney L, Yang JYH, Zhang J: **Bioconductor: open software development for computational biology and bioinformatics.** *Genome Biol* 2004, **5:**R80.
18. Smyth GK, Speed T: **Normalization of cDNA microarray data.** *Methods (San Diego, Calif)* 2003, **31:**265–273.
19. Subramanian A, Tamayo P, Mootha VK, Mukherjee S, Ebert BL, Gillette MA, Paulovich A, Pomeroy SL, Golub TR, Lander ES, Mesirov JP: **Gene set enrichment analysis: a knowledge-based approach for interpreting genome-wide expression profiles.** *Proc Natl Acad Sci U S A* 2005, **102:**15545–15550.
20. Mootha VK, Lindgren CM, Eriksson K-F, Subramanian A, Sihag S, Lehar J, Puigserver P, Carlsson E, Ridderstråle M, Laurila E, Houstis N, Daly MJ, Patterson N, Mesirov JP, Golub TR, Tamayo P, Spiegelman B, Lander ES, Hirschhorn JN, Altshuler D, Groop LC: **PGC-1alpha-responsive genes involved in oxidative phosphorylation are coordinately downregulated in human diabetes.** *Nat Genet* 2003, **34:**267–273.
21. Kanehisa M, Goto S, Sato Y, Furumichi M, Tanabe M: **KEGG for integration and interpretation of large-scale molecular data sets.** *Nucleic Acids Res* 2012, **40**(Database issue):D109–D114.
22. Matthews L, Gopinath G, Gillespie M, Caudy M, Croft D, de Bono B, Garapati P, Hemish J, Hermjakob H, Jassal B, Kanapin A, Lewis S, Mahajan S, May B, Schmidt E, Vastrik I, Wu G, Birney E, Stein L, D'Eustachio P: **Reactome knowledgebase of human biological pathways and processes.** *Nucleic Acids Res* 2009, **37**(Database issue):D619–D622.
23. Kruschke JK: **Bayesian estimation supersedes the t test.** *J Exp Psychol Gen* 2013, **142:**573–603.
24. Anderson RA, Sciorio R, Kinnell H, Bayne RAL, Thong KJ, de Sousa PA, Pickering S: **Cumulus gene expression as a predictor of human oocyte fertilisation, embryo development and competence to establish a pregnancy.** *Reproduction (Cambridge, England)* 2009, **138:**629–637.
25. Adriaenssens T, Segers I, Wathlet S, Smitz J: **The cumulus cell gene expression profile of oocytes with different nuclear maturity and potential for blastocyst formation.** *J Assist Reprod Genet* 2011, **28:**31–40.
26. Feuerstein P, Puard V, Chevalier C, Teusan R, Cadoret V, Guerif F, Houlgatte R, Royere D: **Genomic assessment of human cumulus cell marker genes as predictors of oocyte developmental competence: impact of various experimental factors.** *PLoS One* 2012, **7:**e40449.
27. Wathlet S, Adriaenssens T, Segers I, Verheyen G, Janssens R, Coucke W, Devroey P, Smitz J: **New candidate genes to predict pregnancy outcome in single embryo transfer cycles when using cumulus cell gene expression.** *Fertil Steril* 2012, **98**(2):432–439.
28. Ekart J, McNatty K, Hutton J, Pitman J: **Ranking and selection of MII oocytes in human ICSI cycles using gene expression levels from associated cumulus cells.** *Hum Reprod* 2013, **28:**2930–2942.
29. Wathlet S, Adriaenssens T, Segers I, Verheyen G, Van Landuyt L, Coucke W, Devroey P, Smitz J: **Pregnancy prediction in single embryo transfer cycles after ICSI using QPCR: validation in oocytes from the same cohort.** *PLoS One* 2013, **8:**e54226.
30. May-Panloup P, Ferré-L'Hôtellier V, Morinière C, Marcaillou C, Lemerle S, Malinge M-C, Coutolleau A, Lucas N, Reynier P, Descamps P, Guardiola P: **Molecular characterization of corona radiata cells from patients with diminished ovarian reserve using microarray and microfluidic-based gene expression profiling.** *Hum Reprod* 2012, **27:**829–843.
31. Fragouli E, Wells D, Iager AE, Kayisli UA, Patrizio P: **Alteration of gene expression in human cumulus cells as a potential indicator of oocyte aneuploidy.** *Hum Reprod* 2012, **27:**2559–2568.
32. Ouandaogo ZG, Haouzi D, Assou S, Dechaud H, Kadoch IJ, De Vos J, Hamamah S: **Human cumulus cells molecular signature in relation to oocyte nuclear maturity stage.** *PLoS One* 2011, **6:**e27179.
33. Van Montfoort APA, Dumoulin JCM, Kester ADM, Evers JLH: **Early cleavage is a valuable addition to existing embryo selection parameters: a study using single embryo transfers.** *Hum Reprod* 2004, **19:**2103–2108.
34. Gebhardt KM, Feil DK, Dunning KR, Lane M, Russell DL: **Human cumulus cell gene expression as a biomarker of pregnancy outcome after single embryo transfer.** *Fertil Steril* 2011, **96:**47–52. e2.

35. Assou S, Haouzi D, De Vos J, Hamamah S: **Human cumulus cells as biomarkers for embryo and pregnancy outcomes.** *Mol Hum Reprod* 2010, **16**:531–538.

36. Iager AE, Kocabas AM, Otu HH, Ruppel P, Langerveld A, Schnarr P, Suarez M, Jarrett JC, Conaghan J, Rosa GJM, Fernández E, Rawlins RG, Cibelli JB, Crosby JA: **Identification of a novel gene set in human cumulus cells predictive of an oocyte's pregnancy potential.** *Fertil Steril* 2013, **99**:745–752. e6.

37. Wissing ML, Kristensen SG, Andersen CY, Mikkelsen AL, Høst T, Borup R, Grøndahl ML: **Identification of new ovulation-related genes in humans by comparing the transcriptome of granulosa cells before and after ovulation triggering in the same controlled ovarian stimulation cycle.** *Hum Reprod* 2014, **29**:997–1010.

38. Agca C, Yakan A, Agca Y: **Estrus synchronization and ovarian hyper-stimulation treatments have negligible effects on cumulus oocyte complex gene expression whereas induction of ovulation causes major expression changes.** *Mol Reprod Dev* 2012, **80**:102–117.

39. Devjak R, Fon Tacer K, Juvan P, Virant Klun I, Rozman D, Vrtačnik Bokal E: **Cumulus cells gene expression profiling in terms of oocyte maturity in controlled ovarian hyperstimulation using GnRH agonist or GnRH antagonist.** *PLoS One* 2012, **7**:e47106.

40. Harshman SW, Young NL, Parthun MR, Freitas MA: **H1 histones: current perspectives and challenges.** *Nucleic Acids Res* 2013, **41**:9593–9609.

41. Plumb M, Marashi F, Green L, Zimmerman A, Zimmerman S, Stein J, Stein G: **Cell cycle regulation of human histone H1 mRNA.** *Proc Natl Acad Sci U S A* 1984, **81**:434–438.

42. Hao Z, Zhang H, Cowell J: **Ubiquitin-conjugating enzyme UBE2C: molecular biology, role in tumorigenesis, and potential as a biomarker.** *Tumour Biol* 2012, **33**:723–730.

43. Lee B-K, Bhinge AA, Iyer VR: **Wide-ranging functions of E2F4 in transcriptional activation and repression revealed by genome-wide analysis.** *Nucleic Acids Res* 2011, **39**:3558–3573.

6

The correlation of aromatase activity and obesity in women with or without polycystic ovary syndrome

Jie Chen[1,2†], Shanmei Shen[3†], Yong Tan[1*], Dong Xia[2], Yanjie Xia[2], Yunxia Cao[4], Wenjun Wang[5], Xiaoke Wu[6], Hongwei Wang[2], Long Yi[2], Qian Gao[2] and Yong Wang[2*]

Abstract

Background: This study aimed to investigate the effect of polycystic ovary syndrome (PCOS) on the association of aromatase activity assessed by estradiol-to-testosterone ratio (E_2/T) with body mass index (BMI) in women.

Methods: This was a cohort study in five centers for reproductive medicine in China. Data were collected from July 2012 to December 2013. PCOS patients (n = 785) and non PCOS, healthy, age-matched controls (n = 297) were included. Plasma sex hormones including estradiol (E_2), testosterone (T), follicle stimulating hormone (FSH), and luteinizing hormone (LH) were measured by ELISA, together with BMI and E_2/T being calculated, on the third day of the menstrual cycle. Aromatase activity in PCOS patients with different BMI, T and E_2 levels were compared.

Results: E_2/T was significantly lower ($P < 0.05$) while BMI was significantly increased ($P < 0.05$) in PCOS than non-PCOS. No significant difference was observed in E_2/T among different BMI subgroups of either PCOS or control. Ovarian aromatase activity was decreased in PCOS patients which was independent of BMI. Hyperestrogen promoted ovarian aromatase activity, while hyperandrogen inhibited such activity, both in a dose-dependent, biphasic manner.

Conclusions: Ovarian aromatase activity was lower in PCOS, which was independent of BMI. New therapeutic strategies can be developed by targeting aromatase activity for treating PCOS women, especially those with obesity.

Keywords: PCOS, Aromatase activity, Obesity, Estradiol, Testosterone

Background

Polycystic ovary syndrome (PCOS) is a heterogeneous disorder characterized by dysfunction of gonadal axis and systemic nerve endocrine metabolic network [1], with a prevalence of up to 10% in women of reproductive age [2,3]. Furthermore, this number may underestimate the severity of the situation as many women with PCOS in the community remain undiagnosed [4]. PCOS has significant and diverse clinical implications including reproductive, endocrine and metabolic abnormalities such as hyperandrogenism and obesity [3]. Obesity, particularly abdominal obesity, is one of the independent factors aggravating the PCOS endocrine disorders, as subcutaneous abdominal adipose tissues and the liver tissues contribute to extragonadal aromatization [5].

Aromatase, a product of the CYP19 gene [6], is a member of the cytochrome P450 family [7]. Aromatase is a rate-limiting enzyme that catalyzes the conversion of androgens (androstenedione and testosterone) to estrogens (estrone and estradiol) during steroidogenesis [8]. In ovaries, estradiol is generated by converting C19 androgens derived from theca cells under the influence of aromatase produced by granulosa cells [9]. Consequently, the ratio of estradiol (E_2) to testosterone (T) has been used to evaluate aromatase activity [10,11]. Multiple studies have reported a dysfunctional P450-aromatase activity in PCOS women. However, whether the abnormality is caused by hyperfunction or insufficiency of the enzyme remains unknown [12-16]. The nature of the interaction between ovarian aromatase activity and PCOS in women has been controversial, and the impact of weight gain on aromatase activity as well as E_2 levels is unknown.

* Correspondence: xijun1025@163.com; yongwang@nju.edu.cn
†Equal contributors
[1]First Clinical Medicine College, Nanjing University of Chinese Medicine, Nanjing 210046, China
[2]State Key Laboratory of Chemistry for Life Science and Jiangsu Key Laboratory of Molecular Medicine, Medical School of Nanjing University, Nanjing 210093, China
Full list of author information is available at the end of the article

The objective of this study was to investigate the association and interaction between aromatase activity and levels of body mass index (BMI) from a reproductive hormone perspective in a group of women with or without PCOS.

Methods
Case origin
We designed a cohort study which included 1082 individuals from five clinical centers (785 PCOS and 297 age-matched non-PCOS) from July 2012 to December 2013. The study was approved by the Medical Ethics Committee of the Medical School of Nanjing University, Nanjing, China.

Inclusion and exclusion criteria
PCOS was diagnosed according to the 2006 Rotterdam criteria [17]. PCOS may be confirmed if any two out of the following three criteria are met and any other diseases that cause anovulation or hyperandrogenism can be excluded: (1) Oligovulation or anovulation, (2) Clinical manifestation or biochemical evidence of hyperandrogenism, (3) Occurrence of PCO (at least 12 antral follicles measuring 2–9 mm in diameter or the enlargement of an ovarian volume to more than 10 ml by transvaginal ultrasound). The non-PCOS women were selected from infertile couples if the infertility was attributed to male factors in the study period. All the subjects were between 20 and 35 years of age who had not been taking hormone drugs such as contraceptives, ovulation drugs, corticosteroids three months prior to inclusion and who did not have serious heart, liver, renal, and hematopoietic system diseases or malignant tumors.

Controls were recruited from healthy women with a regular menstrual cycle, normal basal sex hormones levels and absence of PCO on sonography.

Clinical and hormonal analyses
BMI was calculated as weight in kilograms divided by the square of height in metres (kg/m^2). Peripheral blood samples were taken between 08:00–09:00 A.M. on the third day of the menstrual cycle from all subjects after overnight fasting and frozen at −80°C until assayed. Sex hormones including E_2, T, luteinizing hormone (LH) and follicle-stimulating hormone (FSH) were measured by ELISA (Beijing North Institute of Biological Technology of China and the CIS Company of France). Intra- and inter-assay coefficients of variation were 10% for all the assays.

Grouping
Both the PCOS patients and non-PCOS subjects were allocated to one of the three subgroups, namely the obese subgroup (BMI $\geq$ 23 kg/m^2), the normal-weight

subgroup (18.5 kg/m^2 $\leq$ BMI < 23 kg/m^2) and the underweight subgroup (BMI < 18.5 kg/m^2), based on WHO recommendations for the Asia-Pacific region [18].

PCOS patients were also divided into subgroups based on the levels of T (T $\geq$ 2.44 nmol/L or T < 2.44 nmol/L) and E_2 levels (E_2 > 293.6 pmol/L, 146.8 $\leq$ E_2 $\leq$ 293.6 pmol/L, or E_2 < 146.8 pmol/L). The cuts-off were defined by normal laboratory reference values of reproductive medicine centers.

Statistics
SAS version 9.0 (USA) software was used to match cases and controls based on age. SPSS version 17 (SPSS, Chicago, IL, USA) was used to process the data. Parameters were described using mean ± standard deviation, or median ± quartiles (for data not normally distributed) and the statistical analyses were carried out by t-test and the rank-sum test, respectively. Subgroup differences were calculated by single-factor ANOVA. P < 0.05 was considered statistically significant.

Results
Aromatase activity in PCOS
The base sex hormone differences between the PCOS and non-PCOS subjects are summarized in Table 1. PCOS patients showed significantly increased levels of BMI, E_2, T and LH, while their E_2/T, FSH and FSH/LH values were decreased compared with the non-PCOS group.

Aromatase activity in women with different BMI with or without PCOS
All the three PCOS subgroups manifested lower levels of aromatase activity as compared to the corresponding non-PCOS subgroups (Tables 1 and 2). Furthermore, no significant differences in E_2/T were observed in both PCOS and non-PCOS subjects who had higher BMI values. However, there were trends demonstrating rising

Table 1 Biochemical data from PCOS and non-PCOS groups

	P (n = 785)	non P (n = 297)	P
BMI (kg/m^2)	23.87 ± 4.85[a]	22.30 ± 3.27	<0.001
E_2 (pmol/L)	254.81 ± 169.20[a]	219.73 ± 166.32	0.002
T (nmol/L)	2.60 ± 1.58[a]	1.20 ± 0.70	<0.001
E_2/T	0.10 (0.06-0.16)[a]	0.16 (0.10-0.29)	<0.001
FSH (mIU/L)	5.98 ± 2.93[a]	6.43 ± 2.17	0.006
LH (mIU/L)	11.90 ± 8.31[a]	5.37 ± 3.80	<0.001
FSH/LH	0.53 (0.36-0.91)[a]	1.41 (1.02-2.05)	<0.001

Data is shown as means ± SD or median and interquartile ranges.
[a]PCOS group compared with non-PCOS group, P < 0.05 suggests significantly different.
P: PCOS group, non P: non-PCOS group, BMI: body mass index, E_2: estradiol, T: testosterone, FSH: follicle-stimulating hormone, LH: luteinizing hormone.

Table 2 Biochemical data of the subjects by BMI

	$BMI \geq 23$ kg/m^2			18.5 kg/m$^2 \leq BMI < 23$ kg/m^2			$BMI < 18.5$ kg/m^2		
	P (n = 388)	Non P (n = 103)	P	P (n = 343)	Non P (n = 174)	P	P (n = 54)	Non P (n = 20)	P
BMI (kg/m^2)	$27.46 \pm 4.39^{a,b,d}$	$25.86 \pm 2.66^{a,b}$	0.001	20.79 ± 1.24^{c}	20.73 ± 1.23^{c}	0.574	17.54 ± 0.87	17.67 ± 0.95	0.567
E$_2$ (pmol/L)	247.95 ± 161.61^{d}	213.98 ± 164.51	0.048	258.49 ± 174.83^{d}	222.07 ± 166.43	0.023	280.72 ± 185.52	228.93 ± 182.02	0.287
T (nmol/L)	2.60 ± 1.66^{d}	1.23 ± 0.64^{b}	<0.001	2.57 ± 1.45^{d}	1.21 ± 0.74^{c}	<0.001	2.81 ± 1.80^{d}	0.86 ± 0.53	<0.001
E$_2$/T	$0.10 (0.06-0.15)^{d}$	$0.15 (0.09-0.24)$	0.001	$0.10 (0.06-0.16)^{d}$	$0.17 (0.10-0.33)$	<0.001	$0.09 (0.06-0.16)^{d}$	$0.20 (0.11-0.65)$	<0.001
FSH (mIU/L)	$5.74 \pm 2.80^{a,d}$	6.40 ± 2.47	0.027	6.19 ± 2.79^{d}	6.44 ± 2.06	0.045	6.40 ± 4.29	6.50 ± 1.46	0.916
LH (mIU/L)	$10.16 \pm 7.24^{a,b,d}$	5.22 ± 3.82	<0.001	$13.24 \pm 8.94^{b,d}$	5.39 ± 3.75	<0.001	15.90 ± 8.52^{d}	5.98 ± 4.15	<0.001
FSH/LH	$0.63 (0.42-1.03)^{b,d}$	$1.46 (1.00-2.11)$	<0.001	$0.47 (0.34-0.79)^{d}$	$1.40 (1.05-2.01)$	<0.001	$0.36 (0.36-0.51)^{d}$	$1.38 (0.87-1.75)$	<0.001

Data is shown as means ± SD or median and interquartile ranges.
P: PCOS group compared with non-PCOS group.
[a]$BMI \geq 23$ kg/m^2 subgroup compared with $18.5 \leq BMI < 23$ kg/m^2 subgroup, P < 0.05 means significantly different.
[b]$BMI \geq 23$ kg/m^2 subgroup compared with $BMI < 18.5$ kg/m^2 subgroup, P < 0.05 means significantly different.
[c]$18.5 \leq BMI < 23$ kg/m^2 subgroup compared with $BMI < 18.5$ kg/m^2 subgroup, P < 0.05 means significantly different.
[d]PCOS/non PCOS subgroups compared in the same BMI degree, P < 0.05 means significantly different.
P: PCOS group, non P: non PCOS group, BMI: body mass index, E2: estradiol, T: testosterone, FSH: follicle-stimulating hormone, LH: luteinizing hormone.

T levels and decreasing E$_2$/T and E$_2$ levels when BMI values were increased.

Aromatase activity in PCOS patients with different E$_2$ levels
Higher E$_2$ levels correlated with a relatively enhanced E$_2$/T as well as T and LH levels but reduced BMI, FSH and FSH/LH levels in women with PCOS (Table 3).

Aromatase activity in PCOS patients with different T levels
Hyperandrogenic PCOS patients had increased E$_2$ levels but their aromatase activity was markedly inhibited independent of their BMI values. The gonadotropins FSH and LH were both increased in people with higher T levels. More precisely, a more pronounced increase of LH was observed compared with FSH increase (Table 4).

Discussion
The human aromatase gene contains 10 exons and one of them encodes nine alternative promoters to regulate tissue-specific expression, and the other nine are the protein-coding exons [19]. Aromatase is expressed in specific cell populations of a variety of estrogen-producing tissues, including placenta, ovaries, testes, skin, adipose tissue, bone, brain, and vascular smooth muscle cells [19]. Importantly, aromatase in ovarian granulosa and luteinized granulosa cells plays an important role for women of reproductive age.

In this study, we aimed to discover the association between aromatase activity, obesity and sex hormones in a large, well-described cohort of PCOS patients. However, there is certain controversy regarding the correlation of ovarian aromatase activity with PCOS [16]. The E$_2$/T ratio provides important information about aromatase activity because conversion of androgens to estrogens is mediated by CYP19, suggesting that the E$_2$/T ratio may be a direct marker of aromatase activity [20]. Based on our data, PCOS is manifested by a typical abnormal hormone pattern where the increase of LH, testosterone,

Table 3 Biochemical data of PCOS patients by E$_2$ levels

	P (n = 785)			
	E$_2$ > 293.6 pmol/L (n = 233)	$146.8 \leq$ E$_2 \leq 293.6$ pmol/L (n = 348)	E$_2$ < 146.8 pmol/L (n = 204)	P
BMI (kg/m^2)	23.32 ± 4.58^{b}	23.92 ± 4.90	24.40 ± 5.03	0.034
E$_2$ (pmol/L)	$455.73 \pm 169.42^{a,b}$	212.23 ± 40.01^{c}	97.96 ± 29.27	<0.001
T (nmol/L)	$2.97 \pm 1.53^{a,b}$	2.59 ± 1.55^{c}	2.19 ± 1.59	<0.001
E$_2$/T	$0.15 (0.11-0.24)^{a,b}$	$0.09 (0.06-0.14)^{c}$	$0.05 (0.03-0.09)$	<0.001
FSH (mIU/L)	5.64 ± 3.60^{a}	6.21 ± 2.55	5.97 ± 2.63	<0.001
LH (mIU/L)	12.76 ± 9.97^{b}	12.12 ± 7.30^{c}	10.55 ± 7.71	<0.001
FSH/LH	$0.49 (0.33-0.73)^{b}$	$0.52 (0.37-0.86)^{c}$	$0.64 (0.41-1.15)$	<0.001

Data is shown as means ± SD or median and interquartile ranges.
P: compare in the three subgroups.
[a]E$_2$ > 293.6 pmol/L subgroup compared with $146.8 \leq$ E$_2 \leq 293.6$ pmol/L subgroup, P < 0.05 means significantly different.
[b]E$_2$ > 293.6 pmol/L subgroup compared with E$_2$ < 146.8 pmol/L subgroup, P < 0.05 means significantly different.
[c]$146.8 \leq$ E$_2 \leq 293.6$ pmol/L subgroup compared with E$_2$ < 146.8 pmol/L subgroup, P < 0.05 means significantly different.
P: PCOS group, non P: non PCOS group, BMI: body mass index, E2: estradiol, T: testosterone, FSH: follicle stimulating hormone, LH: luteinizing hormone.

Table 4 Biochemical data of the PCOS patients by T levels

	P (n = 785)		
	T ≥ 2.44 nmol/L (n = 364)	T < 2.44 nmol/L (n = 421)	P
BMI (kg/m^2)	23.35 ± 4.16	24.31 ± 5.34	0.076
E$_2$ (pmol/L)	289.41 ± 179.69[a]	224.89 ± 153.62	<0.001
T (nmol/L)	3.85 ± 1.46[a]	1.52 ± 0.55	<0.001
E$_2$/T	0.07(0.05-0.11)[a]	0.13 (0.09-0.20)	<0.001
FSH (mIU/L)	6.29 ± 2.84[a]	5.71 ± 2.98	0.006
LH (mIU/L)	14.03 ± 9.03[a]	10.06 ± 7.15	<0.001
FSH/LH	0.48 (0.34-0.73)[a]	0.59 (0.39-1.10)	<0.001

Data is shown as means ± SD or median and interquartile ranges.
[a]T ≥ 2.44 nmol/L subgroup compared with T < 2.44 nmol/L subgroup of PCOS, $P < 0.05$ means significantly different.
P: PCOS group, non P: non PCOS group, BMI: body mass index, E2: estradiol, T: testosterone, FSH: follicle-stimulating hormone, LH: luteinizing hormone.

and estradiol is accompanied with reduced levels of FSH, FSH/LH, and E$_2$/T. We found a significant decrease of ovarian aromatase activity in women with PCOS as compared to controls which is consistent with previous work [8,16,21]. In the polycystic ovary, theca cells synthesize more androgens than the corresponding cells in a normal ovary. In contrast, granulosa cells in the polycystic ovary have a lower aromatase activity, which results in an imbalance in the production of estrogen and androgen. An earlier research by Soderlund and co-workers found no gross deletions or insertions after PCR amplification of the nine exons of the P450 arom gene from the peripheral blood leukocytes of 25 PCOS patients [22]. But this cannot preclude the importance of an aromatase disorder in the etiology of PCOS, as there may exist causative mutations in the untranslated regions or within introns.

There is evidence that obesity, particularly abdominal obesity, exacerbates both the clinical and endocrine features of PCOS [23] which demonstrates significantly more serious insulin resistance in these individuals than normal-weight counterparts [24]. Although obesity is not included in the diagnostic criteria for PCOS, 35% to 80% of PCOS women, depending on the setting of the study and the ethnic characteristics of the patients, are commonly overweight (BMI above 25 kg/m^2) or obese (BMI above 30 kg/m^2) [25]. Our findings associated higher BMI with PCOS but no concomitant change of E$_2$/T was observed. It is reported that estrogen has the capacity to favorably regulate body composition and glucose homeostasis to prevent diet-induced obesity [26].

Aromatase expression in the ovarian follicle is also responsible for the cyclic changes in serum estradiol levels and the modulation of the structure and function of the female reproductive tract and is essential for the survival, fertilization and implantation of oocytes. PCOS promotes a hyperestrogenic state. In this research, PCOS

with high estradiol levels led to more serious hyperandrogenism but with relatively elevated levels of E$_2$/T. This is consistent with a previous study showing that higher estradiol levels are caused by increased RNA expression of granulosa cell aromatase and its activity [27].

Nevertheless, high testosterone levels of PCOS inhibited aromatase activity. We hypothesize that androgen can dose-dependently affect aromatase activity directly, or indirectly by regulating other factors such as E$_2$ and LH. One report suggests that early exposure of females to androgen induces sex-specific organizational changes of aromatase expression in the preoptic area [28].

Hyperinsulinemia and insulin resistance play a role in the pathogenesis of PCOS. Analyzing existing studies, the relationship between insulin and activity of cytochrome P450 family has been explored. La Marca gave a direct demonstration that decreasing insulin with metformin led to a reduction in stimulated ovarian P450c17α activity in PCOS and Nestler JE's study showed the similar result in lean PCOS [29,30]. Whether P450 aromatase activity may be dependent on insulin resistance will be investigated in our follow-up work.

PCOS is a common ovulatory disorder in young women, which affects 5-10% of the population and results in infertility due to anovulation [31]. Although the pathogenesis of PCOS is still unclear, the role of hyperandrogenism in the pathophysiology of PCOS has been established but not clearly. Oral contraceptives, such as ethinylestradiol and cyproterone acetate tablets, drospirenone and ethinylestradiol tablets, have been used in the clinic to reduce hyperandrogen and to suppress follicular development. Letrozole, an aromatase inhibitor, can induce ovulation in PCOS so that a normal serum androgen level can be maintained by blocking the early low estrogen negative feedback. Generation and metabolism of androgen is directly related to aromatase activity. Along this line, aromatase-agonist-like-drugs perhaps can directly induce follicular development and shorten the treatment course of PCOS women irrespective of the original hyperandrogen state.

Study limitation
We checked controls for PCOS features (PCOM, hyperandrogenism, oligo-anovulation) in this study. Testosterone was the only androgen that was measured in our study and other androgens such as androstenedione and dehydroepiandrosterone sulfate do not be analyzed because of the limitation of research funding.

Conclusion
Taken together, our results showed that ovarian aromatase activity in PCOS was decreased which was independent of BMI. Hyperestrogen promoted ovarian aromatase activity which could be inhibited by hyperandrogenism in a dose-

dependent manner demonstrating a complex biphasic correlation.

In both normal women and PCOS patients, estrogen levels negatively correlated to BMI. Aromatase, the master convertor of androgen to estrogen, can regulate the estradiol-to-testosterone ratio and thereby regulates BMI. Thus, enhancing aromatase activity may become an optimized strategy for developing therapies for PCOS women, especially those with obesity.

Competing interests
The authors declare that they have no competing interests.

Authors' contributions
JC and SS participated in the study design, method investigation, experiment performance and the preparation of the manuscript. YT, YC, WW and XW participated in the clinical management and contributed with acquisition and interpretation of data. DX and YJX conducted the laboratory experiments and performed the statistical evaluations. HW, LY and QG participated in the study design and project coordination and helped to revise the article. YW conceived and directed the study, and assisted in manuscript drafting. All authors read and approved the final manuscript.

Acknowledgements
We would like to extend our sincere thanks to all those who participated in the study, especially those healthy controls.

Fundings
This study was supported by the National Natural Science Foundation of China (814714222, 81373683, 81170541), Science and Technology Project of Jiangsu Province of China (SBL201320056), the Ph.D. Program Foundation of the Ministry of Education of China (20123237110004) and the Ordinary University Graduate Practice Innovation Plan of Jiangsu Province, China (SJZZ_0123).

Author details
[1]First Clinical Medicine College, Nanjing University of Chinese Medicine, Nanjing 210046, China. [2]State Key Laboratory of Chemistry for Life Science and Jiangsu Key Laboratory of Molecular Medicine, Medical School of Nanjing University, Nanjing 210093, China. [3]Divisions of Endocrinology, the Affiliated Drum Tower Hospital, Medical School, Nanjing University, Nanjing 210093, China. [4]Department of Obstetrics and Gynecology, Anhui Medical University, Hefei 230022, China. [5]Centre of Reproduction, Department of Obstetric and Gynaecology, Memorial Hospital of Sun Yat-Sen University, Guangzhou 510120, China. [6]Department of Obstetrics and Gynecology, the First Affiliated Hospital, Heilongjiang University of Chinese Medicine, Harbin 150040, China.

References
1. Fauser BC, Tarlatzis BC, Rebar RW, Legro RS, Balen AH, Lob R. Consensus on women's health aspects of polycystic ovary syndrome (PCOS): the Amsterdam ESHRE/ASRM-Sponsored 3rd PCOS Consensus Workshop Group. Fertil Steril. 2012;97:28–38.
2. Hart R, Hickey M, Franks S. Definitions, prevalence and symptoms of polycystic ovaries and polycystic ovary syndrome. Best Pract Res Clin Obstet Gynaecol. 2004;18:671–83.
3. Goodarzi MO, Dumesic DA, Chazenbalk G, Azziz R. Polycystic ovary syndrome: etiology, pathogenesis and diagnosis. Nat Rev Endocrinol. 2011;7:219–31.
4. March WA, Moore VM, Willson KJ, Phillips DI, Norman RJ, Davies MJ. The prevalence of polycystic ovary syndrome in a community sample assessed under contrasting diagnostic criteria. Hum Reprod. 2010;25:544–51.
5. Cupisti S, Kajaia N, Dittrich R, Duezenli H, Beckmann MW, Mueller A. Body mass index and ovarian function are associated with endocrine and metabolic abnormalities in women with hyperandrogenic syndrome. Eur J Endocrinol. 2008;158:711–9.
6. Ma CX, Adjei AA, Salavaggione OE, Coronel J, Pelleymounter L, Wang L. Human aromatase: gene resequencing and functional genomics. Cancer Res. 2005;65:11071–82.
7. Bulun SE, Sebastian S, Takayama K, Suzuki T, Sasano H, Shozu M. The human CYP19 (aromatase P450) gene:update on physiologic roles and genomic organization of promoters. J Steroid Biochem Mol Biol. 2003;86:219–24.
8. Lesley J, Millsa, Ruth E, Gutjahr G, Gerald E, Zaroogiana, et al. Modulation of aromatase activity as a mode of action for endocrine disrupting chemicals in a marine fish. Aquat Toxicol. 2014;147:140–50.
9. Leandros L, Nectaria X, Elissavet H, Atsushi T, Apostolos K, Georgios M, et al. CYP19 gene variants affect the assisted reproduction outcome of women with polycystic ovary syndrome. Gynecol Endocrinol. 2013;29:478–82.
10. Jiang J, Tang NL, Ohlsson C, Eriksson AL, Vandenon Put L, Chan FW, et al. Association of genetic variations in aromatase gene with serum estrogen and estrogen/testosterone ratio in Chinese elderly men. J Clin Chim Acta. 2010;411:53–8.
11. Jakimiuk AJ, Weitsman SR, Brzechffa PR, Magoffin DA. Aromatase mRNA expression in individual follicles from polycystic ovaries. Mol Hum Reprod. 1998;4:1–8.
12. Barnes RB, Rosenfield RL, Burstein S, Ehrmann DA. Pituitary-ovarian responses to nafarelin testing in the polycystic ovary syndrome. N Engl J Med. 1989;320:559–65.
13. Suikkari AM, McLachlan V, Montalto J, Calderon I, Healy DL, McLachlan RI. Ultrasonographic appearance of polycystic ovaries is associated with exaggerated ovarian androgen and estradiol responses to gonadotrophin-releasing hormone agonist in women undergoing assisted reproduction treatment. Hum Reprod. 1995;10:513–9.
14. Ibanez L, Hall JE, Potau N, Carrascosa A, Prat N, Taylor AE. Ovarian 17-hydroxyprogesterone hyperresponsiveness to gonadotropin-releasing hormone (GnRH) agonist challenge in women with polycystic ovary syndrome is not mediated by luteinizing hormone hypersecretion: evidence from GnRH agonist and human chorionic gonadotropin stimulation testing. J Clin Endocrinol Metab. 1996;81:4103–7.
15. Fulghesu AM, Villa P, Pavone V, Guido M, Apa R, Caruso A, et al. The impact of insulin secretion on the ovarian response to exogenous gonadotropins in polycystic ovary syndrome. J Clin Endocrinol Metab. 1997;82:644–8.
16. la Marca A, Morgante G, Palumbo M, Cianci A, Petraglia F, De Leo V. Insulin-lowering treatment reduces aromatase activity in response to follicle-stimulating hormone in women with polycystic ovary syndrome. Fertil Steril. 2002;78:1234–9.
17. Rotterdam ESHRE/ASRM-Sponsored PCOS Consensus Workshop Group. Revised 2003 consensus on diagnostic criteria and long-term health risks related to polycystic ovary syndrome. Fertil Steril. 2004;81:19–25.
18. International Diabetes Institute World Health Organization, West Pacific Region. The Asia Pacific Perspective: redefining obesity and its Treatment. In: International Association for the Study of Obesity and International Obesity Task Force. 2000.
19. Bulun SE, Lin Z, Imir G, Amin S, Demura M, Yilmaz B, et al. Regulation of aromatase expression in estrogen-responsive breast and uterine disease: from bench to treatment. Pharmacol Rev. 2005;57:359–83.
20. Jin JL, Sun J, Ge HJ, Cao YX, Wu XK, Liang FJ, et al. Association between CYP19 gene SNP rs2414096 polymorphism and polycystic ovary syndrome in Chinese women. BMC Med Genet. 2009;10:139.
21. Kirilovas D, Chaika A, Bergström M, Bergstrom-Petterman E, Carlström K, Nosenko J, et al. Granulosa cell aromatase enzyme activity: effects of follicular fluid from patients with polycystic ovary syndrome, using aromatase conversion and [11C]vorozole-binding assays. Gynecol Endocrinol. 2006;22:685–91.
22. Soderlund D, Canto P, Carranza-Lira S, Mendez JP. No evidence of mutations in the P450 aromatase gene in patients with polycystic ovary syndrome. Hum Reprod. 2005;20:965–9.
23. Kaya C, Cengiz SD, Satiroglu H. Obesity and insulin resistance associated with lower plasma vitamin B12 in PCOS. Reprod Biomed Online. 2009;19:721–6.
24. Morales AJ, Laughlin GA, Bützow T, Maheshwari H, Baumann G, Yen SS. Insulin, somatotropic, and luteinizing hormone axes in lean and obese women with polycystic ovary syndrome: common and distinct features. J Clin Endocrinol Metab. 1996;81:2854–64.
25. Hahn S, Tan S, Sack S, Kimmig R, Quadbeck B, Mann K, et al. Prevalence of the metabolic syndrome in German women with polycystic ovary syndrome. Exp Clin Endocrinol Diabetes. 2007;115:130–5.
26. Barrera J, Chambliss KL, Ahmed M, Tanigaki K, Thompson B, McDonald JG, et al. Bazedoxifene and conjugated estrogen prevent diet-induced obesity,

hepatic steatosis and type 2 diabetes in mice without impacting the reproductive tract. Am J Physiol Endocrinol Metab. 2014;307:E345-54.

27. Shaw ND, Srouji SS, Welt CK, Cox KH, Fox JH, Adams JM, et al. Evidence that increased ovarian aromatase activity and expression account for higher estradiol levels in African American compared with Caucasian women. J Clin Endocrinol Metab. 2014;99:1384–92.

28. Gonzalez B, Ratner LD, Scerbo MJ, Di Giorgio NP, Poutanen M, Huhtaniemi IT, et al. Elevated hypothalamic aromatization at the onset of precocious puberty in transgenic female mice hypersecreting human chorionic gonadotropin: effect of androgens. Mol Cell Endocrinol. 2014;390:102–11.

29. La Marca A, Egbe TO, Morgante G, Paglia T, Cianci A, De Leo V. Metformin treatment reduces ovarian cytochrome P-450c17alpha response to human chorionic gonadotrophin in women with insulin resistance-related polycystic ovary syndrome. Hum Reprod. 2000;5:21–3.

30. Nestler JE, Jakubowicz DJ. Lean women with polycystic ovary syndrome respond to insulin reduction with decreases in ovarian P450c17 alpha activity and serum androgens. J Clin Endocrinol Metab. 1997;82:4075–9.

31. Asuncion M, Calvo RM, San Millan JL, Sancho J, Avila S, Escobar-Morreale HF. A prospective study of the prevalence of the polycystic ovary syndrome in unselected Caucasian women from Spain. J Clin Endocrinol Metab. 2000;85:2434–8.

7

Polycystic ovarian syndrome is accompanied by repression of gene signatures associated with biosynthesis and metabolism of steroids, cholesterol and lipids

Dessie Salilew-Wondim[1], Qi Wang[2,3], Dawit Tesfaye[1], Karl Schellander[1], Michael Hoelker[1], Md Munir Hossain[4] and Benjamin K Tsang[2,3,5]*

Abstract

Background: Polycystic ovarian syndrome (PCOS) is a spectrum of heterogeneous disorders of reproduction and metabolism in women with potential systemic sequel such as diabetes and obesity. Although, PCOS is believed to be caused by genetic abnormalities, the genetic background that can be associated with PCOS phenotypes remains unclear due to the complexity of the trait. In this study, we used a rat model which exhibits reproductive and metabolic abnormalities similar to the human PCOS to unravel the molecular mechanisms underlining this complex syndrome.

Methods: Female Sprague–Dawley rats were randomly assigned to DHT and control (CTL) groups. Rats in the DHT group were implanted with a silicone capsule continuous-releasing 83 μg 5α-dihydrotestosterone (DHT) per day for 12 weeks to mimic the hyperandrogenic state in women with PCOS. The animals were euthanized at 15 weeks of age and the pairs of ovaries were excised and the ovarian cortex tissues were used for gene expression analysis. Total RNA was from the ovarian cortex was amplified, labeled and hybridized to the Affymetrix GeneChip® Rat Genome 230 2.0 Array. A linear model system for microarray data analysis was used to identify genes affected in DHT treated rat ovaries and the molecular pathway of those genes were analyzed using the Database for Annotation, Visualization and Integrated Discovery (DAVID) analysis tool.

Results: A total of 573 gene transcripts, including *CPA1, CDH1, INSL3, AMH, ALDH1B1, INHBA, CYP17A1, RBP4, GAS6, GAS7* and *GATA4*, were activated while 430 others including *HSD17B7, HSD3B6, STAR, HMGCS1, HMGCR, CYP51, CYP11A1 and CYP19A1* were repressed in DHT-treated ovaries. Functional annotation of the dysregulated genes revealed that biosynthesis and metabolism of steroids, cholesterol and lipids to be the most top functions enriched by the repressed genes. However, cell differentiation/proliferation, transcriptional regulation, neurogenesis, cell adhesion and blood vessel development processes were enriched by activated genes.

(Continued on next page)

* Correspondence: btsang@ohri.ca
[2]Reproductive Biology Unit and Division of Reproductive Medicine, Department of Obstetrics & Gynecology and Cellular & Molecular Medicine, Interdisciplinary School of Health Sciences, University of Ottawa, Ottawa K1H 8L6, ON, Canada
[3]Chronic Disease Program, Ottawa Hospital Research Institute, The Ottawa Hospital (General Campus), Critical Care Wing, 3rd Floor, Room W3107, 501 Smyth Road, Ottawa K1H 8L6, ON, Canada
Full list of author information is available at the end of the article

(Continued from previous page)

Conclusion: The dysregulation of genes associated with biosynthesis and metabolism of steroids, cholesterol and lipids, cell differentiation/proliferation in DHT- treated ovaries could be a molecular clue for abnormal steroidogenesis, estrous cycle irregularity, abnormal folliculogenesis, anovulation and lipid metabolism in PCOS patients.

Keywords: Polycystic ovarian syndrome, Anovulation, Gene expression, Ovary

Introduction

The ovary is a key organ in the female reproductive system and its malfunction due to endocrine abnormalities could result in female infertility. Polycystic ovarian syndrome (PCOS) is one of the common hormonal and metabolic disorders in women of reproductive age [1]. However, due to its heterogeneity and complexity, universally accepted clinical definition of PCOS remains ambiguous [2,3]. Indeed, the presence of polycystic ovarian morphology is one of the common phenomena that can occur in the majority of PCOS patients. About 95% of women with PCOS at their early follicular phase could have polycystic ovaries and reduced level of follicle stimulating hormone [4] which may lead to antral follicle growth arrest and increased luteinizing hormone level [5]. In addition, PCOS is also associated with hyperandrogenism, menstrual dysfunction, oligo-ovulation and insulin resistance [6]. In this context, PCOS is considered as a complex androgen excess accompanied by different degrees of gonadotropic and metabolic dysregulation controlled by multiple gene interaction and environmental factors [7]. However, to what extent this trait is transmitted to the next generation and the intrinsic molecular factors underlining the occurrence of PCOS is unclear.

Although, the genetic basis of abnormal follicular development, anovulation, metabolic disorder and other heterogenous clinical abnormalities of PCOS patients seems to require detailed investigation, it is suggested that daughters from women exhibiting a characteristics of PCOS could have a higher chance of acquiring hyperandrogenism and other PCOS phenotypes [8]. Moreover, single nucleotide polymorphism in thyroid adenoma associated (*THADA)*, DENN/MADD domain containing 1A (*DENND1A)*, interleukin 6 (*IL6)* and adiponectin genes has been suggested to be the genetic causes of PCOS [9-11]. In addition, in vitro studies also showed altered expression of *CYP11A* and *CYP17* genes in theca cell derived from PCOS woman [12]. Furthermore, changes in the granulosa and theca cell gene expression have been reported in women with PCOS [13-15]. Although these association studies were performed using the samples of PCOS patients, the majority of gene expression studies were based on the cell culture models which may not necessarily represent and describe the

biological and molecular networks governing its complex phenotype. Indeed, this can in part be due to the availability and accessibility of the human sample or small sample size of the study populations [7] and the complexity of the trait between individuals. However, to addresse the clinical heterogeneity of PCOS, animal models have been described to be the best option to investigate the pathophysiologic mechanisms associated with the etiology of PCOS [16-21]. Therefore, to uncover the broad basis of molecular mechanisms associated with physiological and anatomical changes induced by PCOS, we generated a rat PCOS model that exhibit both polycystic ovaries (PCO) and metabolic abnormalities by implanting silastic capsules containing 5α-dihydrotestosterone (DHT) into their ovary in similar way as previously described by others [22]. Using this rat PCOS model that exhibits both polycystic ovaries (PCO) and metabolic abnormalities, we have previously demonstrated altered expression of 89 miRNAs following chronic androgen treatment [23]. However, the genes that are activated or repressed as well as their molecular functions, gene networks and molecular pathways associated with PCOS phenotypes, remained unclear. Therefore, this study was conducted to gain insight into the genes that are associated with follicular arrest, abnormal steroid and metabolite biosynthesis and metabolism, insulin resistance and ovarian dysfunction.

Materials and methods

Details of the materials and methods used in the present study have been described in our previous publication [23]. Briefly, female Sprague–Dawley rats were randomly assigned to DHT and control (CTL) groups. Rats in the DHT group were implanted with a silicone capsule continuous-releasing 83 μg 5α-dihydrotestosterone (DHT) per day for 12 weeks to mimic the hyperandrogenic state in women with PCOS, whose plasma DHT levels are approximately 1.7-fold higher than those of healthy control and those in CTL group received empty capsule [22]. The animals were euthanized at 15 weeks of age, ovaries were excised and extraneous tissues carefully removed. Corpus luteum (CL) was present in most of control rat ovaries while none or very few CL were observed in DHT-treated rat ovaries. Ovarian cortex tissues were snap-frozen in liquid nitrogen and stored at −80°C for further analysis. The PCOS phenotypic characteristics of DHT-treated rats have been described [23].

Gene expression analysis using GeneChip@rat genome array

Total RNAs were isolated from 3 independent DHT and CTL rat ovaries using miRNeasy mini kit (Qiagen, Hilden, Germany). Genomic DNA contamination was removed from the RNA samples using TURBO DNA-free™ kit (Ambion, Foster City, CA). The concentration of the RNA was analyzed using the Nanodrop 8000 Spectrophotometer (Thermo Fisher Scientific Inc, DE, USA). The RNA integrity and quality was evaluated using Agilent 2100 Bioanalyzer with RNA 6000 Nano LabChip® Kit (Agilent Technologies Inc, CA, USA).

RNA amplification

250 ng of total RNAs from DHT-treated or CTL rat groups in four replicates was amplified and labeled as per the GeneChip®3′ IVT Express Kit (Affymetrix, CA, USA). Eukaryotic poly-A RNA control kit (Affymetrix, CA, USA) was used as a SPIKE-IN control to monitor the entire target labeling process. Following amplification, the biotin labeled amplified RNA (aRNA) was purified and fragmented. The distribution of aRNA fragments were evaluated using Agilent 2100 bioanalyzer with RNA 6000 Nano LabChip® Kit (Agilent Technologies Inc, CA, USA).

Sample hybridization, array washing, staining and scanning

Prior to hybridization, the fragmented and biotin labelled cRNA from each rat ovary was mixed with control oligonucleotide B2 (3 nM), 20× eukaryotic hybridization controls (bioB, bioC, bioD, cre) (Affymetrix, CA, USA), 2× hybridization mix and DMSO. The hybridization cocktail were then incubated at 99°C (5 min) and subsequently at 45°C (5 min). Each sample was then transferred to independent GeneChip® Rat Genome 230 2.0 Array chip. Three biological replicates and one technical replicate (pool of three biological replicates) were hybridized for each rat group for 16 h. The array slides were washed and stained using the Fluidics Station 450/250 (Affymetrix, CA, USA), according to the GeneChip® expression user manual (P/N 702232 Rev. 3). Arrays were scanned with the GeneChip™ 3000 laser confocal slide scanner (Affymetrix, CA, USA) integrated with GeneChip® Operating System (GCOS).

Array data analysis and visualization

The array data was normalized by integrating the bioconductor packages (http://bioconductor.org) in R environment (www.r-project.org), using GC robust multi-array average analysis [24]. Briefly, the cell intensity (CELL) files were imported into R software after loading bioconductor packages (http://bioconductor.org) that suit to the Rat GeneChip affymetrix array. The normalized data and the CELL files are stored in the Gene Expression Omnibus (GEO; http://www.ncbi.nlm.nih.gov/geo/, series entry number GSM1437398). The linear models for microarray data analysis system (LIMMA) [25] and the Benjamini–Hochberg procedure of false discovery rate adjustment [26] were employed to discriminate the gene expression profile between the samples. The differentially expressed genes were tested for their gene ontology (GO) terms for over- or under-representation, using a classical hypergeometric test [27]. The molecular pathway enriched by differentially expressed genes were obtained from the Kyoto Encyclopedia of Genes and Genomes (KEGG) and Panther pathway data bases, using The Database for Annotation, Visualization and Integrated Discovery (DAVID) analysis tool [28]. The heatmaps and clustering of differentially expressed genes were constructed using Bioconductor (http://www.bioconductor.org) in R software environment http://www.r-project.org/ and/or PermutMatrix [29].

Table 1 Gene specific primers used for validation of differentially expressed genes

Gene bank acc. No	Gene symbol	Primer 5′ to 3′	bp
NM_012536	CTRB1	F: CTGAAGATCGCACAGGTCTTT	185
		R: TCTTGAGGGCATTGTATTTGG	
NM_017239	MYH6	F: AAGCTGCAGTTGAAGGTGAAG	214
		R: TGGACAGGTTATTCCTCATCG	
NM_013085	PLAU	F: GAGGGTGCTTGTCCAATATGA	189
		R: CAGGAATACACCAGCTTTGCT	
NM_207602	ST3GAL6	F: TGCGTATCACAATCTGACTGC	200
		R: AATCACCAGGCAGCAACAG	
NM_017128	INHBA	F: TAGGCAGTCTGAAGACCATCC	199
		R: TGAGTGGAAGGAGAGTGAGGA	
NM_031558	STAR	F: CTCACGTGGCTGCTCAGTAT	221
		R: CTTGGCTGAAGGTGAACAGA	
NM_017235	HSD17B7	F: CTTTTAGTCCCAGCGAGGAG	188
		R: TGGCCCAAACACAAACATAC	
NM_138504	OSGIN1	F: CAATCCCTGAGGAGGAAGAG	217
		R: CCCCTCTGGTCTATGGCTAC	
NM_013413	RLN1	F: CGTTCCCAGAGCTACAACAAC	249
		R:CCATTAGCTCCGTATCAGCAG	
NM_031144	ACTB	F: ACTGGGACGATATGGAGAAGA	202
		R:AGAGGCATACAGGGACAACAC	

(bp = number of base pairs).

Validation of differentially expressed genes

Some of the differentially expressed genes were randomly selected for validation, using SYBR Green based quantitative real time polymerase chain reaction (qPCR) and with sequence specific primers designed online (http://frodo.wi.mit.edu/primer3/; Table 1). The specificity and identity of each primer pair was confirmed by sequencing with the GenomeLab™ GeXP Genetic Analysis System (Beckman Coulter). The mRNA level was subsequently quantified using the cDNAs obtained from reverse transcription of total RNA samples used for microarray study. The qPCR was then performed in 20 µl reaction volume containing iTaq SYBR Green Supermix with ROX (Bio-Rad laboratories, Munich, Germany), the cDNA samples of DHT or CTL samples and the specific forward and reverse primer in the StepOnePlus™ Real-Time PCR Systems (Applied Biosystems, Foster City, CA). The presence of specific amplification was monitored by evaluating the dissociation curve. The abundance of each transcript was determined using the comparative threshold cycle (ΔCT) method. Data were analyzed after normalizing the Ct value of the target genes against the housekeeping gene β actin (β-actin). The Student's t-test or least significant difference test procedures was employed to detect differences in mRNA levels between samples. The level of activation or repression of a gene in DHT relative to CTL was determined using the formula $2^{-\Delta\Delta CT}$. Differences with $p < 0.05$ were considered significant.

Results

Ovarian polycystic syndrome is associated with dysregulation of gene expression

This study was a part of our previously published results and thus a detailed description of the PCOS phenotypic data has been provided [23]. The DHT- treated rats had higher body weight, oestrous cycle irregularity and reduced insulin sensitivity. Ovaries from these rats had lower weight and exhibited absence of corpus luteum, higher percentage of follicle cysts, relatively thin membrane granulosa and theca hyperplasia. Thus, to unravel the genes that are abnormally activated or repressed due to PCOS, the ovarian transcriptome profile of DHT-treated and CTL rats were compared using the GeneChip @rat Genome array. The genes of which the pattern of expression was different between the DHT and CTL groups were identified by a linear model described in the LIMMA pipeline and bioconductor packages. 1774 of the 31046 gene transcripts available in GeneChip® Rat Genome 230 2.0 A array showed ≥ 2 fold change dysregulation in DHT-treated rat ovaries compared to CTL group (data not shown). However, using a stricter selection criteria (fold change ≥ 2, $p \leq 0.01$ and false discovery rate (FDR) ≤ 10%), a total of 1003 transcripts were dysregulated in DHT-treated compared to CTL group (Figure 1A and B). Hierarchical clustering of the dysregulated genes exhibited a similar expression pattern within biological replicates and distinct differences between the groups (Figure 1C).

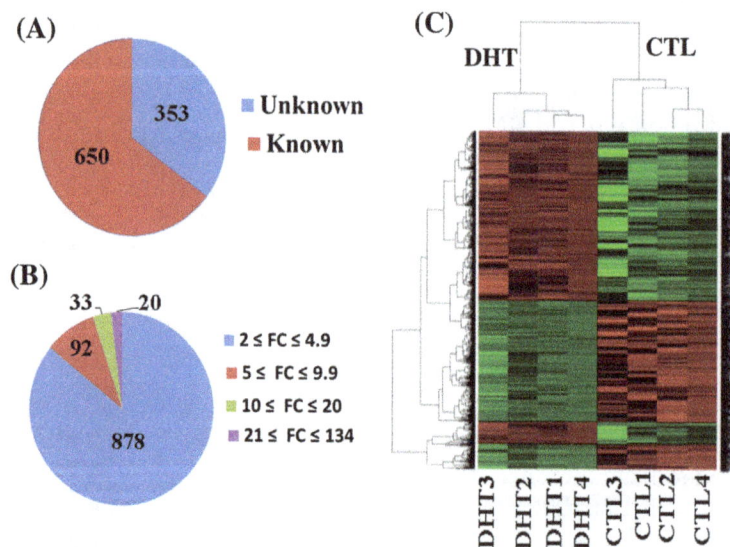

Figure 1 Ovarian transcriptome profile differences between DHT-treated and CTL rat groups. **(A)** The number of annotated (with known gene symbol) and non-annotated (unknown gene symbol) dysregulated genes in DHT rat groups. **(B)** The fold change (FC) distribution of dysregulated genes. **(C)** The heatmap showing the expression pattern of differentially expressed genes within and between biological replicates. DHT represents biological replicates in DHT-treated rat groups while CTL represents biological replicates in rats received an empty silastic capsule. Heatmap was generated using normalized log$_2$ transformed values and the normalized log$_2$ transformed expression values are described by pseudo color scale with red indicating the activated transcript level while the green color shows repressed expression pattern of a specific gene.

Gene transcripts repressed in DHT-treated rats

Following identification of differentially expressed genes between DHT-treated and CTL groups, the genes of which their transcript level was significant reduced by ≥ 2 folds changes in DHT compared to CTL were considered as repressed genes. However, those genes which showed by ≥ 2 folds reduction but displayed a false discovery rate higher that 0.1 were excluded in the analysis. Based on these stringent criteria, including 123 express sequence tags (ESTs), a total of 430 gene transcripts were found to be repressed in the DHT-treated ovaries. Of all the repressed genes, 320 transcripts displayed fold changes between 2 and 5 whereas the expression level of 110 genes was dysregulated between 5 and 134 folds in the DHT group. The list and expression pattern of genes repressed by 11.9 or more folds are described in Figure 2. Among the top repressed genes, the expression pattern of relaxin 1 (RLN1), Phospholipase A2 (*PLA2G1B*), x-prolyl amino-peptidase (*XPNPEP2*), Alpha-2-macroglobulin (*A2M*) and fatty acid binding protein 6 (*FABP6*) was repressed by 133.9, 70.6, 61.6, 58 and 45.8 folds, respectively. In addition, genes involved in steroid and lipid biosynthesis and metabolism, including hydroxysteroid (17-beta) dehydrogenase 7 (*HSD17B7*), hydroxy-delta-5-steroid dehydrogenase 3 beta- and steroid delta-isomerase 6 (*HSD3B6*), steroidogenic acute regulatory protein (*STAR*), 3-hydroxy-3-methylglutaryl-coenzyme A synthase 1 (*HMGCS1*), 3-hydroxy-3-methylglutaryl-coenzyme reductase (*HMGCR*) and cytochrome P450 (*CYP51, CYP11A1, CYP19A1*) were repressed in DHT-treated ovaries.

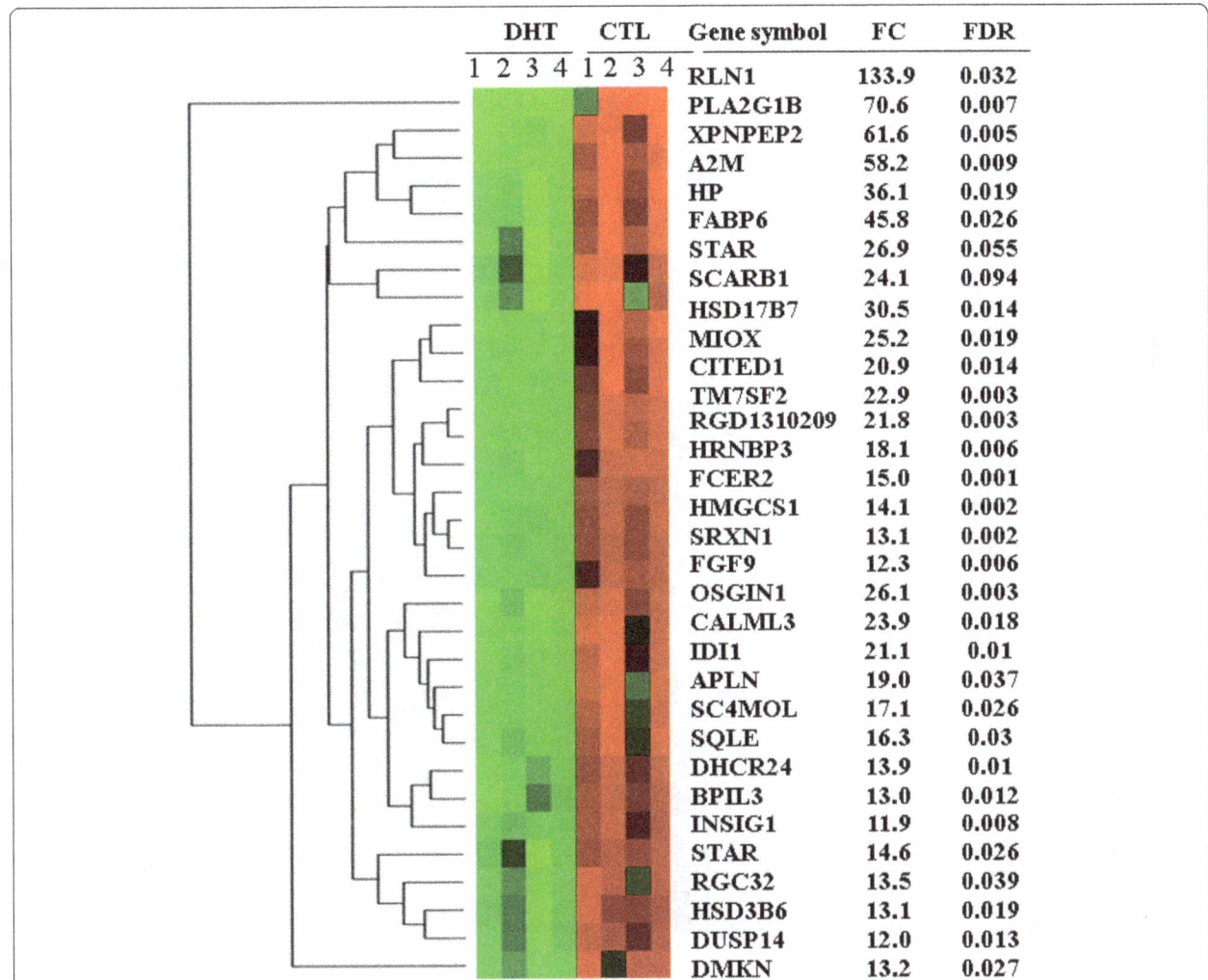

Gene symbol	FC	FDR
RLN1	133.9	0.032
PLA2G1B	70.6	0.007
XPNPEP2	61.6	0.005
A2M	58.2	0.009
HP	36.1	0.019
FABP6	45.8	0.026
STAR	26.9	0.055
SCARB1	24.1	0.094
HSD17B7	30.5	0.014
MIOX	25.2	0.019
CITED1	20.9	0.014
TM7SF2	22.9	0.003
RGD1310209	21.8	0.003
HRNBP3	18.1	0.006
FCER2	15.0	0.001
HMGCS1	14.1	0.002
SRXN1	13.1	0.002
FGF9	12.3	0.006
OSGIN1	26.1	0.003
CALML3	23.9	0.018
IDI1	21.1	0.01
APLN	19.0	0.037
SC4MOL	17.1	0.026
SQLE	16.3	0.03
DHCR24	13.9	0.01
BPIL3	13.0	0.012
INSIG1	11.9	0.008
STAR	14.6	0.026
RGC32	13.5	0.039
HSD3B6	13.1	0.019
DUSP14	12.0	0.013
DMKN	13.2	0.027

Figure 2 Significantly repressed genes by ≥ 11.9 folds in DHT-treated rat ovaries. The hierarchical clustering, the expression pattern, the average fold change (FC) and the false discovery rate of significantly highly repressed genes in DHT treated rat ovaries. DHT represents biological replicates in DHT-treated rat groups while CTL represents biological replicates in rats received an empty silastic capsule. The red color indicates the activated transcript level in CTL groups while the green color shows repressed expression pattern of a specific gene in DHT treated rat ovaries.

Functional classification of the genes repressed in ovaries of DHT-treated rats

To understand the biological processes and molecular function over- or under-represented in ovaries associated with repressed genes in the DHT-treated rats, the functional annotation of the repressed genes were interrogated using the DAVID bioinfomatic tool and the result revealed a total 31 crucial biological processes to be repressed in DHT-treated ovaries (Additional file 1: Table S1). Most importantly, closely interlinked biosynthetic and metabolic functions, namely the biosynthesis and metabolism of sterols/steroids, cholesterol, isoprenoids and lipids, were the top significant biological processes enriched by repressed genes (Figure 3). In addition, the repressed genes were also found to be associated with oxidation/reduction, reactive oxygen species, metabolism and immune processes. Moreover, categorization of the repressed genes into their corresponding activities (molecular functions) revealed that 28% of them were known to be involved in catalytic activity, whereas 15% of the repressed genes are associated with binding of cofactors, coenzymes, irons, carbohydrates, SH3 domains, FADs, heparins, glycosaminoglycans, NADPs/NADPHs, cholesterols, glucoses, immunoglobulins and sterols (Figure 4, Additional file 2: Table S2). Moreover, 34 repressed genes, including *IDH1*, *ME1*, *NSDHL*, *FASN*, *GPD1*, *CYBB*, *FDXR*, *ALDH3B1* and *ACAD9*, are believed to regulate oxidoreductase activity (Figure 4, Additional file 2: Table S2).

Gene transcripts activated in ovaries of DHT-treated rats

To identify the transcripts activated in rat ovaries by DHT treatment, genes of which the expression was increased by ≥ 2-fold (p ≤ 0.01, FDR < 0.1) were investigated, using bioinformatic tools and literature mining. A total of 573 gene transcripts (57.1% of the total

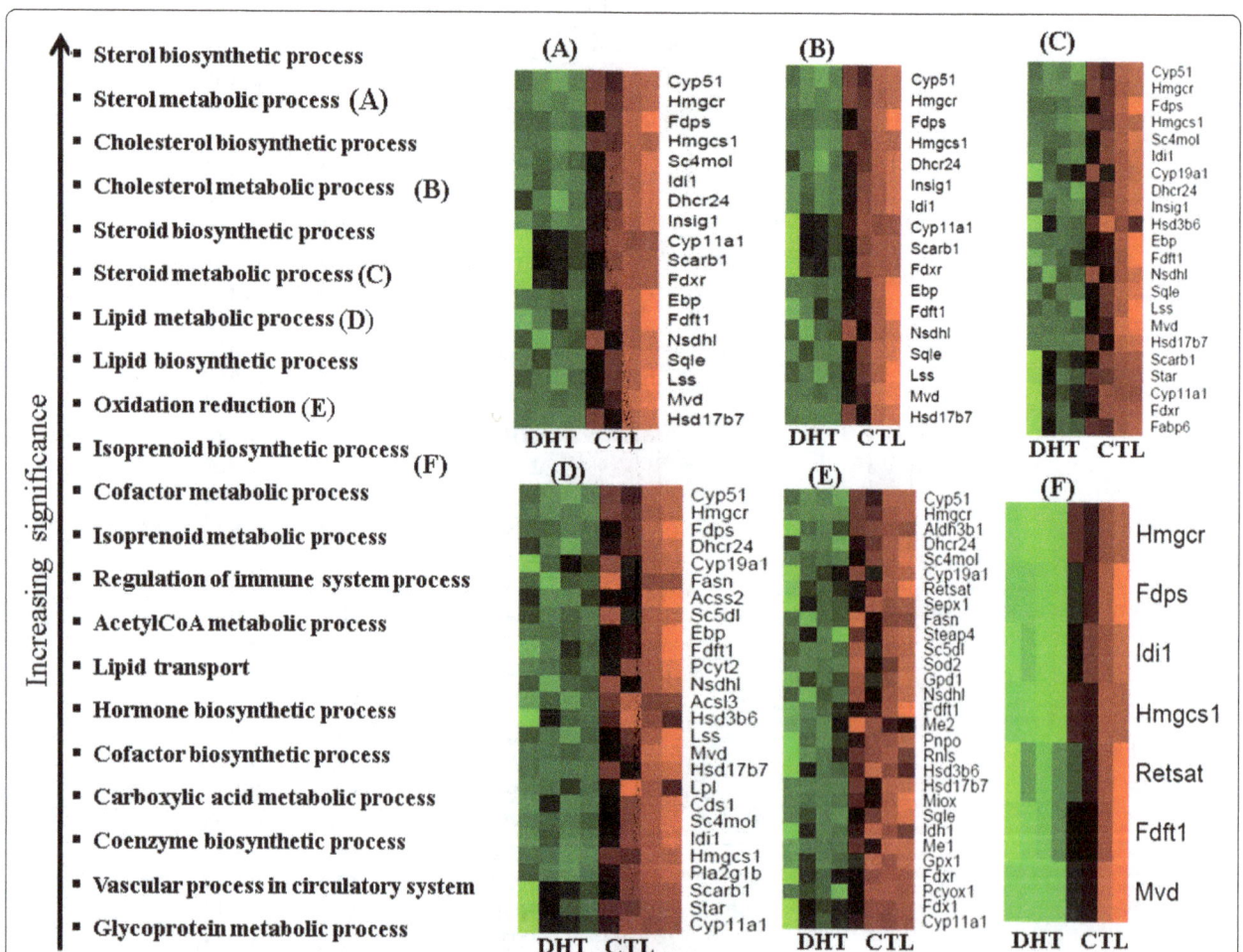

Figure 3 The top biological processes enriched by genes which were repressed in DHT-treated rat ovaries. The heatmaps on the right (**A, B, C, D, E, F**) describe clusters of genes involved in a particular function described by **A, B, C, D, E, F** on the left. The Heatmaps were generated using normalized log$_2$ transformed values and the normalized log$_2$ transformed expression values are described by pseudo color scale with red in CTL groups indicating the activated transcript level while the green color in DHT shows the repressed expression pattern of a specific gene. DHT represents biological replicates in DHT-treated ovaries while CTL represents biological replicates in rats which receive an empty silastic capsule.

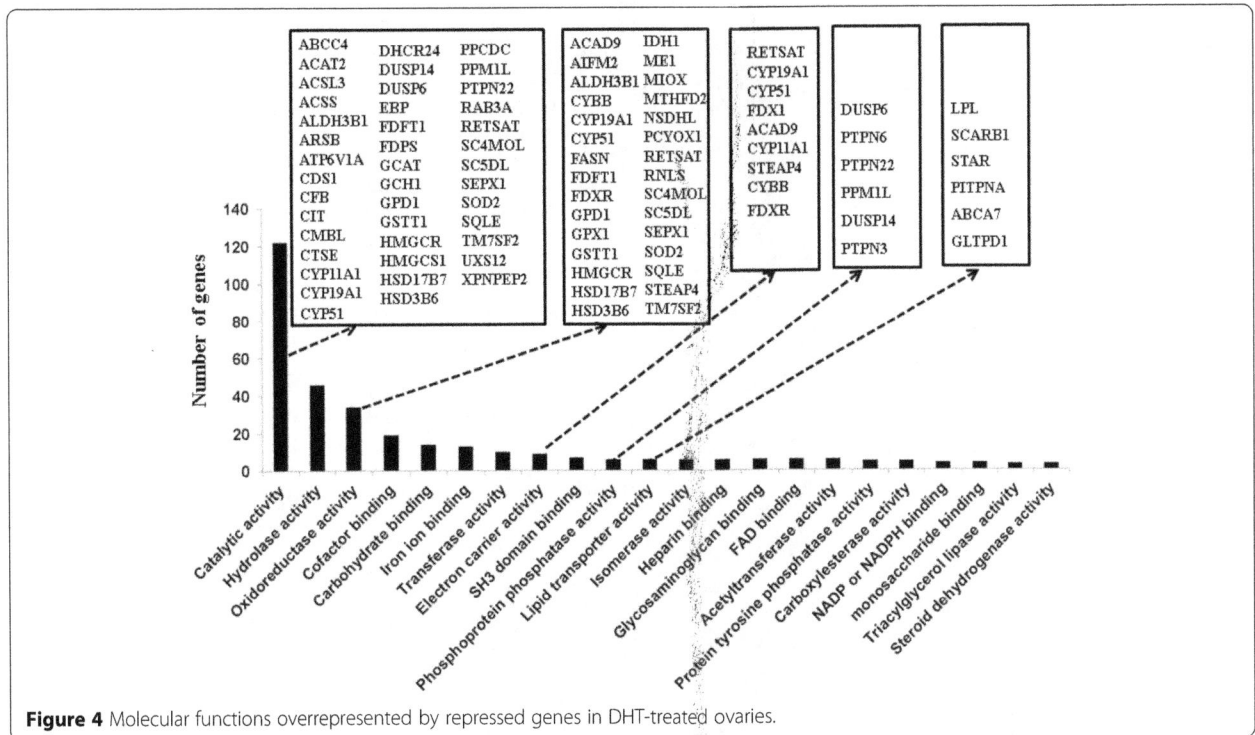

Figure 4 Molecular functions overrepresented by repressed genes in DHT-treated ovaries.

dysregulated genes) were activated in ovaries of DHT-treated rats. The list of top activated genes (with ≥ 4 fold changes) and their expression pattern within and between biological replicates is provided in Figure 5. The most activated genes (between 8- and 35-fold change) include carboxypeptidase A1 (*CPA1*), chymotrypsinogen B1 (*CTRB1*), myosin heavy chain (*MYH6*), carboxypeptidase A2 (*CPA2*), dual specificity phosphatase 27 (*DUSP27*) and cadherin 1 (*CDH1*). In addition, increased expression of genes involved in follicular growth and function was also evident in DHT-treated ovaries, including, anti-Mullerial hormone (*AMH*), aldehyde dehydrogenase 1B1 (*ALDH1B1*), inhibins (*INHBA, INHBB, INHA*), *CYP17A1*, retinol binding protein (*RBP4*), growth arrest specific (*GAS6, GAS7*) and *GATA* binding protein 4 (*GATA4*).

Molecular functions activated in ovaries of DHT-treated rats

Gene set enrichment analysis showed 18 candidate biological processes, including cell differentiation/proliferation, transcriptional regulation/gene expression, neurogenesis, cell adhesion, RNA metabolism, macromolecule biosynthesis and blood vessel development processes to be affected in DHT-treated ovaries due to gene activation (Figure 6). Moreover, the activated genes known to be involved in selective and non-covalent binding of zinc ions, receptors, growth factors, protein phosphatases, DNA secondary structure and peptide

antigens. In addition, some of the activated genes are known to be involved in growth factor activity, initiating for cell growth or proliferation and transcription corepressor activity (Table 2).

Molecular pathways activated or repressed in DHT-treated rats

In addition to their biological or molecular functions, an important and significantly dysregulated molecular interactions and relations associated with the activated or repressed genes were identified using KEGG and Panther gene enrichment analysis. The studies suggest 19 molecular pathways being affected in DHT-treated group (Table 3). Among these, cholesterol and trepenoid biosynthesis pathways, citrate cycle, androgen and estrogen metabolism were enriched by repressed genes while several metabolic pathways including glycolysis/gluconeogenesis, fatty acid metabolism, pyruvate metabolism, butanoate metabolism, lysine, leucine, valine and isoleucine degradation and glutathione metabolic pathways were enriched by both activated and repressed genes (Table 3).

Validation of microarray data using real time quantitative PCR (qPCR)

To validate the expression data generated by microarray analysis, the expression level of 5 activated (*CTRB1, MYH6, PLAU, ST3GAL6* and *INHBA*) and 4 repressed

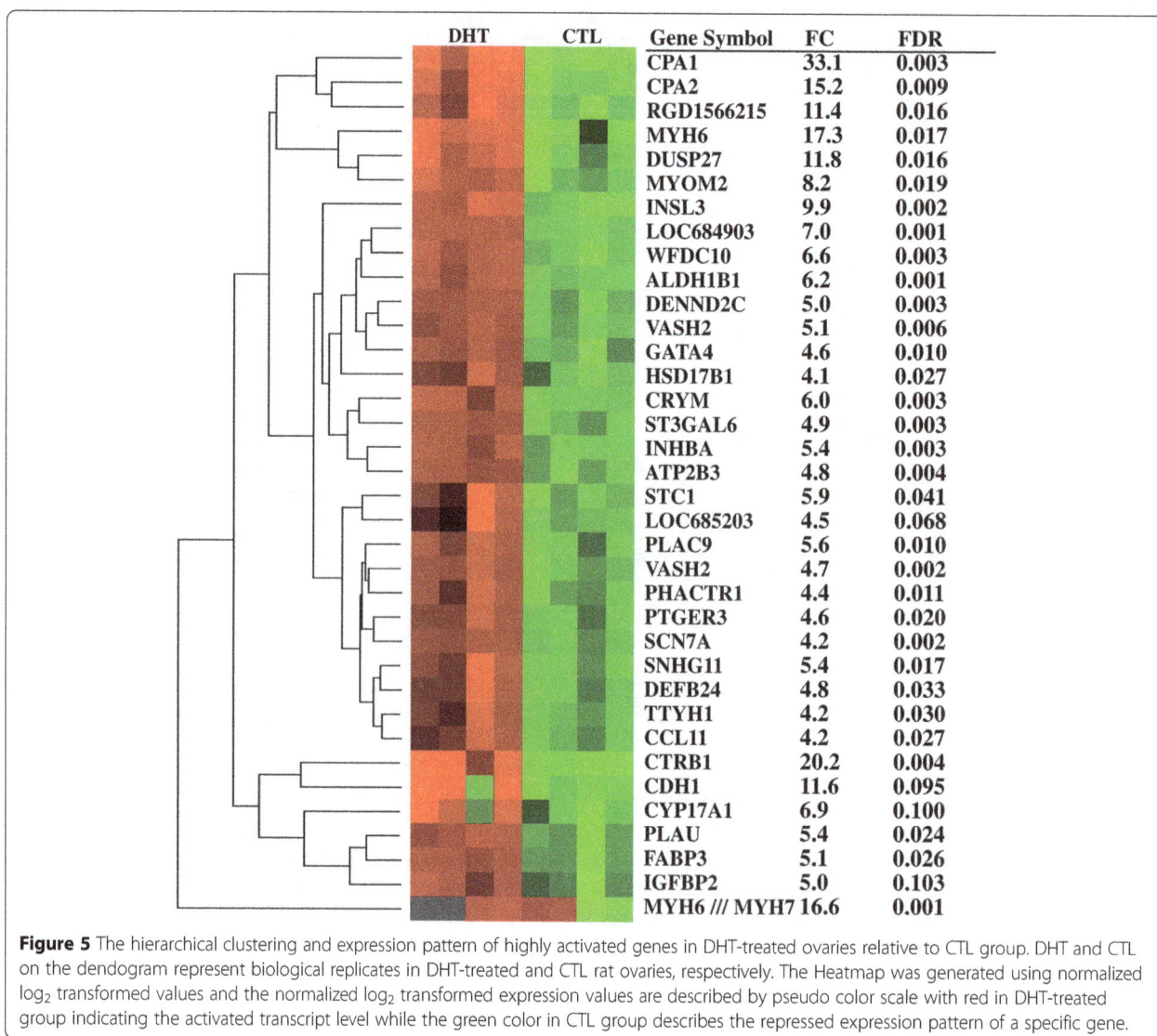

Gene Symbol	FC	FDR
CPA1	33.1	0.003
CPA2	15.2	0.009
RGD1566215	11.4	0.016
MYH6	17.3	0.017
DUSP27	11.8	0.016
MYOM2	8.2	0.019
INSL3	9.9	0.002
LOC684903	7.0	0.001
WFDC10	6.6	0.003
ALDH1B1	6.2	0.001
DENND2C	5.0	0.003
VASH2	5.1	0.006
GATA4	4.6	0.010
HSD17B1	4.1	0.027
CRYM	6.0	0.003
ST3GAL6	4.9	0.003
INHBA	5.4	0.003
ATP2B3	4.8	0.004
STC1	5.9	0.041
LOC685203	4.5	0.068
PLAC9	5.6	0.010
VASH2	4.7	0.002
PHACTR1	4.4	0.011
PTGER3	4.6	0.020
SCN7A	4.2	0.002
SNHG11	5.4	0.017
DEFB24	4.8	0.033
TTYH1	4.2	0.030
CCL11	4.2	0.027
CTRB1	20.2	0.004
CDH1	11.6	0.095
CYP17A1	6.9	0.100
PLAU	5.4	0.024
FABP3	5.1	0.026
IGFBP2	5.0	0.103
MYH6 /// MYH7	16.6	0.001

Figure 5 The hierarchical clustering and expression pattern of highly activated genes in DHT-treated ovaries relative to CTL group. DHT and CTL on the dendogram represent biological replicates in DHT-treated and CTL rat ovaries, respectively. The Heatmap was generated using normalized $\log_2$ transformed values and the normalized $\log_2$ transformed expression values are described by pseudo color scale with red in DHT-treated group indicating the activated transcript level while the green color in CTL group describes the repressed expression pattern of a specific gene.

(*STAR*, *HSD17B7*, *OSGIN1* and *RLN1*) genes were assessed by qPCR. The validation result shows that all the randomly selected genes displayed a similar trend to the microarray data, thus confirming the validity of the microarray results (Table 4).

Discussion

Using a rat PCOS model, we have previously reported altered ovarian expression pattern of 83 miRNAs following DHT treatment [23]. In this study, we investigated the gene expression profile of the same ovarian samples and identified 573 activated and 430 repressed gene transcripts in DHT-treated rats, suggesting the presence of transcriptome profile dysregulation due to hyperandrogenism. In addition, the cellular localization of the products of the activated or repressed gene showed 180 of the dysregulated ones were present in the nucleus while the majority were localized in the cytoplasm (Additional

file 3: Figure S1), suggesting a possible dysregulation of genes function associated with specific ovarian subcellular localization.

The number of dysregulated ovarian genes in the DHT-treated rats appeared consistent with an earlier report by human ovarian cDNA microarray [30] in which the number of up-regulated genes (n = 88) was relatively higher than the down-regulated ones (n = 31) in ovaries of PCOS women compared to the non-PCOS subjects. However in another study where the GeneChips HG_U133A and HG_U133B arrays from Affymetrix used, majority of the dysregulated genes in PCOS were found to be down-regulated [31]. Although the reasons for these apparent discrepancies are not clear, the possibility that this could be due to the differences in tissue sampling, the microarray platform used and the statistical analysis cannot be excluded. To evaluate whether altered ovarian genes in DHT-treated rat resemble those of PCOS women, we

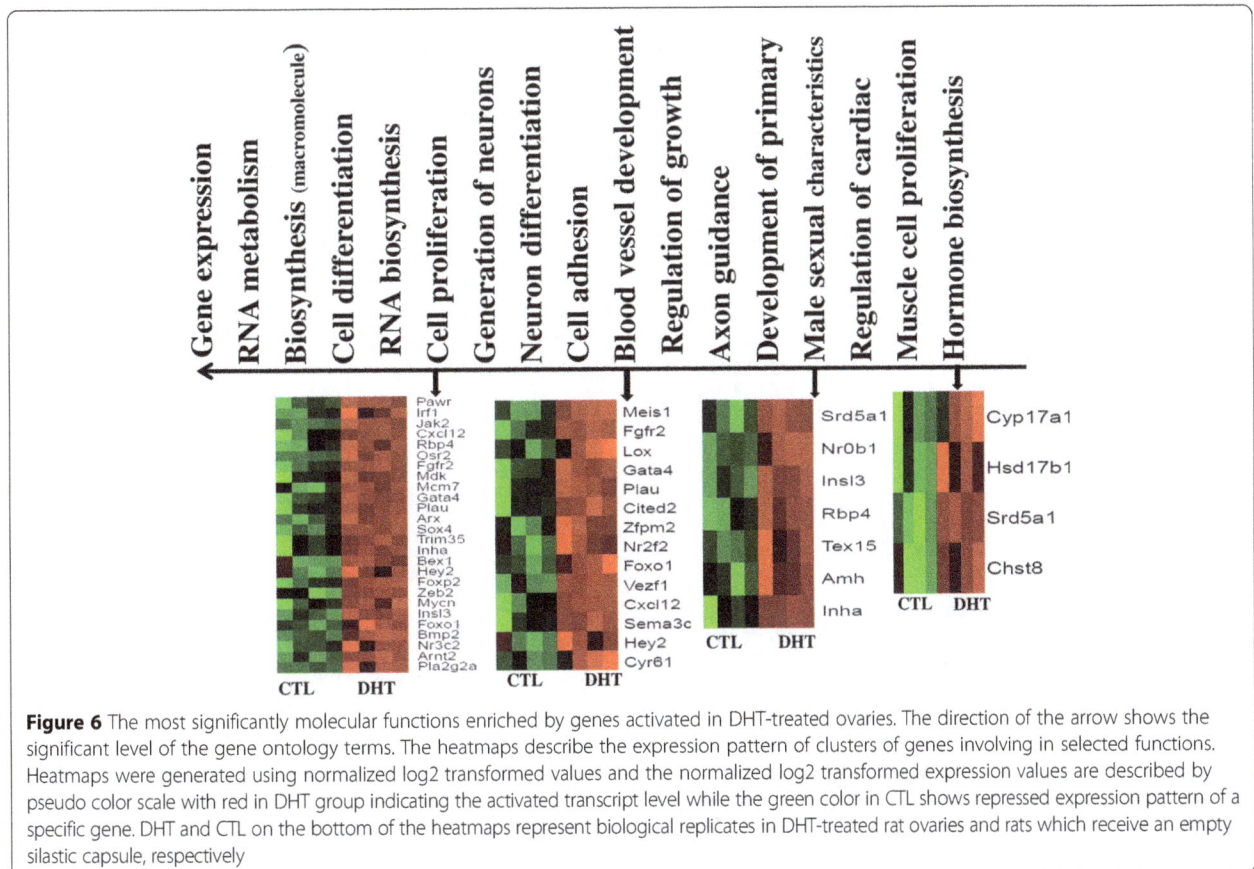

Figure 6 The most significantly molecular functions enriched by genes activated in DHT-treated ovaries. The direction of the arrow shows the significant level of the gene ontology terms. The heatmaps describe the expression pattern of clusters of genes involving in selected functions. Heatmaps were generated using normalized log2 transformed values and the normalized log2 transformed expression values are described by pseudo color scale with red in DHT group indicating the activated transcript level while the green color in CTL shows repressed expression pattern of a specific gene. DHT and CTL on the bottom of the heatmaps represent biological replicates in DHT-treated rat ovaries and rats which receive an empty silastic capsule, respectively

merged our data with the supplemental data previously reported [31] and noted that 160 dysregulated genes were observed in ovaries of both DHT-rats and PCOS women (Additional file 4: Table S3).

In the current study, we have described the key biological processes, molecular functions and pathways affected by dysregulated genes in DHT-treated rats. While the text mining approach would shed light on the relevance of the dysregulated genes with respect to the PCOS phenotype, the present global approach involving pathway analysis and molecular functions provided a more comprehensive understanding of the potential genetic mechanism underling PCOS phenotypes. Our findings also demonstrated ovarian cell type-specific changes in expression of genes involved in granulosa cell proliferation and progesterone biosynthesis [*AMH, RBP4* and cytochrome P450s (*CYP51, CYP19A1, CYP11A1* and *CYP17A1*) and dysregulation of the genes associated with cholesterol biosynthesis and metabolism (acetyl-CoA acetyltransferases enzymes, *ACTAs* and *HMGCR*) in DHT-treated ovaries. These findings are consistent with the dependence of granulosa cell progesterone biosynthesis on the de novo cholesterol synthesis [32].

More importantly, the action of *HMGCR* is believed to be the rate limiting step in cholesterol biosynthesis [33,34].

Our present findings suggest that the dysregulation of the isoprene pathway in cholesterol biosynthesis, leading to abnormal accumulation of cholesterol precursors in hyperandrogenic state. Moreover, down-regulation of cholesterol biosynthesis may limit the amount of cholesterol influx and in turn affect ovarian cellular functions including fertility in DHT-treated rats. Here, a series of the enzymes involving in the conversion of mevalonate to arnesyl-diphosphate, isoprepene to saquale, and squalene in cholesterol were also repressed in ovaries of DHT-treated rats (Figure 7).

One of the major functions of the ovary is the production of steroid hormone [35]. Here, we identified dysregulation of several genes associated with steroidogenesis in ovaries of DHT-treated rats, including repression of cytochrome P450s, STAR and 3β-hydroxysteroid dehydrogenases (Figure 8). The repression of STAR in DHT-treated group suggests a reduced level of cholesterol influx for downstream steroidogenesis. In addition, the down-regulation of *CYP11A1* and CYP19A1 in DHT-treated ovaries was consistent with our previous publication showing decreased aromatase expression and estradiol secretion in granulosa cells from DHT-treated rats [36].

Table 2 List of molecular functions containing genes with increased level of mRNA in DHT treated compared to CTL rat groups

Zinc ion binding	NR2F2,MAP3K1,PTGR1,CPA1,VEZF1, ACY3,SLC39A8,CPA2,RBM5,ZFP278, ZNF574, ZEB2, JARID1A, PHC1, ZCCHC11, KLF11, ZFPM2, OSR2, MSL2L1, TRIM37, PAN3, ZC3H11A, RGNEF, CRYZ, SIVA1, ZFP26, TRIM35, ZFP61, FOXP2, DTX3, ZNF292, GATA4, KLF15, RNF138, MMP23
Transcription regulator activity	NR2F2, CITED2, CRYM, ARNT2, NFIA, NR3C2, BMP2, SMARCD3, RPL7, MYCN, ZFP278, ZEB2, KLF11, ZFPM2, ARX, TLE1, FOXP2, ZNF292, GATA4, NR0B1, RBPJ, MEIS1, HOXD9, CDH1, FOXO1, TWIST, KLF15
Receptor binding	INSL3, INHA, JAK2, AKAP9, CXCL12, INHBB, ARNT2, INHBA, PENK, BMP2, SMARCD3, SEMA3C, EPHA4,SEMA6A, SIVA1, NR0B1, GAS6, ANGPTL1, MDK, STC1, IRS3
Protein dimerization activity	INHA, INHBB, GHR, ARNT2, NR3C2, SHMT1, INHBA, BMP2, MYH6, MYH7, RPL7, PON3, GUCY1A3, FOXP2, NR0B1, MEIS1, ROBO2
Growth factor activity	INHA, JAK2, INHBB, INHBA, BMP2, GAS6, MDK
Carboxylic acid transmembrane transporter activity	SLCO1A4, SLC13A5, SLC1A3, SLC7A5, SLC7A8
Growth factor binding	FGFR2, IGFBP6, CRIM1,HTRA3, CYR61
Insulin-like growth factor binding	IGFBP6, CRIM1, HTRA3, CYR61
Protein phosphatase binding	GHR, PHACTR1, JUP, CDH1
Extracellular matrix binding	VTN, RPSA, CYR61
L-amino acid transmembrane transporter activity	SLC1A3,SLC7A5, SLC7A8
Semaphorin receptor binding	SEMA3C, SEMA6A
Protein tyrosine phosphatase-like protein binding	JUP, CDH1
Actin-dependent atpase activity	MYH6, MYH7
Glycine hydroxyl methyltransferase activity	SHMT1, GART
Peptide antigen binding	SLC7A5, SLC7A8
Metallocarboxypeptidase activity	CPA1, CPA2

Table 3 List of molecular pathways containing genes with activated (↑) and repressed (↓) level of mRNA in DHT treated compared to CTL rat ovary groups

Biosynthesis of steroids	↓CYP51, ↓HMGCR, ↓SQLE, ↓HSD17B7, ↓FDFT1, ↓LSS, MVD, ↓FDPS, ↓IDI1, ↓SC5DL, ↓EBP, ↓SC4MOL, ↓TM7SF2, ↓DHCR24, ↓NSDHL
TGF-beta signaling pathway	↑INHBB, ↑INHBA, ↑AMH, ↑BMP2, ↑FOXO1, ↑FOXP2, ↓FKBP1A,↑ INHA, ↑BAMBI, ↑CITED1, ↓CITED2
Leukocyte transendothelial migration	↑CXCL12, ↓THY1, ↓BCAR1, ↓PECAM1, ↓ CXCR4, ↑CLDN11, ↑MYL9, ↓SIPA1
Cholesterol biosynthesis	↓MVD, ↓HMGCR, ↓HMGCS1, ↓FDPS, ↓IDI1, ↓FDFT1
Pyruvate metabolism	↓ME1, ↓DLAT, ↑ALDH1B1, ↓ME2, ↓ACAT2, ↓ACSS2, ↑ME3
Glycerophospholipid metabolism	↓PLA2G1B, ↑PLA2G2A, ↓GPD1, ↓CDS1, ↓ PCYT2, ↑ETNK2, ↑CRLS1
Complement and coagulation cascades	↓A2M, ↓C2, ↓PLAU, ↑TFPI, ↑MASP1, ↓ CFB, ↓C1QA
Glycolysis/ Gluconeogenesis	↓HK1, ↓HK2, ↓DLAT, ↑FBP2, ↑ALDH1B1, ↓ACSS2
Adipocytokine signaling pathway	↑JAK2, ↓NFKBIB, ↑IRS3, ↓ACSL3, ↓ADIPOR, ↑STK11
Butanoate metabolism	↓HMGCS1, ↓AACS, ↑ALDH1B1, ↓ACAT2, ↑ACSM5
Terpenoid biosynthesis	↓SQLE, ↓FDFT1, ↓FDPS, ↓IDI1
Ether lipid metabolism	↓PLA2G1B, ↑PLA2G2A, ↑PAFAH1B3, ↑ENPP6
Citrate cycle (TCA cycle)	↓ACLY, ↓IDH1, ↓DLAT, ↓DLST
Androgen and estrogen metabolism	↑SRD5A1, ↓ HSD17B1, ↓HSD17B7, ↓HSD3B6
Androgen/estrogene/ progesterone biosynthesis	↓HSD3B6, ↓CYP11A1, ↓NSDHL, ↓CYP19A1
Glutathione metabolism	↓GPX1, ↓IDH1, ↓GSTT1, ↑GPX7
Lysine degradation	↑ALDH1B1, ↓DLST, ↓ACAT2, ↑MGC109340
Fatty acid metabolism	↑ACSL3, ↓ACAA2, ↑ALDH1B1, ↓ACAT2
Valine, leucine and isoleucine degradation	↓HMGCS1, ↓ACAA2, ↑ALDH1B1, ↓ACAT2

Therefore, the dysregulation of genes associated with steroidogenesis in DHT-treated rats could result in abnormal sex hormone levels and ultimately PCOS phenotypes, including cycle irregularity, abnormal folliculogenesis and anovulation.

Women with PCOS may have higher abdominal body fat distribution, due to hyperandrogenism and insulin resistance [37]. This phenomenon may be attributed by increased level of lactate, long-chain fatty acids and triglyceride [38-40]. We have previously demonstrated that the rats treated with DHT exhibited higher body weight compared to control [23]. Although data regarding the total fat content of the ovary is lacking, examination into the gene set enrichment analysis revealed 42 genes associated with lipid metabolism and biosynthesis were repressed in DHT-treated rats. Among those, 26 genes including acyl-CoA synthetase and fatty acid synthase are known to be involved in dual roles of lipid synthesis and metabolism, while 16 other genes were related only to lipid metabolism.

Table 4 The array and qPCR results for selected differentially expressed genes

Gene name	Gene symbol	Acess. No	Array result		qPCR result	
			FC	P value	FC	P value
Chymotrypsinogen b1	CTRB1	NM_012536	20 (↑)	0.00003	27.3 (↑)	0.0023
Myosin, heavy chain 6, cardiac muscle, alpha	MYH6	NM_017239	17 (↑)	0.0004	14 0 (↑)	0.06
Plasminogen activator, urokinase	PLAU	NM_013085	5.37 (↑)	0.0008	5.56 (↑)	0.13
St3 beta-galactoside alpha-2,3-sialyltransferase 6	ST3GAL6	NM_207602	4.9 (↑)	0.0126	5.28 (↑)	0.05
Inhibin beta-a	INHBA	NM_017128	5.43(↑)	0.002	28.9 (↑)	0.04
Steroidogenic acute regulatory protein	STAR	NM_031558	14.57 (↓)	0.001	25.5 (↓)	0.0018
Hydroxysteroid (17-beta) dehydrogenase 7	HSD17B7	NM_017235	30.52 (↓)	0.0003	47.67 (↓)	0.006
Oxidative stress induced growth inhibitor 1	OSGIN1	NM_138504	26.98 (↓)	0.000022	21.57 (↓)	0.0047
Relaxin 1	RLN1	NM_013413	133.9 (↓)	0.0014	255.8 (↓)	0.019

FC = Fold change, ↑ and ↓ indicate the activated and repressed genes in DHT treated compared to CTL rat groups, $p \leq 0.05$ considered as significant.

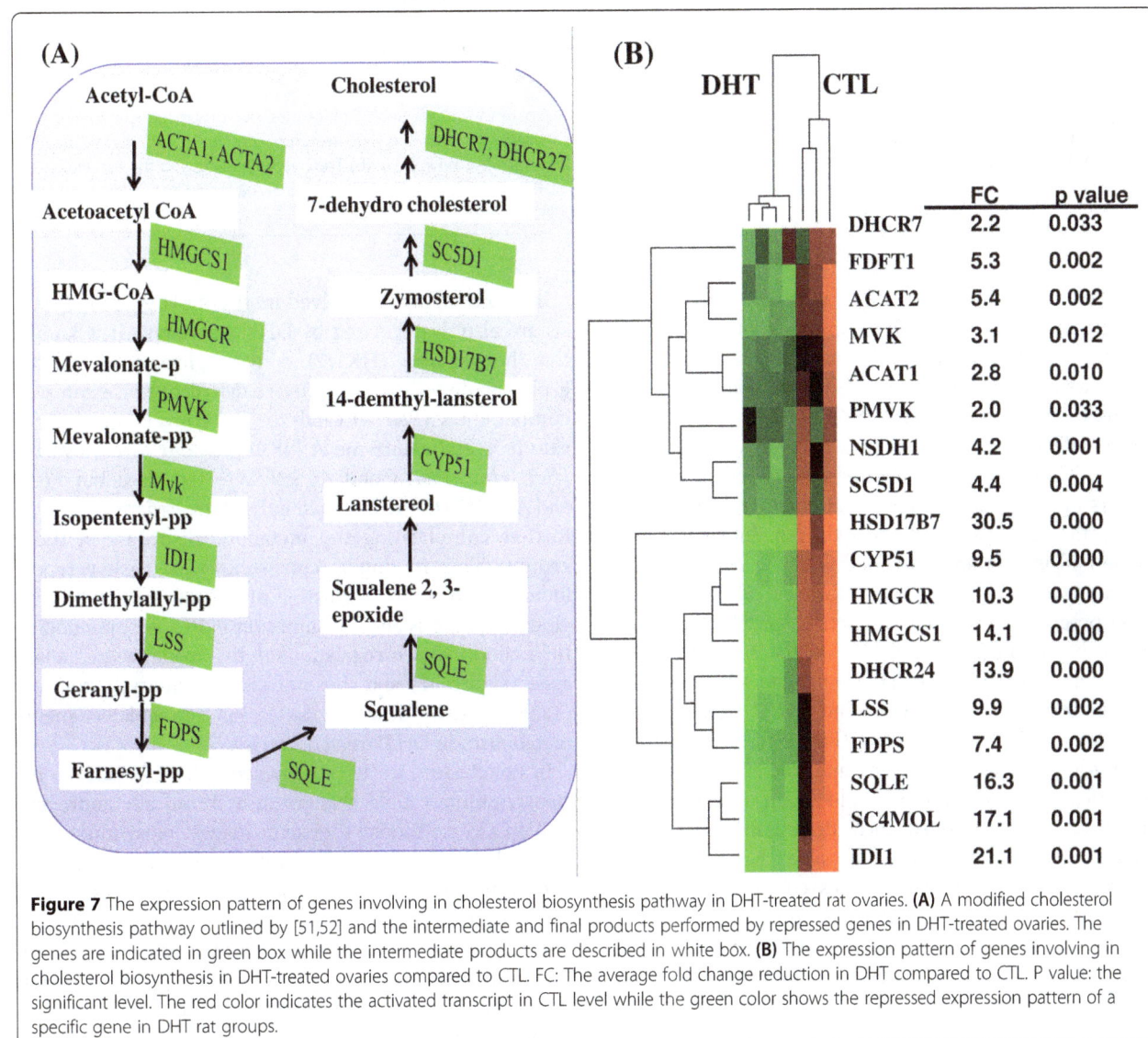

Figure 7 The expression pattern of genes involving in cholesterol biosynthesis pathway in DHT-treated rat ovaries. **(A)** A modified cholesterol biosynthesis pathway outlined by [51,52] and the intermediate and final products performed by repressed genes in DHT-treated ovaries. The genes are indicated in green box while the intermediate products are described in white box. **(B)** The expression pattern of genes involving in cholesterol biosynthesis in DHT-treated ovaries compared to CTL. FC: The average fold change reduction in DHT compared to CTL. P value: the significant level. The red color indicates the activated transcript in CTL level while the green color shows the repressed expression pattern of a specific gene in DHT rat groups.

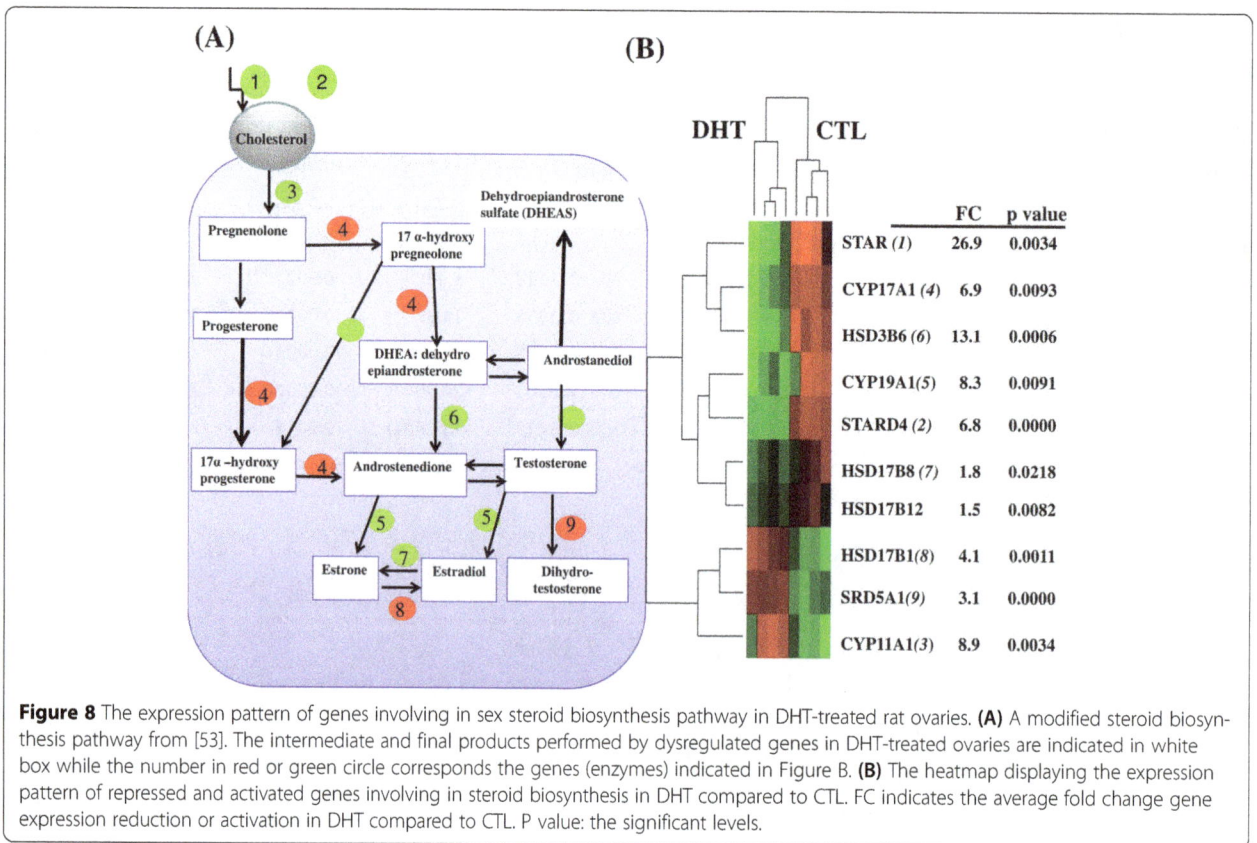

Figure 8 The expression pattern of genes involving in sex steroid biosynthesis pathway in DHT-treated rat ovaries. **(A)** A modified steroid biosynthesis pathway from [53]. The intermediate and final products performed by dysregulated genes in DHT-treated ovaries are indicated in white box while the number in red or green circle corresponds the genes (enzymes) indicated in Figure B. **(B)** The heatmap displaying the expression pattern of repressed and activated genes involving in steroid biosynthesis in DHT compared to CTL. FC indicates the average fold change gene expression reduction or activation in DHT compared to CTL. P value: the significant levels.

The dysregulation of genes involving *de novo* lipid synthesis and metabolism in the DHT group may result in the accumulation of lipid precursors or lack of essential fatty acids which are required for normal ovarian physiology.

One of the characteristics of PCOS is the presence of atretic follicles or premature growth arrest without atresia [41,42]. These phenotypic manifestations could be due to defects in steroid biosynthesis and energy metabolism. In line with this notion, excess androgen, luteinizing hormone and insulin are associated with the recruitment of several but small preovulatory follicles [5]. Indeed, cell cycle progression and proliferation is thought to be controlled by several regulators [43]. In the current study, a total of 45 genes that associated with cell proliferation and differentiation, including *AMH* and *BMP2*, were activated in ovaries of DHT-treated rats (Figure 6). *AMH* inhibits primordial follicle recruitment and decreases the sensitivity of growing follicles to FSH [44]. *AMH* nulls and heterozygous mice exhibited early depletion of primordial follicles [45]. Similarly, it is possible that *BMP2* gene activated in DHT-treated ovaries could participate in the regulation of folliculogenesis and luteinization by modulating gonadotropin receptor expression [46]. Activation of these genes may induce small follicle growth but dominant follicle growth arrest in DHT-treated rats, although this possibility needs further investigation.

In addition, genes involved in glycolysis/gluconeogenesis are also dysregulated by DHT treatment. It is known that hexokinases (HK1/2) convert glucose to glucose 6-phosphate [47] while pyruvate dehydrogenase complex component x (*PDHX*) catalyzes the conversion of pyruvate to acetyl coenzyme A [48,49]. In our study, ovarian *HK1*, *HK2*, *PDHX* and *ACSS2* were repressed but *FBP2* and *ALDH1B1* were activated in DHT-treated rats (Table 3), further complicating the metabolic disorders in those groups. This finding is consistent with earlier report indicating the down-regulation of several genes regulating glucose synthesis and consumption in PCOS patients [50]. In addition, down-regulation of the oxidative reductase gene (Figure 3E) and those of citrate acid cycle pathway (Table 3) adds further evidence for dysregulated energy metabolism in DHT-treated ovaries.

In conclusion, we have provided detailed evidence for transcriptome profile changes in a chronically androgenized PCOS rat model. Our data suggest biosynthesis and metabolism of cholesterol, sterols/steroids, lipids and oxidation/reduction are key molecular functions associated with repressed gene expression in DHT-treated rats. On the other hand, cell differentiation/proliferation, transcriptional regulation, neurogenesis, cell adhesion and blood vessel development were enriched by activated genes in this animal model. It is therefore conceivable that these molecular functional alterations could be a molecular clue for abnormal steroidogenesis, estrous cycle irregularity, abnormal folliculogenesis, anovulation, and disorders in carbohydrate regulation and lipid metabolism occurring in PCOS patients. This study contributes significantly to our understanding of the ovarian transcriptome profile and associated molecular functional alterations in DHT-treated rats, and provides the basis for future in-depth functional and mechanistic studies that to shed light on the pathophysiologic significance of the current findings in PCOS.

Competing interests
The authors declare that they have no competing interests.

Authors' contributions
DSW performed the array hybridization, array data analysis, interpreting the results and drafting and writing the manuscript. QW prepared the PCOs rat model and revised the manuscript. DT assisted in the interpretation of the results, revised the manuscript and supervised the microarray data processing. KS supervised the gene expression analysis and revised the manuscript. MH revised the manuscript. MMH performed total RNA isolation, assisted in array hybridization and interpretation of the results and BKT conceived and oversaw the whole study, revised the manuscript and served as the corresponding author. All authors read and approved the final manuscript.

Acknowledgements
This work was supported by grants from the Canadian Institutes of Health Research (MOP-119381) and the World Class University (WCU) program through the Ministry of Education, Science and Technology and funded by the National Research Foundation of Korea (R31-10056) and research training awards [CIHR-REDIH Doctoral Scholarship and CIHR-QTNPR Doctoral Scholarship (QW)].

Author details
[1]Institute of Animal Science, Animal Breeding and Husbandry Group, University of Bonn, Endenicher Allee 15, Bonn 53115, Germany. [2]Reproductive Biology Unit and Division of Reproductive Medicine, Department of Obstetrics & Gynecology and Cellular & Molecular Medicine, Interdisciplinary School of Health Sciences, University of Ottawa, Ottawa K1H 8L6, ON, Canada. [3]Chronic Disease Program, Ottawa Hospital Research Institute, The Ottawa Hospital (General Campus), Critical Care Wing, 3rd Floor, Room W3107, 501 Smyth Road, Ottawa K1H 8L6, ON, Canada. [4]Department of Animal Breeding and Genetics, Bangladesh Agricultural University, Mymensingh 2202, Bangladesh. [5]Department of Agricultural Biotechnology, World Class University Major in Biomodulation, College of Agriculture and Life Sciences, Seoul National University, Seoul 151-921, South Korea.

References
1. Azziz R, Woods KS, Reyna R, Key TJ, Knochenhauer ES, Yildiz BO. The prevalence and features of the polycystic ovary syndrome in an unselected population. J Clin Endocr Metab. 2004;89:2745–9.
2. Legro RS. Diagnostic criteria in polycystic ovary syndrome. Sem Reprod Med. 2003;21:267–75.
3. Lujan ME, Chizen DR, Pierson RA. Diagnostic criteria for polycystic ovary syndrome: pitfalls and controversies. JOGC. 2008;30:671–9.
4. Legro RS, Chiu P, Kunselman AR, Bentley CM, Dodson WC, Dunaif A. Polycystic ovaries are common in women with hyperandrogenic chronic anovulation but do not predict metabolic or reproductive phenotype. J Clin Endocrinol Metab. 2005;90:2571–9.
5. Franks S, Stark J, Hardy K. Follicle dynamics and anovulation in polycystic ovary syndrome. Hum Reprod Update. 2008;14:367–78.
6. Azziz R, Carmina E, Dewailly D, Diamanti-Kandarakis E, Escobar-Morreale HF, Futterweit W, et al. The androgen excess and PCOS Society criteria for the polycystic ovary syndrome: the complete task force report. Fertil Steril. 2009;91:456–88.
7. Goodarzi MO. The genetic basis of the polycystic ovary syndrome. In Androgen excess disorders in women. Springer; 2007. p. 223-33.
8. Welt CK, Carmina E. Lifecycle of Polycystic Ovary Syndrome (PCOS): From In Utero to Menopause. J Clin Endocrinol Metab. 2013;98:4629–38.
9. Cui L, Zhao H, Zhang B, Qu Z, Liu J, Liang X, et al. Genotype-phenotype correlations of PCOS susceptibility SNPs identified by GWAS in a large cohort of Han Chinese women. Hum Reprod. 2013;28:538–44.
10. Tumu VR, Govatati S, Guruvaiah P, Deenadayal M, Shivaji S, Bhanoori M. An interleukin-6 gene promoter polymorphism is associated with polycystic ovary syndrome in South Indian women. J Assist Reprod Genet. 2013;30:1541–6.
11. Radavelli-Bagatini S, de Oliveira IO, Ramos RB, Santos BR, Wagner MS, Lecke SB, et al. Haplotype TGTG from SNP 45 T/G and 276G/T of the adiponectin gene contributes to risk of polycystic ovary syndrome. J Endocrinol Invest. 2013;36:497–502.
12. Nelson VL, Legro RS, Strauss 3rd JF, McAllister JM. Augmented androgen production is a stable steroidogenic phenotype of propagated theca cells from polycystic ovaries. Mol Endocrinol. 1999;13:946–57.
13. Catteau-Jonard S, Jamin SP, Leclerc A, Gonzales J, Dewailly D, di Clemente N. Anti-Mullerian hormone, its receptor, FSH receptor, and androgen receptor genes are overexpressed by granulosa cells from stimulated follicles in women with polycystic ovary syndrome. J Clin Endocrinol Metab. 2008;93:4456–61.
14. Wood JR, Nelson VL, Ho C, Jansen E, Wang CY, Urbanek M, et al. The molecular phenotype of polycystic ovary syndrome (PCOS) theca cells and new candidate PCOS genes defined by microarray analysis. J Biol Chem. 2003;278:26380–90.
15. Meng Y, Qian Y, Gao L, Cai LB, Cui YG, Liu JY. Downregulated expression of peroxiredoxin 4 in granulosa cells from polycystic ovary syndrome. PLoS One. 2013;8, e76460.
16. Abbott DH, Nicol LE, Levine JE, Xu N, Goodarzi MO, Dumesic DA. Nonhuman primate models of polycystic ovary syndrome. Mol Cell Endocrinol. 2013;373:21–8.
17. Maliqueo M, Benrick A, Stener-Victorin E. Rodent models of polycystic ovary syndrome: phenotypic presentation, pathophysiology, and the effects of different interventions. Sem Reprod Med. 2014;32:183–93.
18. McNeilly AS, Duncan WC. Rodent models of polycystic ovary syndrome. Mol Cell Endocrinol. 2013;373:2–7.
19. Padmanabhan V, Veiga-Lopez A. Animal models of the polycystic ovary syndrome phenotype. Steroids. 2013;78:734–40.
20. Shi D, Vine DF. Animal models of polycystic ovary syndrome: a focused review of rodent models in relationship to clinical phenotypes and cardiometabolic risk. Fertil Steril. 2012;98:185–93.
21. Walters KA, Allan CM, Handelsman DJ. Rodent models for human polycystic ovary syndrome. Biol Reprod. 2012;86:149. 141-112.
22. Manneras L, Cajander S, Holmang A, Seleskovic Z, Lystig T, Lonn M, et al. A new rat model exhibiting both ovarian and metabolic characteristics of polycystic ovary syndrome. Endocrinology. 2007;148:3781–91.
23. Hossain MM, Cao M, Wang Q, Kim JY, Schellander K, Tesfaye D, et al. Altered expression of miRNAs in a dihydrotestosterone-induced rat PCOS model. J Ovarian Res. 2013;6:36.
24. Gharaibeh RZ, Fodor AA, Gibas CJ. Background correction using dinucleotide affinities improves the performance of GCRMA. BMC Bioinformatics. 2008;9:452.

25. Smyth GK. Limma: linear models for microarray data. In: Gentleman R, Carey V, Dudoit S, Irizarry R, Huber W, editors. Bioinformatics and computational biology solutions using R and Bioconductor. New York: Springer; 2005. p. 397–420.

26. Benjamini Y, Hochberg Y. Controlling the false discovery rate: a practical and powerful approach to multiple testing. Roy Statist Soc Ser B. 1995;57:289–300.

27. Falcon S, Gentleman R. Using GOstats to test gene lists for GO term association. Bioinformatics. 2007;23:257–8.

28. Da Wei Huang BTS, Lempicki RA. Systematic and integrative analysis of large gene lists using DAVID bioinformatics resources. Na Protoc. 2008;4:44–57.

29. Caraux G, Pinloche S. PermutMatrix: a graphical environment to arrange gene expression profiles in optimal linear order. Bioinformatics. 2005;21:1280–1.

30. Diao FY, Xu M, Hu Y, Li J, Xu Z, Lin M, et al. The molecular characteristics of polycystic ovary syndrome (PCOS) ovary defined by human ovary cDNA microarray. J Mol Endocrinol. 2004;33:59–72.

31. Jansen E, Laven JS, Dommerholt HB, Polman J, van Rijt C, van den Hurk C, et al. Abnormal gene expression profiles in human ovaries from polycystic ovary syndrome patients. Mol Endocrinol. 2004;18:3050–63.

32. Baranao JL, Hammond JM. FSH increases the synthesis and stores of cholesterol in porcine granulosa cells. Mo Cel Endocrinol. 1986;44:227–36.

33. Tobert JA. Lovastatin and beyond: the history of the HMG-CoA reductase inhibitors. Nat Rev Drug Discov. 2003;2:517–26.

34. Olivier LM, Krisans SK. Peroxisomal protein targeting and identification of peroxisomal targeting signals in cholesterol biosynthetic enzymes. Biochim Biophys Acta. 2000;1529:89–102.

35. Sanderson JT. The steroid hormone biosynthesis pathway as a target for endocrine-disrupting chemicals. Toxico Sci. 2006;94:3–21.

36. Wang Q, Kim JY, Xue K, Liu JY, Leader A, Tsang BK. Chemerin, a novel regulator of follicular steroidogenesis and its potential involvement in polycystic ovarian syndrome. Endocrinology. 2012;153:5600–11.

37. Diamanti-Kandarakis E. Role of obesity and adiposity in polycystic ovary syndrome. Int J Obes. 2007;31:S8–13.

38. Cullberg G, Hamberger L, Mattsson LA, Mobacken H, Samsioe G. Lipid metabolic studies in women with a polycystic ovary syndrome during treatment with a low-dose desogestrel-ethinylestradiol combination. Acta Obstet Gynecol Scand. 1985;64:203–7.

39. Mattsson LA, Cullberg G, Hamberger L, Samsioe G, Silfverstolpe G. Lipid metabolism in women with polycystic ovary syndrome: possible implications for an increased risk of coronary heart disease. Fertli Steril. 1984;42:579–84.

40. Zhao Y, Fu L, Li R, Wang LN, Yang Y, Liu NN, et al. Metabolic profiles characterizing different phenotypes of polycystic ovary syndrome: plasma metabolomics analysis. BMC Med. 2012;10:153.

41. Tamura T, Kitawaki J, Yamamoto T, Osawa Y, Kominami S, Takemorit S, et al. Immunohistochemical localization of 17α-hydroxylase/C17-20 lyase and aromatase cytochrome P-450 in polycystic human ovaries. J Endocrinol. 1993;139:503–9.

42. Townson DH, Combelles CM. Ovarian follicular atresia. Basic Gynecology–Some Related Issues, Prof. Atef Darwish (Ed.), ISBN: 978-953-51-0166-6, InTech. doi:10.5772/32465. Available from: http://www.intechopen.com/books/basic-gynecology-some-related-issues/ovarian-follicular-atresia/.

43. Salvetti NR, Stangaferro ML, Palomar MM, Alfaro NS, Rey F, Gimeno EJ, et al. Cell proliferation and survival mechanisms underlying the abnormal persistence of follicular cysts in bovines with cystic ovarian disease induced by ACTH. Anim Reprod Sci. 2010;122:98–110.

44. Durlinger AL, Visser JA, Themmen AP. Regulation of ovarian function: the role of anti-Mullerian hormone. Reproduction. 2002;124:601–9.

45. Durlinger AL, Kramer P, Karels B, de Jong FH, Uilenbroek JT, Grootegoed JA, et al. Control of primordial follicle recruitment by anti-Mullerian hormone in the mouse ovary. Endocrinology. 1999;140:5789–96.

46. Shi J, Yoshino O, Osuga Y, Koga K, Hirota Y, Nose E, et al. Bone morphogenetic protein-2 (BMP-2) increases gene expression of FSH receptor and aromatase and decreases gene expression of LH receptor and StAR in human granulosa cells. Am J Reprod Immunol. 2011;65:421–7.

47. Walsh Jr CT, Spector LB. The glucose-glucose 6-phosphate exchange catalyzed by yeast hexokinase. Arch Biochem Biophys. 1971;145:1–5.

48. Harris RA, Bowker-Kinley MM, Huang B, Wu P. Regulation of the activity of the pyruvate dehydrogenase complex. Adv Enzyme Regul. 2002;42:249–59.

49. Liu S, Gong X, Yan X, Peng T, Baker JC, Li L, et al. Reaction mechanism for mammalian pyruvate dehydrogenase using natural lipoyl domain substrates. ArchBbioche Biophys. 2001;386:123–35.

50. Kim JY, Song H, Kim H, Kang HJ, Jun JH, Hong SR, et al. Transcriptional profiling with a pathway-oriented analysis identifies dysregulated molecular phenotypes in the endometrium of patients with polycystic ovary syndrome. J Clin Endocrinol Metab. 2009;94:1416–26.

51. Liscurn L. Cholesterol biosynthesis. In: Biochemistry of lipids, lipoproteins and membranes. 4th ed. New York, N: Elsevier; 2002. p. 409–31.

52. Waterham HR. Defects of cholesterol biosynthesis. FEBS Lett. 2006;580:5442–9.

53. Chen ZT, Wang IJ, Liao YT, Shih YF, Lin LL. Polymorphisms in steroidogenesis genes, sex steroid levels, and high myopia in the Taiwanese population. Mol Vis. 2011;17:2297–310.

8

An association study between *USP34* and polycystic ovary syndrome

Shigang Zhao[1,2,3,4,5†], Ye Tian[1†], Wei Zhang[6†], Xiuye Xing[2,3,4,5], Tao Li[2,3,4,5], Hongbin Liu[2,3,4,5], Tao Huang[2,3,4,5], Yunna Ning[2,3,4,5], Han Zhao[2,3,4,5*] and Zi-Jiang Chen[1,2,3,4,5]

Abstract

Background: Polycystic ovary syndrome (PCOS) is a complex multifactor disorder and genetic factors have been implicated in its pathogenesis. Our previous genome-wide association study (GWAS) had identified allele frequencies in several single nucleotide polymorphisms (SNPs) in gene *USP34* (Ubiquitin-Specific Protease 34) were significantly different between PCOS cases and controls. This study was aimed to replicate the previous results in another independent cohort.

Methods: One thousand two hundred eighteen PCOS cases and 1057 controls were recruited. Genotyping of two SNPs (rs17008097 and rs17008940) in *USP34* gene were performed by TaqMan-MGB probe assay and genotype-phenotype analysis was conducted subsequently.

Results: The differences of allele or genotype frequencies were not significant statistically between PCOS and controls, even after age and BMI adjustment. For clinical and metabolic features (LH, T and HOMA-IR) analysis in PCOS cases, no statistical differences among three genotypes of rs17008097 and rs17008940 were found. However, rs17008940 was shown to be slightly associated with BMI in PCOS cases rather than in controls, even after age adjustment (TC vs CC $P = 0.006$, $OR = 1.042$, 95% CI 1.012–1.073; TT vs CC $P = 0.037$, $OR = 1.050$, 95% CI 1.003–1.100).

Conclusions: *USP34* gene polymorphisms (rs17008097 and rs17008940) may not be associated with PCOS in the Han Chinese women.

Keywords: Polycystic ovary syndrome, USP34, SNPs, Association

Background

Polycystic ovary syndrome (PCOS) is a kind of reproductive and metabolic disorder characterized by hyper-androgen and insulin resistance, which affects 6–8 % of reproductive-aged women in Caucasian and 5.6 % in Chinese [1–3]. Clinical diagnosis of PCOS is made on the basis of at least two following criteria after excluding other related diseases: oligo- or anovulation, clinical or biochemical hyperandrogenism and polycystic ovaries under ultrasound [4]. The etiology of PCOS is not well understood yet. However, it's now widely accepted that genetic factors play an indispensable role in the development of PCOS [5] and several candidate genes have been reported recently [6, 7]. We performed the first GWAS for PCOS which followed by replication studies only for SNPs with p value less than 10e-6, and finally identified three susceptibility loci (2p16.3, 2p21 and 9q33.3) [6]. However, other loci with p value around 10e-5 in GWAS, such as SNPs in gene *USP34*, remain intriguing and might also be potential risk factors of PCOS.

The *USP34* gene is located on chromosome 2p15 and encodes a kind of deubiquitinating enzyme, which belongs to ubiquitin-specific protease family. Data obtained from COSMIC database [8] shows that somatic variations of *USP34* are related to ovary tumor. Moreover, USP34 positively regulates Wnt signaling pathway [9], which plays an important role in gender differentiation, folliculogenesis, ovulation and other biological processes in reproduction [10]. The expression patterns of several genes in Wnt pathway are altered in PCOS (such as DKK1, a negative

* Correspondence: hanzh80@yahoo.com
†Equal contributors
²Center for Reproductive Medicine, Provincial Hospital Affiliated to Shandong University, Jinan, China
³National Research Center for Assisted Reproductive Technology and Reproductive Genetics, Jinan, China
Full list of author information is available at the end of the article

regulator of Wnt pathway) [11–13]. Taken together, it is assumed that *USP34* may also have relationship with PCOS. As an extension of GWAS, here we conducted an independent case-control replication study to evaluate the association between *USP34* and PCOS susceptibility.

Methods

This study was approved by Institutional Review Board for Reproductive Medicine of Shanghai Jiaotong University and Shandong University. A total of 1218 PCOS cases and 1057 unrelated controls were recruited consecutively from 2009 to 2013 at the Center for Reproductive Medicine, Renji Hospital, School of Medicine, Shanghai Jiaotong University and the Center for Reproductive Medicine, Provincial Hospital Affiliated to Shandong University. Among them, 94 PCOS cases, also born from Northern China, were collected at Renji Hospital from 2012 to 2013. Signed informed consent was obtained from each participant of this study.

PCOS diagnosis was based on the 2003 Rotterdam PCOS consensus criteria and other related diseases (such as congenital adrenal hyperplasia, Cushing's syndrome, androgen-secreting tumors, thyroid disease and hyperprolactinaemia) were excluded. In detail, PCOS can be diagnosed if at least two of the following three features are met: oligo- or anovulation, clinical and/or biochemical signs of hyperandrogenism and polycystic ovaries. Oligo- or anovulation was referred to menstrual cycles of more than 35 days in length or a history of ≤ 8 menstrual cycles in a year [1]; polycystic ovaries was defined as the presence of at least one ovary >10 ml or at least 12 follicles 2–9 mm in diameter by transvaginal ultrasound [4]. Hyperandrogenism was the presence of hirsutism (Ferriman-Gallwey score ≥ 6) [14] or serum total testosterone ≥ 60 ng/dl [15]. The inclusion criteria for the control group were as follows: normal menstrual cycles, no hyperandrogenism and no polycystic ovaries (PCO) under ultrasound. All individuals who were taking medications such as oral contraceptives and metformin during last 3 months were excluded.

Biochemical measurements

Serum luteinizing hormone (LH) and testosterone (T) levels of subjects were measured by a chemiluminescent analyser (Beckman Access Health Company, Chaska, Minnesota, USA). The plasma glucose was measured by AU640 automatic biochemistry analyser (Olympus Company, Hamburg, Germany) and insulin was measured by chemiluminescent analyzer. Insulin resistance was calculated as fasting glucose (mmol/L)*fasting insulin (mIU/L)/22.5 using homeostasis model assessment (HOMA-IR).

SNP selection

SNPs in *USP34* were selected for replication study according to the following criteria: SNPs that exist in Affymetrix

Genome-Wide Human SNP Array 6.0 (Affymetrix, Santa Clara, CA, USA); can stand for a block; minor allele frequency (MAF) > 5 % in Chinese Han population; statistically different ($P < 10e-4$) from our previous GWAS (see Additional file 1, Table S1); r^2 of selected SNPs < 0.8. Ultimately, rs17008097 and rs17008940 were selected to precede further replication study.

SNP genotyping

Genomic DNA was extracted from whole peripheral blood using QIAamp DNA mini kit (Qiagen, Hilden, Germany). Genotyping of SNPs was carried out by TaqMan-MGB probe assay (Invitrogen Trading, Shanghai, China), probes and primers were shown in Additional file 1, Table S2. Then, 5 % of the samples were randomly selected for direct sequencing to validate the genotyping assays.

Statistical analysis

Numerical variables of clinical characteristics of PCOS cases and controls were expressed as mean ± SD. Hardy-Weinberg equilibrium (HWE) and linkage disequilibrium (LD) tests were performed by Haploview software. The case-control genetic power was analyzed by Genetic Power Calculator [16]. A sample size > 721 PCOS cases (case: control = 1) would provide 80 % power ($\alpha = 0.05$), assuming higher risk allele frequency (A) of 0.05 and a genotype relative risk (Aa) of 1.5. Frequencies of genotype and allele between PCOS subjects and controls were compared by Pearson Chi-square test, and the p value was adjusted by logistic regression to eliminate the effect of age and body mass index (BMI) using SPSS v.19.0 (SPSS Inc., Chicago, IL, USA). $P < 0.05$ was considered statistically significant.

For genotype-phenotype analysis in PCOS patients, additive model (+/+ vs +/− vs −/−) was selected after comparison; one-way analysis of variance (ANOVA) test was used for phenotype comparison among different genotypes. Linear regression was used for age and BMI adjustment. Conservative Bonferroni test was used for multiple testing corrections.

Results

As shown in Table 1, the PCOS group was younger than the controls ($P < 0.001$). In addition, PCOS group had higher BMI, LH level and T level than the control group

Table 1 Characteristics of PCOS cases and controls

	PCOS	Control	p value
Age (years)	28.55 ± 3.72	31.84 ± 4.74	<0.001
BMI (kg/m²)	25.12 ± 4.35	22.78 ± 3.25	<0.001
LH (IU/L)	10.03 ± 5.93	4.76 ± 2.23	<0.001
T (ng/dl)	51.69 ± 21.00	42.35 ± 18.46	<0.001

BMI: body mass index; LH: Luteinizing hormone; T: testosterone

Table 2 Genotype and allele frequencies of *USP34* in PCOS and controls

			PCOS	Control	P	P adjusted	OR/95 % CI
rs17008097	Genotype	CC	548(45 %)	484(45.8 %)	0.807	0.791	
		GC	531(43.6 %)	447(42.3 %)			
		GG	139(11.4 %)	126(11.9 %)			
	Allele	C	1627(66.8 %)	1415(66.9 %)	0.918	0.791	0.993 (0.878–1.124)
		G	809(33.2 %)	699(33.1 %)			
rs17008940	Genotype	CC	575(47.2 %)	505(47.8 %)	0.948	0.862	
		TC	513(42.1 %)	438(41.4 %)			
		TT	130(10.7 %)	114(10.8 %)			
	Allele	C	1663(68.3 %)	1448(68.5 %)	0.869	0.862	0.990 (0.873–1.122)
		T	773(31.7 %)	666(31.5 %)			

P adjusted: adjust the p value by age and BMI; OR: Odd Ratio; CI: Confidence Interval

($P < 0.001$). In PCOS group, 90 patients present with hyperandrogenism and oligo-anovulation (HA + OA, 9.44 %), 10 patients present with hyperandrogenism and polycystic ovaries (HA + PCO, 1.05 %), 620 patients present with oligo-anovulation and polycystic ovaries (HA + PCO, 65.06 %), and 233 patients present with full-phenotype (HA + OA + PCO, 24.45 %).

The genotype frequencies of the two polymorphisms in PCOS cases and controls were all in Hardy-Weinberg equilibrium ($P > 0.05$). Genotype and allele frequencies were summarized in Table 2 and no significant differences were observed between PCOS and controls. After age and BMI adjustment with logistic regression, no association was found. The minor allele frequencies (MAF) of the 2 SNPs in four subgroups of PCOS were further analyzed. No significant differences of MAF were observed between each subgroup of PCOS and controls in the present study (see Additional file 1, Table S3). Additionally, there was no statistical difference among three genetic models (additive, dominant and recessive) in genotype analysis (see Additional file 1, Table S4), thus additive model of genotype was selected for subsequent phenotype analysis.

In genotype-phenotype analysis, clinical and metabolic features were compared among different genotypes in PCOS subjects, rs17008940 was shown to be associated with BMI ($P = 0.028$) (Table 3), however, the association was not significant after Bonferroni correction for multiple testing. The average level of BMI in TC and TT group was higher than that in CC group after age adjustment (TC vs CC $P = 0.006$, $OR = 1.042$, 95 % CI 1.012–1.073; TT vs CC $P = 0.037$, $OR = 1.050$, 95 % CI 1.003–1.100). But in control group, no significant difference was found in BMI among the three genotypes of rs17008940 ($P = 0.256$). Additionally, there were no significant differences in LH, T or HOMA-IR among the PCOS cases carrying different genotypes of the two SNPs, even after age and BMI adjustment (Table 3, Table 4).

Discussion

As a powerful technique, GWAS shed new light on genetic study for complex diseases. GWAS data is obtained from computing and statistical analyses following SNP chips detection, so the results are bioinformatics rather than biological. However, GWAS itself owns some limitations and it is necessary to be validated through further replication studies. In general, p value of 5*10e-8 was used as significant level for random variations in case-control GWAS with a power of 0.8 [17, 18]. In our previous GWAS, only SNPs with p value < 10e-6 were replicated to confirm the first step results [6]. However, some SNPs with p value around 10e-5 were disputable. Recently we found two novel susceptibility genes *YAP1* and *LPP* for PCOS from these SNPs [7, 19]. So we selected two SNPs with p value around 10e-5 in *USP34* to validate whether *USP34* was associated with PCOS. No association was

Table 3 Clinical and metabolic characteristics of PCOS cases in rs17008940 genotype subgroups

Characteristics	CC(n = 575)	TC(n = 513)	TT(n = 130)	P	P adjusted
Age (years)	28.83 ± 3.73	28.39 ± 3.72	28.02 ± 3.66	0.046	–
BMI (kg/m²)	24.740 ± 4.29	25.418 ± 4.34	25.517 ± 4.51	0.028	–
LH (IU/L)	9.999 ± 6.08	10.028 ± 5.88	10.177 ± 5.44	0.957	0.500
T (ng/dl)	51.17 ± 20.73	51.74 ± 21.41	53.72 ± 20.61	0.485	0.505
HOMA-IR	2.62 ± 2.62	2.70 ± 2.12	2.79 ± 2.32	0.653	0.399

HOMA-IR: homeostasis model assessment; P adjusted: adjust the p value by age and BMI in logistic regression

Table 4 Clinical and metabolic characteristics of PCOS cases in rs17008097 genotype subgroups

Characteristics	CC(n = 548)	GC(n = 531)	GG(n = 139)	P	P adjusted
Age(years)	28.82 ± 3.79	28.44 ± 3.64	27.97 ± 3.73	0.044	–
BMI (kg/m²)	24.824 ± 4.26	25.287 ± 4.37	25.581 ± 4.51	0.106	–
LH (IU/L)	10.000 ± 6.12	9.963 ± 5.81	10.399 ± 5.61	0.746	0.393
T (ng/dl)	51.446 ± 20.14	51.897 ± 21.97	51.868 ± 20.69	0.940	0.904
HOMA-IR	2.642 ± 2.61	2.676 ± 2.19	2.773 ± 2.24	0.800	0.415

HOMA-IR: homeostasis model assessment; P adjusted: adjust the p value by age and BMI in logistic regression

replicated in the present study. Therefore, SNPs with p value around 10e-5 in GWAS were controvertible and demanded for independent and large cohort of samples for verification.

Although rs17008940 was not shown to be related to PCOS, it might confer slight risk to the elevated BMI in PCOS. However, this slightly association possibly results from a selection bias derived from the patients and controls being recruited in an infertility clinical center and not from the general population. Hence, the results need further validation. Higher BMI was one of the important characteristics in PCOS and over 50 % PCOS women were overweight or obesity [20, 21]. Consistent with our results, previous studies also showed FTO and MC4R were associated with increased BMI in PCOS subjects rather than PCOS itself [22]. Abundant evidence have linked Wnt signals to the regulation of adipogenesis [23, 24] and body fat distribution [25]. For example, Christodoulides et al. reported that mutation C256Y in WNT10B was associated with overweight or obesity because the mutation was unable to activate canonical Wnt pathway [26]; and Choi et al. found that indirubin-3′-oxime (I3O), also an activator of the Wnt signaling like USP34, inhibited the development of obesity in high-fat diet fed mice [27]. Moreover, besides acting as an activator of Wnt pathway, USP34 was also found to play a role in NFκB signal regulation in T lymphocytes [28] and DNA damage response control as it was the downstream of ATM/ATR checkpoint kinase [29, 30]. USP34 may indirectly participate in the pathophysiology of PCOS by elevating BMI, but further studies were still needed to evaluate the function of USP34 in the BMI increase among PCOS women.

Some limitations of the present replication study should be mentioned. First, the sample size of this replication study was relatively small (rs17008940, OR = 1.010; rs17008097, OR = 1.007) and this replication study maybe not sufficient to detect the potential association between USP34 gene and PCOS. Second, only 2 SNPs were chosen which may cause incomplete coverage of the gene variations. Third, the recruited subjects were all Han Chinese women and the result could not represent other population.

Conclusions
In conclusion, the present study found that polymorphisms of USP34 gene may not be associated with PCOS women among Han Chinese population. SNPs with p value around 10e-4 ~ 10e-6 in GWAS were disputable and requiring replication studies for validation. Large well-designed and population-based studies are warranted to confirm our findings.

Competing interests
The authors declare that they have no competing interests.

Authors' contributions
SZ, YT and WZ carried out studies, and drafted the manuscript. YN carried out the biochemical measurements. YT, XX and TL participated in the design of the study and performed the statistical analysis. HL and TH helped to select subjects. HZ and ZJC conceived of the study, and participated in its design and coordination and helped to draft the manuscript. All authors read and approved the final manuscript.

Acknowledgements
The authors thank Li You, Jiangtao Zhang, Guangyu Li and Changming Zhang for technical support and sample collection. This work was supported by the National Basic Research Program of China (973 program) (2012CB944700, 2011CB944502), the National Natural Science Foundation of China (31371453, 81430029), the Scientific Research Foundation of Shandong Province of Outstanding Young Scientist (2012BSE27089) and the Doctoral Innovation Fund Projects from Shanghai Jiaotong University School of Medicine (Grant No. BXJ201324).

Author details
[1]Shanghai Key Laboratory for Assisted Reproduction and Reproductive Genetics, Center for Reproductive Medicine, Renji Hospital, School of Medicine, Shanghai Jiaotong University, Shanghai 200135, China. [2]Center for Reproductive Medicine, Provincial Hospital Affiliated to Shandong University, Jinan, China. [3]National Research Center for Assisted Reproductive Technology and Reproductive Genetics, Jinan, China. [4]The Key laboratory for Reproductive Endocrinology of Ministry of Education, Jinan, China. [5]Shandong Provincial Key Laboratory of Reproductive Medicine, Jinan 250021, China. [6]Department of joint and bone oncology, Provincial Hospital Affiliated to Shandong University, Jinan 250021, China.

References

1. Azziz R, Woods KS, Reyna R, Key TJ, Knochenhauer ES, Yildiz BO. The prevalence and features of the polycystic ovary syndrome in an unselected population. J Clin Endocrinol Metab. 2004;89(6):2745–9.
2. Goodarzi MO, Azziz R. Diagnosis, epidemiology, and genetics of the polycystic ovary syndrome. Best Pract Res Clin Endocrinol Metab. 2006;20(2):193–205.
3. Li R, Zhang Q, Yang D, Li S, Lu S, Wu X, et al. Prevalence of polycystic ovary syndrome in women in China: a large community-based study. Hum Reprod. 2013;28(9):2562–9.
4. Rotterdam EA-SPCWG. Revised 2003 consensus on diagnostic criteria and long-term health risks related to polycystic ovary syndrome. Fertil Steril. 2004;81(1):19–25.
5. Calogero AE, Calabro V, Catanuso M, Condorelli RA, La Vignera S. Understanding polycystic ovarian syndrome pathogenesis: an updated of its genetic aspects. J Endocrinol Invest. 2011;34(8):630–44.
6. Chen ZJ, Zhao H, He L, Shi Y, Qin Y, Shi Y, et al. Genome-wide association study identifies susceptibility loci for polycystic ovary syndrome on chromosome 2p16.3, 2p21 and 9q33.3. Nat Genet. 2011;43(1):55–9.
7. Li T, Zhao H, Zhao X, Zhang B, Cui L, Shi Y, et al. Identification of YAP1 as a novel susceptibility gene for polycystic ovary syndrome. J Med Genet. 2012;49(4):254–7.
8. COSMIC database. Wellcome Trust Sanger Institute, England. 2004. http://cancer.sanger.ac.uk/cancergenome/projects/cosmic. Accessed 4 Feb 2004.
9. Lui TT, Lacroix C, Ahmed SM, Goldenberg SJ, Leach CA, Daulat AM, et al. The ubiquitin-specific protease USP34 regulates axin stability and Wnt/beta-catenin signaling. Mol Cell Biol. 2011;31(10):2053–65.
10. Richards JS, Russell DL, Ochsner S, Hsieh M, Doyle KH, Falender AE, et al. Novel signaling pathways that control ovarian follicular development, ovulation, and luteinization. Recent Prog Horm Res. 2002;57:195–220.
11. Corton M, Botella-Carretero JI, Benguria A, Villuendas G, Zaballos A, San Millan JL, et al. Differential gene expression profile in omental adipose tissue in women with polycystic ovary syndrome. J Clin Endocrinol Metab. 2007;92(1):328–37.
12. Jansen E, Laven JS, Dommerholt HB, Polman J, van Rijt C, van den Hurk C, et al. Abnormal gene expression profiles in human ovaries from polycystic ovary syndrome patients. Mol Endocrinol. 2004;18(12):3050–63.
13. Kenigsberg S, Bentov Y, Chalifa-Caspi V, Potashnik G, Ofir R, Birk OS. Gene expression microarray profiles of cumulus cells in lean and overweight-obese polycystic ovary syndrome patients. Mol Hum Reprod. 2009;15(2):89–103.
14. Ferriman D, Gallwey JD. Clinical assessment of body hair growth in women. J Clin Endocrinol Metab. 1961;21:1440–7.
15. Shi Y, Gao X, Sun X, Zhang P, Chen Z. Clinical and metabolic characteristics of polycystic ovary syndrome without polycystic ovary: a pilot study on Chinese women. Fertil Steril. 2008;90(4):1139–43.
16. Purcell S, Cherny SS, Sham PC. Genetic Power Calculator: design of linkage and association genetic mapping studies of complex traits. Bioinformatics. 2003;19(1):149–50.
17. Newton-Cheh C, Hirschhorn JN. Genetic association studies of complex traits: design and analysis issues. Mutat Res. 2005;573(1–2):54–69.
18. Lewis CM. Genetic association studies: design, analysis and interpretation. Brief Bioinform. 2002;3(2):146–53.
19. Zhang B, Zhao H, Li T, Gao X, Gao Q, Tang R, et al. Association study of gene LPP in women with polycystic ovary syndrome. PLoS One. 2012;7(10), e46370.
20. Legro RS, Kunselman AR, Dodson WC, Dunaif A. Prevalence and predictors of risk for type 2 diabetes mellitus and impaired glucose tolerance in polycystic ovary syndrome: a prospective, controlled study in 254 affected women. J Clin Endocrinol Metab. 1999;84(1):165–9.
21. Shi Y, Guo M, Yan J, Sun W, Zhang X, Geng L, et al. Analysis of clinical characteristics in large-scale Chinese women with polycystic ovary syndrome. Neuro Endocrinol Lett. 2007;28(6):807–10.
22. Ewens KG, Jones MR, Ankener W, Stewart DR, Urbanek M, Dunaif A, et al. FTO and MC4R gene variants are associated with obesity in polycystic ovary syndrome. PLoS One. 2011;6(1), e16390.
23. Ross SE, Hemati N, Longo KA, Bennett CN, Lucas PC, Erickson RL, et al. Inhibition of adipogenesis by Wnt signaling. Science. 2000;289(5481):950–3.
24. Bennett CN, Ross SE, Longo KA, Bajnok L, Hemati N, Johnson KW, et al. Regulation of Wnt signaling during adipogenesis. J Biol Chem. 2002;277(34):30998–1004.
25. Gesta S, Bluher M, Yamamoto Y, Norris AW, Berndt J, Kralisch S, et al. Evidence for a role of developmental genes in the origin of obesity and body fat distribution. Proc Natl Acad Sci U S A. 2006;103(17):6676–81.
26. Christodoulides C, Scarda A, Granzotto M, Milan G, Dalla Nora E, Keogh J, et al. WNT10B mutations in human obesity. Diabetologia. 2006;49(4):678–84.
27. Choi OM, Cho YH, Choi S, Lee SH, Wha Seo S, Kim HY, et al. The small molecule indirubin-3'-oxime activates Wnt/beta-catenin signaling and inhibits adipocyte differentiation and obesity. Int J Obes. 2013;38(8):1044–52.
28. Poalas K, Hatchi EM, Cordeiro N, Dubois SM, Leclair HM, Leveau C, et al. Negative regulation of NF-kappaB signaling in T lymphocytes by the ubiquitin-specific protease USP34. Cell Commun Signal. 2013;11(1):25.
29. Mu JJ, Wang Y, Luo H, Leng M, Zhang J, Yang T, et al. A proteomic analysis of ataxia telangiectasia-mutated (ATM)/ATM-Rad3-related (ATR) substrates identifies the ubiquitin-proteasome system as a regulator for DNA damage checkpoints. J Biol Chem. 2007;282(24):17330–4.
30. Sy SM, Jiang J, O WS, Deng Y, Huen MS. The ubiquitin specific protease USP34 promotes ubiquitin signaling at DNA double-strand breaks. Nucleic Acids Res. 2013;41(18):8572–80.

9

Short term monotherapy with GLP-1 receptor agonist liraglutide or PDE 4 inhibitor roflumilast is superior to metformin in weight loss in obese PCOS women: a pilot randomized study

Mojca Jensterle[1], Vesna Salamun[2], Tomaz Kocjan[1], Eda Vrtacnik Bokal[2] and Andrej Janez[1*]

Abstract

Objective: To evaluate whether liraglutide or roflumilast significantly affects body weight when compared to metformin in obese women with PCOS.

Design/main outcome measure: A 12-week prospective randomized open-label study was conducted with 45 obese women with PCOS diagnosed by the ASRM-ESHRE Rotterdam criteria. They were randomized to metformin (MET) 1000 mg BID or liraglutide (LIRA) 1.2 mg QD s.c. or roflumilast (ROF) 500 mcg QD. The primary outcome was change in measures of obesity.

Results: Forty-one patients (aged 30.7 ± 7.9 years, BMI 38.6 ± 6.0 kg/m^2, mean $\pm$ SD) completed the study. Subjects treated with LIRA lost on average 3.1 ± 3.5 kg ($p = 0.006$), on ROF 2.1 ± 2.0 kg ($p = 0.002$) vs. 0.2 ± 1.83 kg in MET group. BMI decreased for 1.1 ± 1.26 kg/m^2 in LIRA ($p = 0.006$), for 0.8 ± 0.99 kg/m^2 in ROF ($p = 0.001$) vs. 0.1 ± 0.67 kg/m^2 in MET. LIRA was superior to MET in reducing weight ($p = 0.022$), BMI ($p = 0.020$), waist circumference ($p = 0.007$). LIRA also resulted in decrease in VAT area ($p = 0.015$) and more favorable dynamics in glucose homeostasis during OGTT. ROF resulted in reduction of waist circumference ($p = 0.023$). In addition, ROF led to testosterone reduction ($p = 0.05$) and increase in menstrual frequencies ($p = 0.009$) when compared to baseline.

Conclusion: Short-term monotherapy with liraglutide or roflumilast was associated with significant weight loss in obese PCOS. Liraglutide was superior to metformin, whereas roflumilast resulted in greater, yet not statistically significant, mean weight loss when compared to metformin. Reduction of body weight with liraglutide resulted in improvement of body composition.

Trial registration: ClinicalTrials.gov NCT02187250.

Keywords: Liraglutide, Metformin, Obesity, PCOS, Roflumilast

Background

Obesity is frequently present in women with polycystic ovary syndrome (PCOS) and aggravates the adverse features of the syndrome [1]. In overweight and obese patients with PCOS, lifestyle changes represent first-line treatment [2]. However, weight loss is frequently unsatisfactory with lifestyle changes alone or in combination with metformin and many women eventually regain weight [3].

In these women, the combination of lifestyle changes with identification of new effective and safe treatment options for weight reduction could be considered.

Pharmacological interventions on incretin system are a novel treatment of type 2 diabetes and proved valuable for weight loss in other obese populations [4]. In addition, obese women with PCOS who have not responded to lifestyle modification and metformin benefit from 12 week treatment with long-acting glucagon-like peptide (GLP)—1 receptor agonist liraglutide as an add-on therapy to metformin [5]. Experiences with the use of GLP-1 receptor agonist regarding weight loss as a primary outcome in

* Correspondence: andrej.janez@kclj.si
[1]Department of Endocrinology, Diabetes and Metabolic Diseases, University Medical Centre Ljubljana, Zaloska 7, SI-1000 Ljubljana, Slovenia
Full list of author information is available at the end of the article

PCOS are still very limited although an essential role of GLP-1 as a multi-targeting regulator of food intake has been recognized also in this population [6].

Less recognized distinct regulatory mechanisms related to the enhancement of GLP-1 mediated action through the inhibition of phosphodiesterase enzymes (PDE) 4 has recently became a reasonable focus of a potential new anti-obesity management. Roflumilast, the first drug specifically targeting PDE4, is well recognized as efficient treatment of chronic inflammatory diseases, primarily chronic obstructive pulmonary disease (COPD) [7, 8]. In addition, the use of roflumilast has shown positive metabolic effects on glucose homeostasis and weight reduction in newly diagnosed type 2 diabetes mellitus (T2DM) [9]. Furthermore, combined therapy of roflumilast and metformin significantly reduced body weight in obese PCOS when compared to metformin, primarily due to a loss of fat mass [10]. The observed beneficial metabolic outcomes of selective PDE4 inhibition by roflumilast are based on the interplay between the PDE4 and the regulation of GLP-1 [11].

No previous studies to date compared the effect of long acting GLP-1 receptor agonist liraglutide and selective PDE4 inhibitor roflumilast that is involved in GLP-1 release on body weight either in PCOS or any other obese population. The aim of this pilot study was to evaluate whether the monotherapy with liraglutide or roflumilast significantly affects body weight when compared to metformin in obese women with PCOS.

The study is registered on www.ClinicalTrials.gov as NCT02187250.

Methods
Study design
The study consists of a 12-week prospective randomized open-label design conducted with 45 obese women with PCOS diagnosed by ASRM-ESHRE Rotterdam criteria. All subjects had type A phenotype of PCOS including concomitant presence of a) hyperandrogenemia on either the biochemical or the clinical level, b) menses abnormalities and c) PCO morphology. They were eligible for enrollment if they were aged 18 years to menopause and obese (body mass index: BMI ≥ 30). Exclusion criteria was history of carcinoma or neuropsychiatric events, personal or familiar history of multiple endocrine neoplasia 2, significant cardiovascular, kidney or hepatic disease and the use of medications known to affect reproductive or metabolic functions within 180 days prior to study entry. Some of them were using oral contraceptives advised by their gynecologists more than 6 month before being recruited.

They were randomized to one of the three treatment arms: metformin (MET) 1000 mg BID or liraglutide (LIRA) 1.2 mg QD s.c. or roflumilast (ROF) 500 mcg

QD. Liraglutide was initiated at a dose of 0.6 mg injected s.c. once per day and increased to 1.2 mg/day after 1 week. Metformin was initiated at a dose of 500 mg once per day and increased by 500 mg every 3 days up to 1000 mg BID. Patients on liraglutide were provided with glucose-monitoring devices and supplies and educated on their use. They were instructed to measure blood glucose levels at any signs and symptoms suggesting low blood glucose. Hypoglycemia was defined according to American Diabetes Association criteria as symptoms suggestive of low blood glucose confirmed by self-monitored blood glucose measurement below 3.9 mmol/l [12]. All women were instructed to report any side effects during the treatment. They were given a general advice on lifestyle intervention. A diet of 500–800 kcal/day reduction made up of 50 % carbohydrates, 20 % proteins and 30 % of fat with increased consumption of fiber, whole grains, cereals, fruits and vegetables along with at least 30 min of moderate intensity physical activity daily had been recommended to all women at the beginning of the study. During the study lifestyle intervention was not again actively promoted.

The primary outcome of the study was mean change in measures of obesity. Secondary outcomes included hormonal and metabolic changes. Post randomization and at study endpoint all patients underwent standard anthropometric measurements: height, weight, waist circumference, blood pressure, measurement of whole-body composition by a Hologic Dual Energy X-ray Absorptiometer (DXA), including visceral adipose tissue (VAT) area. BMI was calculated as the weight in kilograms divided by square of height in meters. Before randomization transvaginal ultrasound scans of the ovaries was performed by an experienced sonographer. The presence of PCO morphology was diagnosed by the presence of 12 or more follicles in each ovary measuring 2–9 mm in diameter and/or increased ovarian volume (>10 cm³).

A fasting blood was drawn for determination of glucose, insulin, luteinizing hormone (LH), follicle stimulating hormone (FSH), androstenedione, dehydroepiandrosterone sulphate (DHEAS), total and free testosterone (T) followed by a standard 75 g oral glucose tolerance test (OGTT) to assess glucose homeostasis. Glucose levels were determined using a standard glucose oxidase method (Beckman Coulter Glucose Analyzer, Beckman Coulter Inc CA, USA). Insulin was determined by immunoradiometric assay (Biosource Europe S.A., Nivelles, Belgium). LH and FSH were determined using an immunometric assay (Diagnostic Products Corporation, LA). Androstenedione and DHEAS were measured by specific double antibody RIA using 125 I-labeled hormones (Diagnostic Systems Laboratories, Webster, Tx). Total and free testosterone levels were measured by coated tube RIA (DiaSorin, S. p. A, Salluggia, Italy and Diagnostic Products Corporation, LA, respectively).

Sex hormone binding globulin (SHBG) was determined with a chemiluminescent immunoassay (Immulite 2000 Analyzer, Siemens Healthcare, Erlangen, Germany). Intraassay variations ranged from 1.6 to 6.3 %, and interassay variations ranged from 5.8 to 9.6 % for the applied methods. Pre- and posttreatment samples from each patient were assayed in the same assay run.

Homeostasis model assessment (HOMA-IR) calculation was applied as a measure for insulin resistance (IR). Safety clinical assessment was performed at the beginning and week 4, 8 and 12 of the treatment period. Pregnancy was excluded by measuring β-human chorionic gonadotropin. Its measurement was repeated during the study whenever pregnancy was clinically possible. Women were advised to strictly use barrier contraception.

Study approval

The study was approved by a National Medical Ethics Committee and conducted in accordance with the Declaration of Helsinki and Good Clinical Practice guidelines. Informed consent was obtained from all patients before participation.

Statistical analysis

The primary endpoint of this study, for which a power calculation was used to determine the sample size, was mean change in weight. We based our calculations on a previous study with comparative treatment intervention [4]. It was determined that 12 patients would be needed per group in order to give a power of 80 % for the detection of a statistically significant difference (alpha = 0.05) of approximately 2.5 % in weight loss and estimated dropout rate of 15 %. The power estimate was performed with the online calculator at http://hedwig.mgh.harvard.edu/sample_size/size.html. A block randomization was used for subject assignment in random block sizes of 3, 6, and 9. A list of random numbers was excel generated and each random number corresponds with 1 of the 3 possible interventions (MET, LIRA, ROF).

Results are presented as mean ± standard deviation (SD). Normal data distribution was checked with the Shapiro-Wilk test. Differences at baseline between the treatment groups were checked with general linear model. The differences between treatment groups were checked and confirmed using ANOVA test. Treatment impact on the primary outcome measure was analyzed with evaluable patients data using repeated-measures linear mixed effects model with time points (baseline, 12 weeks) and therapeutic groups (MET arm, LIRA arm, ROF arm). Multiple testing of secondary outcomes was not performed. P value of less than 0.05 was considered statistically significant. Other than sample size calculation, all statistical analyses were performed using the SPSS 17.0 Statistical Software Package.

Results

Baseline results

The study enrolled 45 participants. Two MET treated patient discontinued the study, one because of diarrhea, one due to protocol violation, one LIRA treated because of nausea and one ROF treated because of headache. Forty-one patients (aged 30.7 ± 7.9 years, BMI 38.6 ± 6.0 kg/m², mean ± SD) completed the study: 13 on MET, 14 on LIRA and 14 on ROF. There were no significant differences at baseline in any of the parameters between the treatment groups. Baseline characteristics of the study outcomes are provided in Tables 1 and 2.

Measures of obesity

Subjects treated with LIRA lost on average 3.1 ± 3.5 kg ($p = 0.006$), on ROF 2.1 ± 2.0 kg ($p = 0.002$) vs 0.2 ± 1.83 kg weight loss in MET group ($p = 0.735$). BMI decreased for 1.1 ± 1.26 kg/m² in LIRA ($p = 0.006$), for 0.8 ± 0.99 kg/m² in ROF ($p = 0.001$) vs 0.1 ± 0.67 kg/m² in MET ($p = 0.731$). LIRA was superior to MET in reducing weight ($p = 0.022$), BMI ($p = 0.020$) and waist circumference ($p = 0.007$). Roflumilast resulted in greater, yet not statistically significant, mean weight loss when compared to metformin ($p = 0.203$). Although the mean weight loss was greater in the LIRA than in the ROF arm the difference was not statistically significant ($p = 0.992$). LIRA resulted in significant decrease in VAT area ($p = 0.015$). Both LIRA and ROF were associated with waist circumference reduction when compared to baseline ($p = 0.009$ and $p = 0.023$, respectively). The mean pre-and post-treatment measures of obesity are presented in Table 1.

Metabolic parameters

HOMA-IR decreased in all treatment arms, although the between treatment difference was not statistically significant yet. There was a statistically significant within-treatment reduction from baseline to last visit in fasting glucose levels and glucose at 30 (from 8.2 ± 2.4 to 7.7 ± 2.1 mmol/l, $p = 0.028$) and 120 min (from 6.7 ± 2.9 to 5.4 ± 1.9 mmol/l, $p = 0.050$) of OGTT in LIRA treated women. Liraglutide was superior to metformin in reducing glucose at 120 min of OGTT ($p = 0.041$). The mean pre-and post-treatment values of fasting glucose, fasting insulin and HOMA-IR are presented in Table 2.

Endocrine parameters

At 12 weeks a significant total T and Free Androgen Index (FAI) reduction were noted in ROF arm when compared to baseline. No statistically significant differences were found in free T, SHBG, androstenedione, DHEAS (Table 2), or in LH and FSH, neither over time nor when analyzing it separately by therapeutic arm.

Table 1 Baseline and 12-week post-treatment measures of obesity

	MET (n = 13)		LIRA (n = 14)		ROF (n = 14)		P values
	Baseline	After therapy	Baseline	After therapy	Baseline	After therapy	
Weight (kg)	108.3 ± 17.0	108.1 ± 17.5	102.8 ± 16.3	99.7 ± 17.2	111.1 ± 16.1	109.0 ± 16.4	T = 0.025 (L vs. M = 0.022); I (L = 0.006; R = 0.002)
BMI (kg/m²)	39.4 ± 6.9	39.3 ± 7.0	36.7 ± 5.6	35.6 ± 5.8	39.9 ± 5.4	39.1 ± 5.7	T = 0.023 (L vs. M = 0.020); I (L = 0.006; R = 0.001)
Waist circumference (cm)	120.5 ± 14.5	121.3 ± 13.2	115.7 ± 12.5	112.6 ± 12.9	123.0 ± 15.9	121.8 ± 16.1	T = 0.009 (L vs. M = 0.007); I (L = 0.009; R = 0.023)
VAT area (cm²)	131 ± 44.5	126.5 ± 48.3	160.3 ± 67.9	140.7 ± 60.8	157.3 ± 36.7	153.7 ± 21.9	I (L = 0.015)

For p values, T = overall effect after all treatments, R = ROF, L = LIRA, M = MET, I = interaction differences between treatment over trials

Table 2 Baseline and 12-week post-treatment metabolic and endocrine parameters

	MET (n = 13)		LIRA (n = 14)		ROF (n = 14)		P values
	Baseline	After therapy	Baseline	After therapy	Baseline	After therapy	
Glu 0 min OGTT (mmol/L)	4.8 ± 0.9	4.4 ± 1.6	5.1 ± 1.1	4.7 ± 0.7	5.1 ± 0.5	5.0 ± 0.4	I (L = 0.048)
Insulin 0 min OGTT (mU/L)	15.5 ± 6.0	12.7 ± 7.0	16 ± 9.3	14.5 ± 9.4	21.0 ± 7.7	21.0 ± 8.7	NS
HOMA-IR	3.3 ± 1.2	2.5 ± 1.9	3.8 ± 2.8	3.2 ± 2.4	4.5 ± 1.7	4.6 ± 2.1	NS
Total T (nmol/L)	1.7 ± 1.1	1.5 ± 1.2	1.7 ± 0.7	1.5 ± 0.6	1.8 ± 0.5	1.5 ± 0.6	I (R = 0.050)
Free T (nmol/L)	3.6 ± 2.6	4.3 ± 3.0	3.7 ± 2.0	3.2 ± 2.0	4.0 ± 2.2	4.0 ± 2.3	NS
SHBG (nmol/L)	28.6 ± 11.1	31.5 ± 5.6	30.5 ± 9.9	32.8 ± 14.2	27.0 ± 11.4	29.1 ± 12.1	NS
FAI	7.6 ± 8.0	4.8 ± 3.6	6.5 ± 3.7	5.4 ± 2.9	8.3 ± 5.9	6.1 ± 4.6	I (R = 0.016)
Androstenedione (nmol/L)	8.9 ± 3.8	10.7 ± 7.0	8.7 ± 3.4	9.0 ± 3.9	9.5 ± 2.5	9.4 ± 3.9	NS
DHEA-S (µmol/L)	5.9 ± 2.5	6.8 ± 3.5	6.6 ± 3.3	6.1 ± 2.4	5.6 ± 2.7	5.2 ± 1.9	NS

For p values, T = overall effect after all treatments, R = ROF, L = LIRA, M = MET, I = interaction differences between treatment over trials
NS not significant

Changes in menstrual pattern

Menstrual frequency increased with all treatments. The increase was shown as being slightly greater in patients treated with ROF (from 0.57 ± 0.40 to 0.88 ± 0.20 per month, p = 0.009), compared with MET (from 0.74 ± 0.30 to 0.92 ± 0.20 per month, p = 0.090) and LIRA (from 0.62 ± 0.30 to 0.74 ± 0.30, p = 0.165). However, the between-treatment differences were not statistically significant yet.

Adverse events

The most commonly reported adverse events in MET group were diarrhea (4/14) and nausea (4/14) that resolved in the first week for 3/14 subjects and within 4 weeks of the study onset for the 1/14 woman. Adverse events associated with LIRA were nausea (4/14), obstipation (2/14), diarrhea (1/14), headache (1/14) and insomnia (1/14). In the ROF group, 5/14 subjects had mild gastrointestinal problems (nausea and diarrhea), 2/14 had mild headache and 1/14 reported mild depression in the last month of the study. Nausea in LIRA arm was present up to 3 days when liraglutide was initiated at a dose of 0.6 mg injected s.c. once per day and if present reappeared for 2 to 3 days when the dose was increased to 1.2 mg/day after 1 week. It was not accompanied with vomiting. Nausea in ROF arm was more persistent when compared to MET yet it was mild and not accompanied with vomiting. Some subjects in all treatment groups had multiple side effects. No side effect was reported by 10/14 women in MET arm, 8/14 in LIRA arm and 8/14 in ROF arm. Hypoglycemic event was not reported in any group. The injection regimen of LIRA did not impair adherence or cause significant withdrawal over ROF and MET during treatment.

Discussion

The comparison of long-acting GLP-1 receptor agonist liraglutide or selective PDE4 inhibitor roflumilast versus metformin on changes of measures of obesity have not yet been evaluated in women with PCOS or any other obese population. To our knowledge, this is the first study to date demonstrating that in a short period of time liraglutide was significantly more effective than metformin regarding weight loss and improvement of body composition in obese PCOS women. Roflumilast resulted in greater, yet not statistically significant, mean weight loss when compared to metformin. In addition, liraglutide treatment was followed with within-treatment favorable improvements in glucose homeostasis during OGTT and in significantly greater reduction of glucose at 120 min of OGTT when compared to metformin, while roflumilast resulted in testosterone reduction and increase in menstrual frequencies when compared to baseline.

Liraglutide resulted in the between-treatment difference of about 3 kg weight lost versus metformin. Although metformin is still widely used in the management of PCOS due to its observed curative and potentially preventive clinical benefits, including body weight reduction and improvement of fat distribution, recent guidelines developed by the Endocrine Society recommended its use only in women with PCOS who are already undergoing lifestyle treatment and do not have improvement in impaired glucose tolerance and in those who have normal weight, but still have impaired glucose tolerance [13]. In fact, its effect on weight reduction and fat distribution in PCOS remains controversial. In accordance with our study, most studies and meta-analysis concluded that as a mono-therapy, metformin does not significantly reduce body weight, although some studies have reported some marginal benefit in longer observation period [14, 15].

Until today, only few studies have addressed the possible use of GLP-1 receptor agonists in women with PCOS, but all with some important methodological limitations regarding the evaluation of their effect on body weight. We previously conducted a study with obese PCOS women who had been pretreated with metformin and had lost less than 5 % of body weight in 6 months with metformin before recruitment. In that study, one group was kept on metformin for 12 more weeks while comparing it for weight loss with other two groups taking liraglutide alone or liraglutide in combination to metformin. Patients on combined treatment lost on average 6.5 kg compared with a 3.8 kg loss in LIRA group, with the between-treatment difference of about 5 and 3 kg, respectively, when compared to metformin mono-therapy [5]. The results are perfectly in line with the findings of this study. However, the main issue of our previous study was inclusion of non-responders for the outcome of interest that could have brought bias from the beginning. Apprised of that limitation the present study was conducted with a much better and fair design that included drug naïve patients. Furthermore, an average weight reduction of 3.0 kg, yet achieved in a longer period of observation and with larger dosage of 1.8 mg QD s.c., was observed also in a 24 week-study that reported the potential impact of liraglutide on markers of liver fibrosis in PCOS [16]. However, the study was not designed to evaluate the change in measures of obesity as a primary outcome of interest. As opposed to long acting GLP-1 agonist liraglutide, the only report using short acting GLP-1 agonist exenatide in treatment-naive overweight patients with PCOS was a 24 week-study conducted to evaluate change in menstrual frequency whereas change in body weight was pre-specified as secondary outcome. Combined treatment with exenatide and metformin was superior to exenatide and metformin mono-therapies resulting in an average weight reduction of 6 kg in combined group compared to 3.2 kg in the exenatide, and of 1.6 kg in metformin group [17]. Weight reduction in our study is of comparable magnitude to the exenatide group, but achieved in a shorter period of time. In addition, we observed small drop out in our study as opposed to relatively large drop out in the study with exenatide, which was probably conditioned by the choice of GLP-1 receptor agonist. It has been demonstrated in individuals with type 2 diabetes mellitus that liraglutide caused less adverse events and therapy discontinuation than exenatide [18].

Contrary to liraglutide acting as a GLP-1 receptor agonist, selective PDE4 inhibitor roflumilast interacts to GLP- mediated effect through completely different pathways. It is involved in the PDE4 regulation of signaling cascades linked to GLP-1 release. In rodent model roflumilast enhanced plasma GLP-1 levels up to 2.5 –fold [11]. In clinical studies, roflumilast was associated with a weight decrease of about 2 kg versus placebo in 12 months in patients with chronic obstructive pulmonary disease (COPD) [7, 8] and with mean weight change of about 2 kg in 12 weeks versus placebo in patients with newly diagnosed type 2 diabetes mellitus without COPD

[9]. We recently reported that in obese women with PCOS, roflumilast added to metformin was superior to metformin alone in reducing mean body weight after 12 weeks, with the between treatment difference of about 5 kg [10]. Referring to the patients' history on pre-treatment with metformin we were cautioned that the study did not have a proper control to draw definitive conclusions solely about the effects of roflumilast in PCOS. Considering the innovative concept that grasps selective PDE4 inhibition as a potential new therapeutic target in obesity associated populations, in the present study we used an upgraded design to further elucidate the potential effect of roflumilast in treatment-naïve obese PCOS population. Treatment with roflumilast resulted in the between-treatment difference of about 2 kg weight lost versus metformin, which is in accordance with the study of the same observational period in patients with newly diagnosed type 2 diabetes mellitus [9]. However, the weight reduction with both liraglutide and roflumilast in the present study was of lesser magnitude when compared to the studies in PCOS population using combined therapies, including combined treatment of GLP-1 receptor agonist [5, 17] and metformin or combination of roflumilast and metformin [10], which might suggest a possible additive role of metformin to GLP-1 mediated effect [19, 20].

Furthermore, the results of this study indicate that liraglutide was superior to roflumilast regarding improvements of measures of obesity and metabolic profile, not being demonstrated with roflumilast. Previously, effects of roflumilast on glucose metabolism has been studied in a 12 week, randomized, double blind, placebo controlled study of patients with newly diagnosed type 2 diabetes mellitus without COPD. Over 12 weeks, HbA1C levels declined substantially in the roflumilast group compared with placebo [9]. The beneficial impact of roflumilast on metabolic parameters has been explained by the same mechanisms mediated through its elevating effect on the GLP-1 incretin hormone levels as being hypothesized to be responsible for its effect on body weight reduction [9]. No study to date directly compared these two therapies and we might only reasonably speculate that the direct enhancement of GLP-1 axis with GLP-1 receptor agonists is more potent than GLP-mediated effect through PDE4 regulation. However, this was a pilot study, not powered for all possible relevant metabolic outcomes, but powered specifically for weight loss.

Surprisingly, despite the superiority of liraglutide in weight reduction and glucose homeostasis, roflumilast resulted in total testosterone and FAI reduction and increase in menstrual frequencies not being demonstrated in liraglutide arm. These observed beneficial trends that obviously went beyond weight reduction effect might be related to the expression of PDE4 enzymes in ovaries and the recognized involvement of PDEs in steroidogenesis. A potential role of roflumilast in direct regulation of ovarian steroidogenesis and in the pathophysiology of PCOS could not be excluded [21, 22]. The improvement of androgen profile tended to be slightly greater also in PCOS patients treated with roflumilast added to metformin in our previous study [10]. Clearly, due to generally known methodological problem for assessment of androgens in PCOS, relatively small study sample size and lack of any data on roflumilast specific effects on PCOS treatment outcomes, our observations in both studies so far do not allow more than a speculation in this regard.

The present study has several limitations. Number of patients in each treatment group was small, partially at the expense of the originality of the comparative design including three treatment arms. The 12-week observation period was too short to assess the efficacy and safety of liraglutide and roflumilast as weight loss drugs in obese women with PCOS. The short-term design was conducted mainly due to insufficient longer-term safety data of liraglutide and roflumilast in women that might still wish to conceive. The importance of lifestyle intervention was introduced at the beginning of the study but not actively promoted over the course of the study, yet such setting had the advantage of being similar to the daily practice. In addition, the open label nature of the study might be further potential limitation with this regard, as women in the LIRA arm would know they were given a drug that has been mentioned in the media as an anti-obesity drug. This could have resulted in a higher motivation to adhere to the lifestyle intervention. However, the main strength of this pilot study was the original concept that grasps inclusion of two agents acting through the GLP-1 axis that had not yet been compared either in PCOS or any other obese population.

Conclusions

Short-term monotherapy with liraglutide or roflumilast was superior to metformin in weight loss in obese PCOS women. Reduction of body weight resulted in improvement of body composition. In addition, liraglutide was associated with beneficial effects on glucose homeostasis, whereas roflumilast resulted in total testosterone reduction and improvement of menstrual frequencies. Considering the recognized role of incretin system and potential role of PDE 4 signaling pathways in the pathophysiology of PCOS further explorations in larger studies of longer duration are needed to assess the effects of both agents in this population providing the possible basis for the clinical approach that could tailor treatment choices to the specific needs of the patient.

The role of metformin in the management of obesity remains unsatisfactory. Following recent clinical practice guidelines metformin should be used in women with PCOS

who are already undergoing lifestyle treatment and do not have improvement in impaired glucose tolerance or in those who have normal body weight but still have impaired glucose tolerance [13]. However, the potential additive efficacy of novel anti-obesity treatment options targeting incretin system in combination to metformin should be a focus of further investigation in PCOS population.

Abbreviations
PCOS: Polycystic ovary syndrome; GLP: Glucagon-like peptide; PDE: Phosphodiesterase enzyme; ASRM-ESHRE: American Society for Reproductive Medicine—European Society of Human Reproduction and Embryology; MET: Metformin treatment arm; LIRA: Liraglutide treatment arm; ROF: Roflumilast treatment arm; DXA: Dual Energy X-ray Absorptiometer; VAT: Visceral adipose tissue; LH: Luteinizing hormone; FSH: Follicle stimulating hormone; DHEAS: Dehydroepiandrosterone sulphate; T: Testosterone; OGTT: Oral glucose tolerance test; HOMA: Homeostasis model assessment; IR: Insulin resistance; COPD: Chronic obstructive pulmonary disease.

Competing interests
AJ has received consulting fee from Takeda Pharmaceutical Company as a member of European advisory board. MJ, VS, TK and EVB have nothing to declare.
The study was supported by the Ministry of Health, Republic of Slovenia, Tertiary Care Scientific grant Number 20120047 of the University Medical Centre Ljubljana. Takeda or Novo Nordisk Pharmaceutical Company did not participate in the study.

Authors' contributions
MJ and AJ designed the study. MJ, VS and AJ conceived and carried out experiments. All authors were involved in writing the paper and had final approval of the submitted and published versions.

Acknowledgements
The authors would like to thank Franci Cucek and Ziga Krizaj for statistical analysis. We appreciate the assistance of Mirela Ozura and Elizabeta Stepanovic, RNs.

Author details
[1]Department of Endocrinology, Diabetes and Metabolic Diseases, University Medical Centre Ljubljana, Zaloska 7, SI-1000 Ljubljana, Slovenia. [2]Department of Obstetrics and Gynecology, Reproductive Unit, University Medical Centre Ljubljana, Zaloska 7, 1525 Ljubljana, Slovenia.

References
1. Yildiz BO, Knochenhauer ES, Azziz R. Impact of obesity on the risk for polycystic ovary syndrome. J Clin Endocrinol Metab. 2008;93:162–8.
2. Domecq JP, Prutsky G, Mullan RJ, Sundaresh V, Wang AT, Erwin PJ, et al. Adverse effects of the common treatments for polycystic ovary syndrome: a systematic review and meta-analysis. J Clin Endocrinol Metab. 2013;98:4655–63.
3. Galani C, Schneider H. Prevention and treatment of obesity with lifestyle interventions: review and meta-analysis. Int J Public Health. 2007;52:348–59.
4. Astrup A, Carraro R, Finer N, Harper A, Kunesova M, Lean ME, et al. Safety, tolerability and sustained weight loss over 2 years with the once-daily human GLP-1 analog, liraglutide. Int J Obes. 2012;36:843–54.
5. Jensterle Sever M, Kocjan T, Pfeifer M, Kravos NA, Janez A. Short-term combined treatment with liraglutide and metformin leads to significant weight loss in obese women with polycystic ovary syndrome and previous poor response to metformin. Eur J Endocrinol. 2014;170:451–9.
6. Aydin K, Arusoglu G, Koksal G, Cinar N, Yazgan Aksoy D, Yildiz BO. Fasting and post-prandial glucagon like peptide 1 and oral contraception in polycystic ovary syndrome. Clin Endocrinol (Oxf). 2014;81:588–92.
7. Calverley PMA, Rabe KF, Goehring U-M, Kristiansen S, Fabbri LM, Martinez FJ, et al. Roflumilast in symptomatic chronic obstructive pulmonary disease: two randomised clinical trials. Lancet. 2009;374:685–94.

8. Fabbri LM, Calverley PMA, Izquierdo-Alonso JL, Bundschuh DS, Brose M, Martinez FJ, et al. Roflumilast in moderate-to-severe chronic obstructive pulmonary disease treated with long-acting bronchodilators: two randomised clinical trials. Lancet. 2009;374:695–703.
9. Wouters EF, Bredenbröker D, Teichmann P, Brose M, Rabe KF, Fabbri LM, et al. Effect of the phosphodiesterase 4 inhibitor roflumilast on glucose metabolism in patients with treatment-naive, newly diagnosed type 2 diabetes mellitus. J Clin Endocrinol Metab. 2012;97:E1720–5.
10. Jensterle M, Kocjan T, Janez A. Phosphodiesterase 4 inhibition as a potential new therapeutic target in obese women with polycystic ovary syndrome. J Clin Endocrinol Metab. 2014;99:E1476–81.
11. Vollert S, Kaessner N, Heuser A, Hanauer G, Dieckmann A, Knaack D, et al. The glucose-lowering effects of the PDE4 inhibitors roflumilast and roflumilast-N-oxide in db/db mice. Diabetologia. 2012;55:2779–88.
12. American Diabetes Association. Standards of medical care in diabetes–2013. Diabetes Care. 2013;36 Suppl 1:S11–66.
13. Legro RS, Arslanian SA, Ehrmann DA, Hoeger KM, Murad MH, Pasquali R, et al. Diagnosis and treatment of polycystic ovary syndrome: an endocrine society clinical practice guideline. J Clin Endocrinol Metab. 2013;98:4565–92.
14. Lord JM, Flight IHK, Norman RJ. Metformin in polycystic ovary syndrome: systematic review and meta-analysis. BMJ. 2003;327:951–3.
15. Nieuwenhuis-Ruifrok AE, Kuchenbecker WKH, Hoek A, Middleton P, Norman RJ. Insulin sensitizing drugs for weight loss in women of reproductive age who are overweight or obese: systematic review and meta-analysis. Hum Reprod Update. 2009;15:57–68.
16. Kahal H, Abouda G, Rigby AS, Coady AM, Kilpatrick ES, Atkin SL. Glucagon-like peptide-1 analogue, liraglutide, improves liver fibrosis markers in obese women with polycystic ovary syndrome and nonalcoholic fatty liver disease. Clin Endocrinol (Oxf). 2014;81:523–8.
17. Elkind-Hirsch K, Marrioneaux O, Bhushan M, Vernor D, Bhushan R. Comparison of single and combined treatment with exenatide and metformin on menstrual cyclicity in overweight women with polycystic ovary syndrome. J Clin Endocrinol Metab. 2008;93:2670–8.
18. Buse JB, Rosenstock J, Sesti G, Schmidt WE, Montanya E, Brett JH, et al. Liraglutide once a day versus exenatide twice a day for type 2 diabetes: a 26-week randomised, parallel-group, multinational, open-label trial (LEAD-6). Lancet. 2009;374:39–47.
19. Maida A, Lamont BJ, Cao X, Drucker DJ. Metformin regulates the incretin receptor axis via a pathway dependent on peroxisome proliferator-activated receptor-α in mice. Diabetologia. 2011;54:339–49.
20. Mannucci E, Tesi F, Bardini G, Ognibene A, Petracca MG, Ciani S, et al. Effects of metformin on glucagon-like peptide-1 levels in obese patients with and without Type 2 diabetes. Diabetes Nutr Metab. 2004;17:336–42.
21. Vezzosi D, Bertherat J. Phosphodiesterases in endocrine physiology and disease. Eur J Endocrinol. 2011;165:177–88.
22. Tsai L-CL, Beavo JA. The roles of cyclic nucleotide phosphodiesterases (PDEs) in steroidogenesis. Curr Opin Pharmacol. 2011;11:670–5.

10

Relative importance of AMH and androgens changes with aging among non-obese women with polycystic ovary syndrome

Vitaly A. Kushnir[1,2*], Noy Halevy[3], David H. Barad[1,4], David F. Albertini[1,5] and Norbert Gleicher[1,4,6]

Abstract

Background: To assess the changes in phenotypes and endocrine profiles of women with polycystic ovary syndrome (PCOS) with advancing age.

Methods: In a cross-sectional study conducted at a private tertiary fertility clinical and research center we identified anonymized electronic records of 37 women who had presented with a prior diagnosis of PCOS. They were stratified as younger (<35 years) and older (≥40 years). As controls, we identified 43 women with age-specific low functional ovarian reserve and 14 young women with normal functional ovarian reserve. Endocrine profiles for each group were evaluated based on total (TT) and free testosterone (FT), anti-Müllerian hormone (AMH) and sex hormone binding globulin (SHBG).

Results: Patients including those with PCOS were mostly non-obese, evidenced by normal BMIs (21.6 ± 6.0) with no differences between study groups. Young PCOS patients presented with a typical pattern of significant hyperandrogenemia and elevated AMH in comparison to young women with normal functional ovarian reserve [TT 44.0 (32.9–58.7) vs. 23.9 (20.3–28.1) ng/dL, ($P<0.05$); and AMH 7.7 (6.2–9.1) vs. 2.5 (2.0–3.0) ng/mL, ($P<0.05$)]. With advancing age, hyperandrogenemia in PCOS diminished in comparison to young women with normal functional ovarian reserve, resulting in similar TT levels [28.6 (19.7–37.5) vs. 23.9 (20.3–28.1) ng/dL]. Though also declining, AMH remained significantly elevated in older PCOS women in comparison to young women with normal functional ovarian reserve [4.0 (2.7–5.2) vs. 2.5 (2.0–3.0) ng/mL, ($P<0.05$)]. Patients with low functional ovarian reserve demonstrated significantly lower AMH at both young and older ages compared to women with normal functional ovarian reserve ($P<0.05$ for both). However, among patients with low functional ovarian reserve no differences were observed at young compared to older ages in TT [17.6 (12.9–24.1) vs. 18.1 (13.6–24.1) ng/dL)] and AMH [0.4 (0.3–0.6) vs. 0.3 (0.2–0.5) ng/mL]. SHBG did not differ significantly between groups but trended opposite to testosterone.

Conclusions: The PCOS population predominantly consisted of non-obese phenotype at both young and advanced ages. This suggests that patients with "classical" obese PCOS phenotype rarely reach tertiary infertility care, while non-obese PCOS patients may be more resistant to lower levels of infertility treatments. PCOS patients also demonstrate more precipitous declines in testosterone then AMH with advancing age. These data support incorporation of AMH as diagnostic criterion for PCOS regardless of age, and imply that testosterone should not be relied upon in the diagnosis of PCOS in older women.

Keywords: Polycystic ovarian syndrome (PCOS), Ovarian reserve, Androgens, Testosterone, Anti-Müllerian hormone (AMH)

* Correspondence: vkushnir@thechr.com
[1]Center for Human Reproduction, 21 East 69th Street, New York, NY 10021, USA
[2]Wake Forest School of Medicine, Winston-Salem, NC, USA
Full list of author information is available at the end of the article

Background

The polycystic ovary syndrome (PCOS) is an amalgam of clinical conditions, to a large degree characterized by a polycystic ovary phenotype (POP) [1]. Various classifications have been proposed to define the syndrome, consensus opinions have been issued [2–7], though none have found universal acceptance. The 2003 Rotterdam criteria for diagnosis of PCOS are, likely, the currently most widely accepted definition of PCOS, including irregular ovulatory function (oligomenorrhea or amenorrhea), evidence of hyperandrogenism (chemical or clinical) and presence of an POP on sonography [2].

Principal reasons for lack of consensus are likely differing etiologies and pathophysiologies leading to PCOS [8]. In addition, increasing evidence suggests that PCOS is not stable and/or static as women advance in age [9].

Many of the typical phenotypic features, especially hyperandrogenism and anovulation, normalize with advancing age [10]. Consequently, women, who may present with fairly typical PCOS at young ages by older ages, when they reach fertility treatments, may no longer exhibit those typical findings. Though their history of PCOS may still have clinical relevance, their PCOS diagnosis may no longer be obvious to treating physicians.

Importance of normal androgen levels for normal follicle growth and maturation and, therefore, for female fertility has been increasingly recognized over the last decade [11]. Declines in androgen levels with advancing age [10, 12], therefore, have the potential of affecting ovarian functions and female fertility. Consequently, androgen supplementation has been utilized in hypoandrogenic infertile women with low functional ovarian reserve (LFOR) [13].

Because PCOS ovaries (and their androgen receptors) may from younger years be used to higher androgen levels, functional hypoandrogenism may be comparatively more pronounced in older PCOS patients than normal older women.

Further complicating diagnosis and classifications of PCOS is that only a fraction of patients exhibit the "classic" PCOS phenotype, characterized by trunkal obesity (high BMI) [4]. A similar percentage of women with PCOS presents without obesity and may also lack other phenotypical characteristics of "classic" PCOS [14, 15].

Whether high BMI and non-obese low BMI PCOS patients differ in their respective ovarian aging patterns is still unknown. Because both start from different endocrine and metabolic baselines, it appears possible that they differ in how they evolve with advancing age.

Androgens characteristically decline with age [12]. In patients with LFOR they are, however, comparatively low at all ages [16]. PCOS patients, in contrast, at young ages are almost uniformly hyperandrogenic.

Hyperandrogenemia, however, usually resolves with advancing age, at times allowing for spontaneous resumption of regular menstruation at relatively advanced reproductive ages [4]. Interestingly, despite similar androgen levels, young non-obese PCOS patients demonstrate fewer signs and symptoms of hyperandrogenism than "classical" PCOS patients. This is likely the consequence of increased bio-availability of androgens in peripheral tissues and enhanced 5α-reductase activity in obese patients [17].

Whether different PCOS phenotypes "age" differently has so far not been studied. Should there be differences, they might have significant clinical consequences. One very obvious one would be the clinical accuracy of diagnosis of PCOS at older ages, based on Rotterdam criteria.

We recently proposed that, functionally, and in hormonal parameters, PCOS and LFOR represent opposing extremes of ovarian function, characterized by hyper- and hypo-androgenemia and hyper- and hypoactive follicle recruitment, respectively [18]. Like in PCOS, the natural history of LFOR over time is, however, largely unknown.

This study, therefore, aimed to improve the understanding of androgen dynamics in women with PCOS and LFOR over advancing age. In completing this study, we gained interesting and, at times surprising, new insights into the non-obese PCOS phenotype. They point toward potential new treatment options, and also allow for the development of new hypotheses about the pathophysiology of PCOS.

Methods

IRB and informed consents

All patients at our center sign at initial consultation an informed consent, which allows use of their medical record data for clinical research as long as their identity remains protected and the medical record remains confidential. Since both of these conditions were met, this study qualified for expedited review and approval by the center's IRB.

Patient populations

All 94 patients investigated in this cross sectional study presented to our fertility center between 2009 and 2014, and were part of an anonymized electronic research database our center has been maintaining. Among those, 37 were study subjects, prior to presentation to our center diagnosed elsewhere with PCOS. To qualify for this study group, they in addition to on medical records review having been formally diagnosed with PCOS, had to have verified histories of oligo/amenorrhea consistent with intermittent anovulation and female infertility.

Two distinct patient groups, during the same time period treated at our center, served as controls. The first control group included 43 women with LFOR, with the diagnosis defined by anti-Müllerian hormone (AMH) below age-specific 95 % CI, as previously reported for our center's patient population [19, 20]. Under age 35 years such patients were classified as premature ovarian aging (POA), by some also given the acronym occult primary ovarian insufficiency (oPOI). Above age 40 years, we consider all patients with LFOR to suffer from physiologic ovarian aging. A second control group involved 14 young women with normal functional ovarian reserve (NFOR), who during the study period had entered fertility treatment for either male factor infertility or tubal disease. These patients were used to establish normal reference values, reflecting young, normal ovaries.

PCOS and LFOR groups were further stratified by age into younger (age <35 years) and older (age ≥40 years) groups, thus yielding a total of five distinct study groups (Table 1).

Laboratory testing

All laboratory tests were performed at time of initial presentation to our center, when patients undergo a first diagnostic evaluation. AMH and serum androgens were performed at random, unrelated to day of menstrual cycle. Laboratory tests were performed via commercial testing (Laboratory Corporation of America). AMH was measured by enzyme-linked immunosorbent, Gen II assay (Beckman Coulter, Inc., Webster, Texas). All androgen levels were measured by liquid chromatography/tandem mass spectrometry.

Statistical analyses

Statistical analyses were performed in MedCalc, Version 14.8.1. (Ostend, Belgium). Normality of data was tested

for all continuous variables. Those not normally distributed were log transformed. Values are, where appropriate, shown as means and 95 % confidence intervals (CI). One-way ANOVA was used to evaluate differences between study groups. Post-hoc analysis was performed with Student-Newman-Keuls (SMK) test for pair wise comparisons. A P-value <0.05 was considered statistically significant.

Results

Table 1 summarizes patient characteristics, including baseline hormone measurements for all study groups. Significant age differences between older and younger patient groups were a feature of study design. However, distribution of age was similar within respective young and older subgroups. Surprisingly, BMI values were practically identical between all five patient groups.

As demonstrated in Fig. 1, young PCOS women presented with a typical pattern of significantly elevated AMH and hyperandrogenism in comparison to young women with NFOR [TT 44.0 (95 % CI, 32.9 to 58.7) vs. 23.9 (95 % CI 20.3 to 28.1) ng/dL, ($P < 0.05$); AMH 7.7 (95 % CI 6.2 to 9.1) vs. 2.5 (95 % CI 2.0 to 3.0) ng/mL, ($P < 0.05$)]. With advancing age, hyperandrogenemia in association with PCOS, however, diminished significantly ($P < 0.05$), resulting in similar TT and FT levels to young women with NFOR [TT 27.8 (95 % CI 21.8 to 35.5) vs. 23.9 (95 % CI 20.3 to 28.1) ng/dL].

AMH, however in older PCOS women remained significantly elevated in comparison to young women with NFOR [4.0 (95 % CI 3.3 to 4.8) vs. 2.5 (95 % CI 2.0 to 3.0) ng/mL, ($P < 0.05$)]. As expected, AMH was significantly lower in older than younger PCOS women ($P < 0.05$; Fig. 1).

Younger and older LFOR patients demonstrated significantly lower AMH levels in comparison to young women with NFOR [0.4 (95 % CI 0.3 to 0.6) and 0.3

Table 1 Patient characteristics and baseline hormone measurements

	Young PCOS	Older PCOS	Young LFOR	Older LFOR	Young NFOR
N	21	16	24	19	14
Age (years)	30.7 (29.3–32.1)	41.6 (40.9–42.4)*	32.9 (31.8–34.1)	41.7 (41.0–42.4)*	31.4 (29.6–33.1)
BMI (kg/m^2)	21.6^a (19.1–24.6)	23.5 (20.4–26.5)	20.8 (18.8–22.7)	24.0^a (21.9–26.3)	21.1 (17.7–24.4)
AMH (ng/mL)	7.7 (6.2–9.1)*	4.0 (3.3–4.8)*	0.4 (0.3–0.6)*	0.3^a (0.2–0.5)*	2.5 (2.0–3.0)
Total Testosterone (ng/dL)	44.0^a (32.9–58.7)*	27.8^a (21.8–35.5)	17.6^a (12.9–24.1)	18.1^a (13.6–24.1)	23.9^a (20.3–28.1)
Free Testosterone (pg/mL)	4.1 (2.2–5.9)*	1.5^a (1.0–2.2)	0.7^a (0.4–1.1)	1.4 (0.9–1.9)	1.6 (1.2–2.0)
DHEA (ng/dL)	398.8 (223.3–574.3)	269.6^a (205.1–354.4)	315.3 (223.3–407.3)	274.6^a (189.2–398.5)	302.8 (211.6–394.1)
DHEA-S (ug/dL)	236.6 (170.6–302.5)	183.9 (124.4–243.5)	130.6 (99.3–171.8)	158.5^a (117.1–214.5)	231.9 (157.3–306.4)
SHBG (nmol/L)	71.0 (26.7–115.2)	86.5 (56.9–116.1)	76.0^a (56.6–102.0)	65.6^a (50.4–85.4)	75.4^a (52.2–109.0)

Data in this table are reported as Mean (95 % Confidence Interval)
^{a}indicates data back-transformed after initial logarithmic transformation
*indicates statistically significant difference ($P < 0.05$) in comparison to Young NFOR group

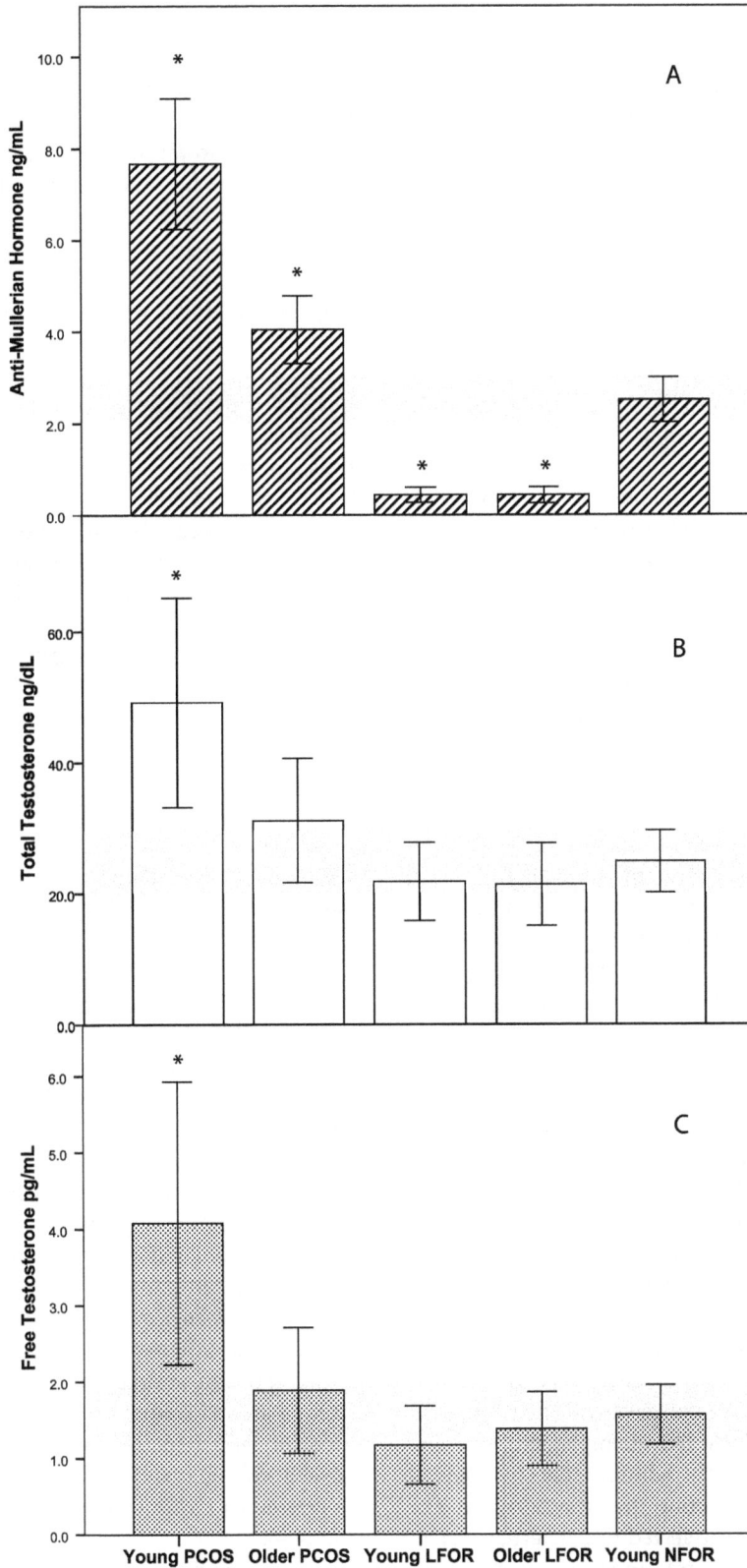

Fig. 1 AMH and testosterone levels in women with PCOS and LFOR stratified by age. **a** AMH levels (ng/mL). **b** Total Testosterone (ng/dL). **c** Free Testosterone (pg/mL); Error bars represent 95 % Confidence Intervals. Shaded area corresponds to the 95 % Confidence Interval of the Young NFOR comparison group. *indicates statistically significant difference ($P < 0.05$) in comparison to Young NFOR group

(95 % CI 0.2 to 0.5) respectively vs. 2.5 (95 % CI 2.0 to 3.0) ng/mL] (both $P < 0.05$). Interestingly, AMH levels did not decrease in older LFOR in comparison to young LFOR patients, possibly because even young LFOR patients already approached lower levels of AMH assay sensitivity [21].

This explanation, however, does not hold up for androgens: as previously reported [16], TT and FT levels even in young LFOR patients trended lower (though, likely due to relatively small sample size, did not reach significance) in comparison to young controls with NFOR. Yet, TT and FT in older women with LFOR also did not further decrease in comparison to young LFOR women [18.1 (95 % CI 13.6 to 24.1) vs. TT 17.6 (95 % CI 12.9 to 24.1) ng/dL], suggesting that whatever causes relative hypoandrogenemia in these patients at already young ages appears to mimic the physiologic hypoandrogenemia of older age. In other words, LFOR at young ages truly appears to reflect "premature ovarian aging".

Since androgen effects on follicle development are primarily mediated by T (via androgen receptor) [11], it is not surprising that DHEA and DHEAS levels were similar among all the groups. Sex hormone binding globulin (SHBG) trended into the opposite direction to T but did not reach statistical significance (Table 1).

Discussion

Despite relatively small patient numbers in all five patient groups, this study produced surprisingly robust statistical data. Likely, the most remarkable finding of the study was the recognition that in identifying established PCOS patients who had sought out fertility treatment at our center, practically all were of the "non-classical," non-obese phenotype.

The study allows for this conclusion for a number of reasons: Based on very high AMH levels and hyperandrogenemia at young ages, here investigated young infertility patients, unquestionably, had been correctly assigned a diagnosis of PCOS. That their BMI was practically identical to the BMI of young controls with NFOR precludes the possibility that this group of PCOS patients to a significant degree represented the "classical" PCOS phenotype.

Infertile women who reach tertiary fertility centers like ours have not only failed to spontaneously conceive but, in most cases, also failed to conceive with first line ovulation inducing medications, like clomiphene citrate and aromatase inhibitors, mostly administered by general gynecologists at earlier infertility treatment stages. The finding that PCOS patients referred to our tertiary fertility center were predominantly non-obese, therefore, defines here investigated PCOS patients as different from average PCOS populations, generally described in the literature [22].

That PCOS patients reaching tertiary infertility care at our center practically exclusively turned out to be non-obese PCOS patients, therefore, suggests that this PCOS phenotype already at young ages may be more resistant to fertility treatments than "classical" PCOS, who likely conceive with lower levels of care.

If confirmed by other studies, this here for the first time reported observation would suggest distinctly different underlying pathophysiology for these two distinct PCOS phenotypes. It would also confirm a recent report from Azziz's group, which suggested that referral biases affect the prevalence of obesity in PCOS patient populations [22].

As Fig. 1 demonstrates, the non-obese PCOS phenotype loses between young and older age, based on AMH levels, approximately 50 % of functional ovarian reserve (FOR). Yet, FOR still remains above what even at young ages is considered a NFOR. Androgens, however, follow a different trajectory: as Fig. 1 demonstrates, TT and FT also decline and, indeed, proportionally decline less than AMH. TT and FT levels, yet, approximated the normal range of young women with NFOR and, indeed, no longer differed statistically.

As AMH is produced in granulosa cells of growing follicles [23], these findings suggest that, considering still ongoing excessive follicle recruitment (i.e., still high AMH levels), non-obese PCOS patients at older ages produce relatively deficient amounts of T in ovarian theca cells and/or adrenals, even though in young controls with NFOR, these T levels would be considered in entirely normal range.

Women with non-obese PCOS, therefore, comparatively suffer from relative hypoandrogenemia because of asynchrony between growing follicle volume and androgen levels. Based on this observation, it is tempting to hypothesize that the reason why women with "classical" PCOS may conceive easier (and earlier) may be that their more pronounced hyperandrogenism may prevent such asynchrony, and the resulting relative hypoandrogenemia with advancing ages, from occurring.

Here observed rather remarkable differences between PCOS and LFOR patients offer further insights into the interplay between growing follicular cell mass and androgen levels. In contrast to significant declines in FOR (i.e., AMH) and androgens (TT and FT) in non-obese PCOS patients, women with LFOR demonstrated practically no detectable changes in both parameters between younger and older ages. They, thus, at both age extremes exhibit a hormonal profile of cellular exhaustion.

This observation strongly supports the contention that, hormonally, POA at young ages presents with a very similar profile to physiological ovarian aging at older age, and explains why androgen supplementation in women with LFOR appears similarly effective in younger and older women [13].

Androgens induce PCOS-like POPs in various animal models [24]. They work synergistically with FSH during small growing follicle stages by enhancing the sensitivity of granulosa cells to follicle stimulating hormone (FSH) [25]. A detailed review on the subject was recently published [11]. We demonstrated that combining androgen supplementation with consecutive FSH exposure in sequential in vitro fertilization cycles improves FOR and improves oocyte yields at advanced ages even in women with severe LFOR [26].

What initiates hyperandrogenism in association with PCOS and relative hypoandrogenism in association with LFOR has so far remained unresolved. We have hypothesized about the existence of a yet undiscovered androgen production factor (APF) of, possibly, immune system origin, which is hyperactive in association with PCOS and hypoactive in LFOR [18].

Here presented data also suggest potential for new clinical therapies. For example, if non-obese PCOS patients despite seemingly normal androgen levels, indeed, suffer from relative hypoandrogenism, as has been reported in LFOR patients [13, 27], androgen supplementation may help in improving oocyte/embryo quality and fertility treatment outcomes.

Here reported data should also lead to better diagnosis of non-obese PCOS in older infertile patients, a diagnosis currently widely overlooked. At young ages, AMH and androgens easily differentiate women with PCOS and LFOR from women with NFOR. At older ages, the differential diagnosis, as Table 1 and Fig. 1 demonstrate becomes significantly more complex.

While TT and FT levels statistically differentiated young PCOS patients from women with LFOR and NFOR, these markers, as here demonstrated, become inadequate at older ages. In contrast, AMH levels appear to maintain their differentiating power even into older age, therefore allowing for the identification of PCOS regardless of age.

AMH, therefore, in PCOS women of advanced reproductive age should be considered a better disease marker than T, supporting the incorporation of AMH levels into updated criteria for the diagnosis of PCOS at all ages [28]. Conversely, T should not be relied upon in the diagnosis of PCOS in older women.

Conclusions

These data suggest that the "classical" PCOS phenotype with elevated BMI only rarely reaches tertiary infertility care. If confirmed, non-obese PCOS patients may be more resistant to lower levels of infertility treatments. They with advancing age also demonstrate more precipitous T than AMH declines. Low and high BMI

PCOS patients may, therefore, reflect distinctively different pathophysiologies. These data also suggest that AMH at all ages is a better diagnostic criterion for PCOS than T.

Abbreviations
PCOS: Polycystic ovary syndrome; LFOR: Low functional ovarian reserve; NFOR: Normal functional ovarian reserve; TT: Total Testosterone; FT: Free testosterone; AMH: Anti-Müllerian hormone; SHBG: Sex hormone binding globulin; POP: Polycystic ovary phenotype; BMI: Body mass index; oPOI: Occult primary ovarian insufficiency; CI: Confidence intervals; SMK: Student-Newman-Keuls; APF: Androgen production factor; FSH: Follicle stimulating hormone; T: Testosterone.

Competing interest
V.A.K and N.H. have no conflicts to report. N.G. and D.H.B. are listed as co-owners of a number of already awarded and still pending U.S. patents, involving androgen supplementation of women with LFOR. N.G. is a shareholder in Fertility Nutraceuticals, LLC and owner of the Center for Human Reproduction (CHR), where this study was conducted. N.G. and D.H.B receive patent royalties from Fertility Nutraceuticals, LLC. This study was supported by intramural funds from The Center for Human Reproduction and financial contributions from The Foundation for Reproductive Medicine, a not-for-profit foundation. Some data in this manuscript were presented at the 2015 Endocrine Society Meeting in San Diego, CA.

Authors' contributions
V.A.K., N.H., D.H.B., and N.G., were responsible for study design; V.A.K. and N.H. acquired the data. D.H.B. and V.A.K. analyzed and interpreted the data; V.A.K. and N.G. wrote the manuscript. D.F.A. contributed to the manuscript. All authors read and approved of the final manuscript.

Author details
[1]Center for Human Reproduction, 21 East 69th Street, New York, NY 10021, USA. [2]Wake Forest School of Medicine, Winston-Salem, NC, USA. [3]Sackler School of Medicine, Tel Aviv University, Tel Aviv, Israel. [4]Foundation for Reproductive Medicine, New York, NY, USA. [5]University of Kansas, Lawrence, KS, USA. [6]Rockefeller University, New York, NY, USA.

References
1. Lujan ME, Jarrett BY, Brooks ED, Reines JK, Peppin AK, Muhn N, et al. Updated ultrasound criteria for polycystic ovary syndrome: reliable thresholds for elevated follicle population and ovarian volume. Hum Reprod. 2013;28:1361–8.
2. Rotterdam ESHRE/ASRM-Sponsored PCOS consensus workshop group. Revised 2003 consensus on diagnostic criteria and long-term health risks related to polycystic ovary syndrome (PCOS). Hum Reprod. 2004;19:41–7.
3. Thessaloniki ESHRE/ASRM-Sponsored PCOS Consensus Workshop Group. Consensus on infertility treatment related to polycystic ovary syndrome. Hum Reprod. 2008;23:462–77.
4. Fauser BC. Consensus on women's health aspects of polycystic ovary syndrome (PCOS): the Amsterdam ESHRE/ASRM-Sponsored 3rd PCOS Consensus Workshop Group. Fertil Steril. 2012;97:28–38.e25.
5. Wild RA. Assessment of cardiovascular risk and prevention of cardiovascular disease in women with the polycystic ovary syndrome: a consensus statement by the Androgen Excess and Polycystic Ovary Syndrome (AE-PCOS) Society. J Clin Endocrinol Metab. 2010;95:2038–49.
6. Azziz R. Positions statement: criteria for defining polycystic ovary syndrome as a predominantly hyperandrogenic syndrome: an Androgen Excess Society guideline. J Clin Endocrinol Metab. 2006;91:4237–45.
7. Azziz R. The Androgen Excess and PCOS Society criteria for the polycystic ovary syndrome: the complete task force report. Fertil Steril. 2009;91:456–88.
8. Balen A. The pathophysiology of polycystic ovary syndrome: trying to understand PCOS and its endocrinology. Best Pract Res Clin Obstet Gynaecol. 2004;18:685–706.
9. Orio F, Palomba S. Reproductive endocrinology: New guidelines for the diagnosis and treatment of PCOS. Nat Rev Endocrinol. 2014;10:130–2.

10. Brown ZA, Louwers YV, Fong SL, Valkenburg O, Birnie E, de Jong FH, et al. The phenotype of polycystic ovary syndrome ameliorates with aging. Fertil Steril. 2011;96:1259–65.

11. Prizant H, Gleicher N, Sen A. Androgen actions in the ovary: balance is key. J Endocrinol. 2014;222:R141–151.

12. Kushnir MM, Blamires T, Rockwood AL, Roberts WL, Yue B, Erdogan E, et al. Liquid chromatography-tandem mass spectrometry assay for androstenedione, dehydroepiandrosterone, and testosterone with pediatric and adult reference intervals. Clin Chem. 2010;56:1138–47.

13. Gleicher N, Kim A, Weghofer A, Shohat-Tal A, Lazzaroni E, Lee HJ, et al. Starting and resulting testosterone levels after androgen supplementation determine at all ages in vitro fertilization (IVF) pregnancy rates in women with diminished ovarian reserve (DOR). J Assist Reprod Genet. 2013;30:49–62.

14. Dewailly D. Definition and significance of polycystic ovarian morphology: a task force report from the Androgen Excess and Polycystic Ovary Syndrome Society. Hum Reprod Update. 2014;20:334–52.

15. Alsamarai S, Adams JM, Murphy MK, Post MD, Hayden DL, Hall JE, et al. Criteria for polycystic ovarian morphology in polycystic ovary syndrome as a function of age. J Clin Endocrinol Metab. 2009;94:4961–70.

16. Gleicher N, Kim A, Weghofer A, Kushnir VA, Shohat-Tal A, Lazzaroni E, et al. Hypoandrogenism in association with diminished functional ovarian reserve. Hum Reprod. 2013;28:1084–91.

17. Kiddy DS. Differences in clinical and endocrine features between obese and non-obese subjects with polycystic ovary syndrome: an analysis of 263 consecutive cases. Clin Endocrinol (Oxf). 1990;32:213–20.

18. Sen A, Kushnir VA, Barad DH, Gleicher N. Endocrine autoimmune diseases and female infertility. Nat Rev Endocrinol. 2014;10(1):37–50.

19. Barad DH, Weghofer A, Gleicher N. Utility of age-specific serum anti-Mullerian hormone concentrations. Reprod Biomed Online. 2011;22:284–91.

20. Gleicher N, Kim A, Kushnir V, Weghofer A, Shohat-Tal A, Lazzaroni E, et al. Clinical Relevance of Combined FSH and AMH Observations in Infertile Women. J Clin Endocrinol Metab. 2013;98:2136–45.

21. Kumar A, Kalra B, Patel A, McDavid L, Roudebush WE. Development of a second generation anti-Mullerian hormone (AMH) ELISA. J Immunol Methods. 2010;362:51–9.

22. Ezeh U, Yildiz BO, Azziz R. Referral bias in defining the phenotype and prevalence of obesity in polycystic ovary syndrome. J Clin Endocrinol Metab. 2013;98:E1088–1096.

23. Pellatt L, Hanna L, Brincat M, Galea R, Brain H, Whitehead S, et al. Granulosa cell production of anti-Mullerian hormone is increased in polycystic ovaries. J Clin Endocrinol Metab. 2007;92:240–5.

24. Shi D, Vine DF. Animal models of polycystic ovary syndrome: a focused review of rodent models in relationship to clinical phenotypes and cardiometabolic risk. Fertil Steril. 2012;98:185–93.

25. Sen A, Prizant H, Light A, Biswas A, Hayes E, Lee HJ, et al. Androgens regulate ovarian follicular development by increasing follicle stimulating hormone receptor and microRNA-125b expression. Proc Natl Acad Sci U S A. 2014;111:3008–13.

26. Barad DH, Kushnir VA, Lee HJ, Lazzaroni E, Gleicher N. Effect of inter-cycle interval on oocyte production in humans in the presence of the weak androgen DHEA and follicle stimulating hormone: a case–control study. Reprod Biol Endocrinol. 2014;12:68.

27. Gleicher N, Barad DH. Dehydroepiandrosterone (DHEA) supplementation in diminished ovarian reserve (DOR). Reprod Biol Endocrinol. 2011;9:67.

28. Pigny P, Jonard S, Robert Y, Dewailly D. Serum anti-Mullerian hormone as a surrogate for antral follicle count for definition of the polycystic ovary syndrome. J Clin Endocrinol Metab. 2006;91:941–5.

11

Effect of oral administration of low-dose follicle stimulating hormone on hyperandrogenized mice as a model of polycystic ovary syndrome

Irene Tessaro[1], Silvia C. Modina[1,2], Federica Franciosi[1], Giulia Sivelli[1], Laura Terzaghi[1], Valentina Lodde[1] and Alberto M. Luciano[1,2*] (iD)

Abstract

Background: Polycystic Ovary Syndrome (PCOS) is a widespread reproductive disorder characterized by a disruption of follicular growth and anovulatory infertility. In women with PCOS, follicular growth and ovulation can be induced by subcutaneous injections of low doses of follicle stimulating hormone (FSH). The aim of this study was to determine the effect of oral administration of recombinant human FSH (rhFSH) on follicle development in a PCOS murine model. Moreover, since it is unlikely that intact rhFSH is present into the circulation after oral administration, the biological activity of a peptide fragment, derived from the predicted enzymatic cleavage sites with the FSH molecule, was investigated *in vitro* on cumulus-enclosed oocytes (COCs).

Methods: Female peripubertal mice were injected with dehydroepiandrosterone (DHEA) diluted in sesame oil for 20 consecutive days and orally treated with a saline solution of rhFSH. A control group received only sesame oil and saline solution. At the end of treatments, blood was analyzed for hormone concentrations and ovaries were processed for morphological analysis. The presumptive bioactive peptide was added during *in vitro* maturation of bovine COCs and the effects on cumulus expansion and on maturation rate were evaluated.

Results: DHEA treatment increased serum levels of testosterone, estradiol and progesterone as well as the percentage of cystic follicles. Orally administered rhFSH restored estradiol level and reduced the percentage of cystic follicles. Despite these results indicating a reduction of the severity of PCOS in the mouse model, the presumptive bioactive peptide did not mimic the effect of rhFSH and failed to induce bovine cumulus expansion and oocyte maturation *in vitro*.

Conclusions: Although further studies are needed, the present data supports the concept that orally administrated FSH could attenuate some of the characteristic of PCOS in the mouse model.

Keywords: Polycystic ovary syndrome, Ovary, Follicle cyst, Mouse, Oral administration, Bioactive peptides, Gonadotropins, Animal model

Background

Polycystic Ovary Syndrome (PCOS) is a widespread reproductive and endocrinologic disorder, which accounts for approximately 80 % of women with anovulatory infertility [1, 2]. PCOS is characterized by hyperandrogenism and

polycystic ovaries, in addition to anovulation [3]. This syndrome can also be associated with metabolic issues including obesity, insulin resistance, hyperinsulinemia, and type 2 diabetes mellitus, besides cardiovascular problems, breast and endometrial cancers, and neurological and psychological effects on quality of life [4, 5].

In affected women, the normal ovarian function is disturbed mostly by hyperandrogenism and by the elevated serum concentrations of luteinizing hormone (LH, [6, 7]), thus resulting in multiple small cysts [8, 9]. A nearly universal finding in PCOS is an increased gonadotropin-releasing hormone (GnRH) pulse frequency, which favors

* Correspondence: alberto.luciano@unimi.it
[1]Reproductive and Developmental Biology Laboratory, Department of Health, Animal Science and Food Safety, Università degli Studi di Milano, Via Celoria 10, Milan 20133, Italy
[2]Interdepartmental Research Centre for the Study of Biological Effects of Nano-concentrations (CREBION), Università degli Studi di Milano, Via Celoria 10, Milan 20133, Italy

LH production over follicle stimulating hormone (FSH) [10, 11]. The increased LH subsequently promotes theca cell production of androgens, while the relative FSH deficiency reduces the ability of granulosa cells to convert androgen into estrogen and impairs follicle maturation and ovulation [12].

Ovulation induction protocols can be used to restore fertility in PCOS patients [13]. One protocol involves ovarian stimulation by subcutaneous FSH injection [13, 14]. However, because of the large number of small antral follicles that are sensitive to FSH [15], women with PCOS have a higher risk in developing ovarian hyper-stimulation syndrome (OHSS) in response to FSH treatment [16]. To reduce this risk, low-dose administrations of injectable FSH have been used [17, 18]. For this purpose, the most appropriate regime is the step-up protocol, in which the FSH dose is gradually increased until follicular development is observed, and then maintained until follicular selection is achieved [19, 20].

Regardless of good pregnancy and live birth rates [17], ovarian stimulation with FSH is actually considered a second-line treatment for the PCOS patients with infertility [13]. This is mainly due to the lack of an oral formulation, the elevated price, and the potentially severe adverse effects, such as multiple pregnancy and OHSS (reviewed in [13]). The basic concern about oral formulation is the low bioavailability of FSH that stem from stomach enzymatic degradation and poor penetration of FSH peptides across the intestinal membrane [21, 22]. As a consequence it is clear that the research leading to improved oral FSH therapy could ultimately lead to the development of innovative and more comfortable treatments for PCOS.

Androgen-treated rodents have been widely used as models to study both reproductive and metabolic deficits of PCOS (reviewed in [23–25]). These studies demonstrate that dihydroepiandrosterone (DHEA) is able to induce many of the salient features of the human PCOS condition, such as hyperandrogenism, insulin resistance, altered steroidogenesis, acyclicity, abnormal maturation of ovarian follicles, and anovulation in rodents models [26–29]. Then the present work aims to assess first of all, the effect of oral administration of low-dose FSH on the morphological and endocrine function of the ovaries of hyperandrogenized mice. Subsequently, since intact FSH is unlikely to be transferred from the gastrointestinal tract into the circulation, the effect of a minimal amino acid sequence, derived from the analysis of the enzymatic cleavage sites, was analyzed on an *in vitro* system of bovine oocyte maturation (IVM). Recombinant human FSH is commonly used in *in vitro* maturation to stimulate meiotic resumption and cumulus expansion both for research purpose and for application in assisted

reproductive technologies in bovine *in vitro* embryo production [30–34] and its effectiveness is sustained by a growing body of literature. Moreover, the bovine IVM model represents a highly standardized protocol [35, 36], particularly efficient and versatile, which allows at the same time to limit the use and sacrifice of experimental animals.

Methods

All procedures were carried out in accredited animal care facilities at the University of Milan, maintained by the Center for Laboratory Animal Care. The experimental protocol was approved by the University of Milan Ethics Committee and by the Responsible for Laboratory Animal Care veterinarian and in accordance with National (Italian DLT 27/01/1992 n. 116) and European (European Directive 86/609/EEC on Animal Care and use for scientific and other experimental purposes) legislation.

The chemicals used in this study were purchased from Sigma Chemical Company (St. Louis, MO, USA) except for those specifically mentioned.

Hyper-androgenization and hormonal treatment

Female Balb/c mice (Charles River Laboratories Italia s.r.l., Calco, LC, Italy) were maintained on 12-h light, 12-h dark cycles and given food and water *ad libitum*.

All experiments were performed using mice at postnatal day 40 and of weight ranging from 14 to 19 g. In order to hyper-androgenize mice, daily subcutaneous (SC) injection of dehydroepiandrosterone (DHEA; 1.2 mg/mouse/day, derived from 6 mg/100 g body weight [37]) dissolved in 0.1 ml sesame oil were performed for 20 consecutive days. To study the effect of oral administration of recombinant human FSH on PCOS-induced animals, three groups of 8 mice each were used (see the Experimental Design in Table 1). Simultaneously to DHEA treatment, one group (DHEA+rhFSH) received 0.02 IU of rhFSH (Gonal-F, Merck-Serono, Darmstradt, Germany) deriving from the dose of 50 IU in women [17] and recalculated according to the body weight average in the mouse in a total volume of 0.1 ml of saline solution,

Table 1 Experimental design

Treatments	SC injection	PO administration		
CTRL	Sesame oil	Saline solution		
DHEA	DHEA (1.2 mg)	Saline solution		
DHEA+rhFSH	DHEA (1.2 mg)	rhFSH		
		1st week	2nd week	3rd week
		0.02 IU	0.03 IU	0.04 IU

Daily sub-cutaneous (SC) injection and *per os* (PO) administration for each experimental group composed of 8 mice. The total volume for both the SC injection and the PO administration is 0.1 ml of sesame oil or of saline solution respectively. The treatment continued for 20 consecutive days administred directly into the stomach of mice via oral gavage, once a day for 1 week, with progressive increases of 50 % of initial dose each week for a total of 3 weeks in a step-up approach (Table 1). A second group (DHEA) was treated only with DHEA by SC administration and saline by oral gavage, as previously described. The last group served as controls (CTRL) and only received sesame oil subcutaneously and saline solution by oral gavage throughout the experiment. The body weight of animals was measured at the beginning and at the end of the 20-days treatments.

Hormonal analysis of serum

After 20 consecutive days of treatments, blood samples were collected from each mouse before sacrifice. To separate serum, blood was kept at 4 °C for 1 h, followed by two consecutive centrifugations for 10 min at 15000 g at 4 °C. Serum was kept at –20 °C until hormonal assay was performed. Analysis of Testosterone (T) was performed employing a competitive inhibition enzyme immunoassay technique (Mouse Testosterone ELISA Kit, CSB-E05101m, Cusabio, Hubei Province, China; minimum detectable concentration (minDC) = 0.1 ng/ml; intra-assay and inter-assay precisions (mean of the percentages of coefficients of variation) are both <15 %). According to the manufacturer's instructions, no significant cross-reactivity or interference between mouse testosterone and analogues was observed. Levels of Progesterone (P4), Estradiol (E2) and LH were measured using a magnetic bead immunoassay based on Luminex Multiplex System (Merck Millipore, Darmstadt, Germany), according to the manufacturer's instructions; respectively E2 and P4 were analyzed by the "Steroid/Thyroid Hormone Magnetic Bead Panel" (# STTHMAG-21K; minDC = 0.02 ng/ml for E2 and 0.09 ng/ml for P4; intra-assay and inter-assay precisions are <10 % for both analytes), while the "Mouse Pituitary Magnetic Bead Panel" (# MPTMAG-49K; minDC = 1.34 pg/ml; intra-assay precision <15 % and inter-assay precision <20 %) was used for LH.

Morphological evaluation of ovaries

The ovaries were collected immediately after sacrifice and fixed in 10 % neutral buffered formalin (Bio-Optica, Milan, Italy) over night. The ovaries were dehydrated in a graded series of ethanol, cleared with xylene, embedded in paraffin (Bio-Optica) and serially sectioned at 4 μm. Slices were placed on glass microscope slides in traceable order, stained with hematoxylin and eosin (DDK Italia, Vigevano, Italy) and finally analyzed under light microscopy to assess follicles diameter and morphological features [38].

In order to select a representative follicular population to be analyzed in each ovary, we considered one slice every 150 μm (i.e. every 37 sections), resulting in a mean of 4 slices for each ovary. These slices were used to identify the antral follicles to be measured. For each follicle, measurements and morphological evaluation were than conducted on the neighboring slices containing the corresponding equatorial section. The follicle diameter was calculated as the mean distance between opposite basal membrane portions, while the wall thickness was calculated as the sum of theca interna and granulosa cell layers. Averages from three different measurements were considered. The follicular population was divided in two classes according to follicle diameter: 150–300 μm (early-small antral follicles) and >300 μm (large antral follicles) [39–41]. Moreover the presence of morphological cystic signs, as previously described [26, 27, 42–44]), were recorded for each antral follicle. Two investigators performed morphological analysis independently.

Immunoexpression of aromatase cytochrome P450

Indirect immunohistochemistry was carried out to evaluate the expression and localization of aromatase cytochrome P450 (P450 arom). Before immunohistochemical staining, sections were routinely deparaffinized, rehydrated and successively heated in a microwave oven in 0.01 M citrate buffer. Then sections were incubated with 10 % (v/v) normal rabbit serum, 0.3 % (v/v) Triton X-100 and 3 % (w/v) bovine serum albumin (BSA) in phosphate buffered saline (PBS) for 30 min to block non-specific binding of secondary antibody. Sections were incubated overnight at 4 °C with 4 μg/ml of polyclonal goat anti-CYP19 (CYP19 (C-16): sc-14245, Santa Cruz Biotechnologies, Inc, Dallas, TX, USA;) diluted in PBS with 1 % (w/v) BSA and 0.3 % (v/v) Triton X-100. Primary antibody was detected by using an Alexa Fluor 488-labeled rabbit anti-goat IgG (diluted 1:1000 in PBS with 1 % (w/v) of BSA. Negative controls were performed by omitting the primary antibody. The sections were mounted with an antifade medium Vecta Shield (Vector Laboratories, Inc., Burlingame, CA, USA) supplemented with 1 μg/ml 4′,6-diamidino-2-phenylindole (DAPI). Samples were analyzed on an epifluorescence microscope (Eclipse E600, Nikon Corp., Tokyo, Japan) at a magnification of 200–400×.

FSH-derived bioactive peptide synthesis

The FSH sequence ([Uniprot: P01225]; www.uniprot.org/uniprot/P01225; www.rcsb.org/pdb/explore/explore.do?structureId=1XWD) was examined for cleavage sites using Peptide Cutter (web.expasy.org; [45]), a tool that predicts potential digestion sites cleaved by pepsin, trypsin and chymotrypsin. This process resulted in the identification of a peptide sequence of the beta-subunit that likely maintains the biological activity of intact FSH and is composed of amino acids 95–121 (Fig. 1 and Additional file 1: Figure S1). This sequence possesses the amino

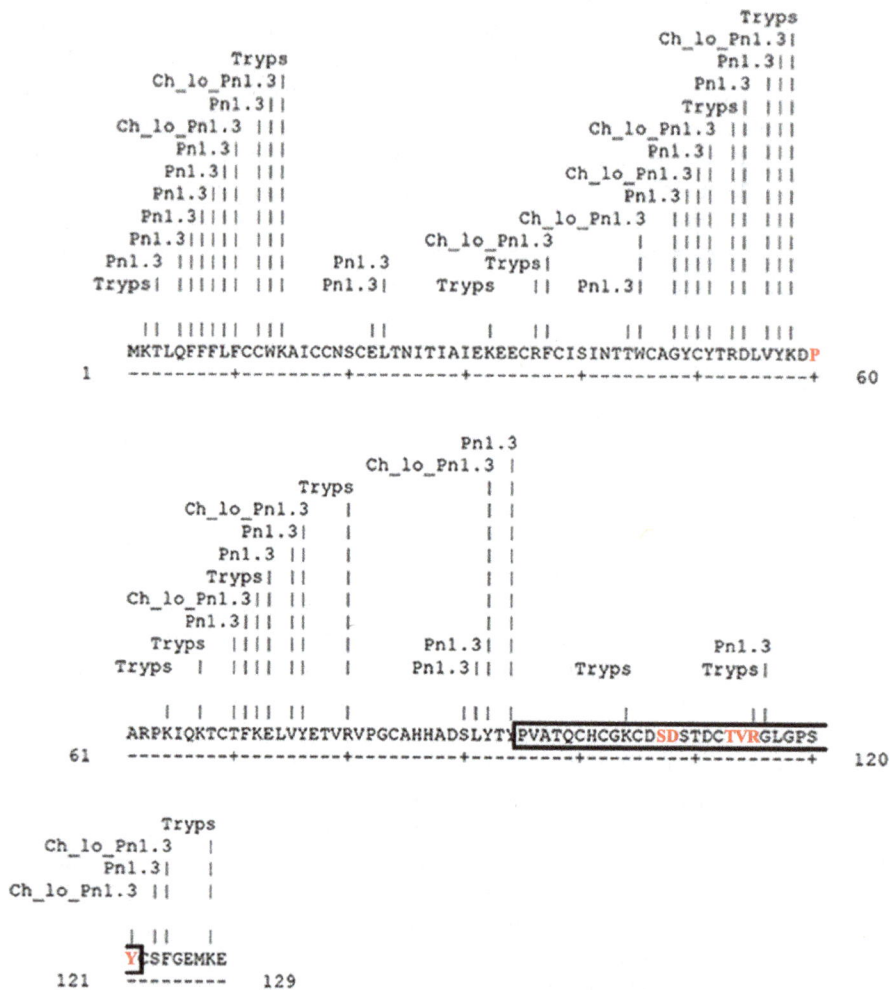

Fig. 1 Map of follitropin beta-subunit cleavage sites from stomach and pancreatic proteases digestion: pepsin, trypsin, chymotrypsin. The image derives from resource web portals *web.expasy.org* and databases for protein sequences www.uniprot.org; www.rcsb.org/pdb/). This tool predicts cleavage sites of selected proteases in a protein sequence, in this case pepsin (*Pn1.3*), trypsin (*Tryps*), chymotrypsin (*Ch_Lo*). In the map, the cleavage probability of trypsin and chymotrypsin is 70 % at least. Cleavage occurs at the right side (C-terminal direction) of the marked amino acid. Specific residues for hFSH-receptor binding in the follitropin beta-subunit [48] are identify in *red*. The highlighted peptide sequence composed of amino acids 95–121 likely maintains the biological activity of intact FSH, based on our in silico analysis, and it was used for *in vitro* assay

acid sequence involved in binding to the FSH receptor [46–48]. The identified peptide of 27 amino acids has been chemically synthetized (PRIMM Biotech, Milan, Italy) at a high degree of purity (>95 %) for subsequent biological evaluations.

Assessment of biological activity of FSH-derived peptide

The activity of the peptide sequence was tested on our standard *in vitro* maturation (IVM) protocol [49]. As biological endpoints, cumulus expansion and meiotic maturation rate were evaluated at the end of IVM period [36].

Bovine ovaries were recovered at the abattoir (INALCA Spa., Ospedaletto Lodigiano, LO, IT 2270M CE, Italy) from pubertal females (4–8 years old) subjected to routine veterinary inspection and in accordance to the specific health requirements stated in Council Directive 89/556/ECC and subsequent modifications. Ovaries were transported to the laboratory within 2 h in sterile saline at 26 °C. All subsequent procedures, unless differently specified, were performed at 35–38 °C and carried out as previously described [50]. Cumulus-oocyte complexes (COCs) were retrieved from mid-sized antral follicles (2–6 mm) with a 16-gauge needle mounted on an aspiration pump (COOK-IVF, Brisbane QLD, Australia) in M199 supplemented with 20 mM HEPES, 1790 units/L heparin and 0.4 % BSA. After examination under a stereomicroscope, only COCs medium-brown in color, with five or more complete layers of cumulus cells enclosing an oocyte with finely granulated homogenous ooplasm were used. Selected COCs were individually cultured for 24 h in M-199 added with 0.68 mM L-glutamine,

25 mM $NaHCO_3$, 0.4 % BSA fatty acid free and 0.2 mM sodium pyruvate in humidified air under 5 % CO_2 at 38.5 °C. The basic culture medium was then supplemented with 10^{-1} IU/ml of rhFSH (as in standard IVM in bovine oocytes [51]) or with the peptide (at the same molar concentration), or not supplemented (control group). A picture for each COC was taken before and at the end of *in vitro* culture and cumulus expansion was calculated as ratio between final cumulus area and initial cumulus area. Cumulus area was measured by ImageJ 1.48v (National Institute of Health, USA; [52]) tools. Oocytes were then mechanically freed from cumulus cells and fixed in 500 μl of 60 % Methanol in Dulbecco's Phosphate Buffered Saline for 30 min at 4 °C. The oocytes were then stained with 0.5 mg/ml of Propidium Iodide to evaluate meiotic stage by observation at 200–400× under fluorescence microscopy [50]. About 30 COCs were analyzed for each group during three different runs.

Statistical analysis
Statistical analyses were performed using Prism Graph-Pad (GraphPad Software, version 6.0f, San Diego, CA, USA). *In vivo* data were analyzed by one-way ANOVA, followed by Fisher's Least Significant Difference (LSD) multiple comparison test. Fisher's exact test was used to compare the percentages of atretic/cystic follicles on the total follicle population. Data of cumulus expansion assay were tested for Gaussian distribution using Kolmogorov-Smirnov test. Since these data were not normally distributed, Kruskal-Wallis test, followed by Dunn's multiple comparison test was used to analyze the cumulus expansion data. Regardless of the test P values <0.05 were considered significant.

Results
Body weight increase
To investigate the effect of different hormonal treatments on the body mass, mice were weighted during experimentation. Before treatment the body mass of

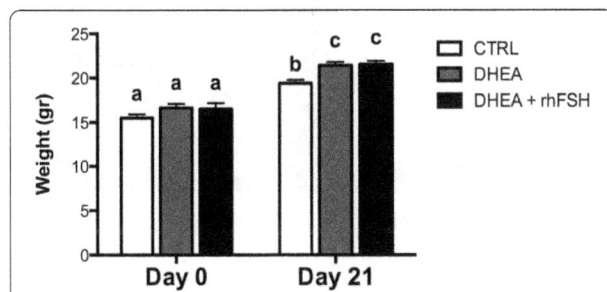

Fig. 2 Effect of different hormonal treatments on body weight of mice at day 0 and 21. Data were analyzed by one-way ANOVA, followed by Fisher's LSD multiple comparison test; different letters indicate significant differences between groups (P <0.05)

animals was not statistically different between groups (Fig. 2). Mice increased in weight during the treatment phase of this experiment but those treated with DHEA gained approximately 10 % more than controls (Fig. 2).

Hormonal analysis of serum
The effect of low dose administration of rhFSH on the serum hormonal profiles was evaluated using immunoassay techniques. Results are illustrated in Fig. 3. Testosterone and P4 concentration were statistically higher in all the PCOS-induced animals (DHEA treated) compared to CTRL, irrespectively to rhFSH administration (Fig. 3a and b respectively). E2 analysis revealed that while DHEA significantly increased serum E2 concentration compared to CTRL, DHEA+rhFSH treatment was able to restore E2 concentration statistically similar to the CTRL (Fig. 3c). Finally DHEA alone or with rhFSH resulted in a statistical decrease of LH concentration respect to CTRL (Fig. 3d).

Morphological evaluation of ovaries
To study the potential role of the oral administration of low doses of rhFSH on follicle development in DHEA-treated animals, the number of follicles 150–300 μm in diameter and of follicles >300 μm in diameter was monitored in each ovary. DHEA statistically reduced the number of small follicles per ovary independently from rhFSH (Fig. 4a). On the other hand, DHEA in the presence or absence of rhFSH importantly increases the number of larger follicles per ovary, but rhFSH attenuated DHEA's actions, significantly reducing large follicle population (Fig. 4b).

The number of granulosa cells as assessed by the thickness of the theca and granulosa cell layers was decreased by DHEA (P <0.05), irrespective of rhFSH administration, in the large (>300 μm) follicles (Fig. 5) but not in 150–300 μm follicles (data not shown).

Finally, morphological signs of progressive follicle atresia and cystic formations were observed (Fig. 6, upper panel). These include granulosa cell pyknosis (Fig. 6b), disruption of the basement membrane (indicated by asterisks in Fig. 6b, c, d) and granulosa cells layers (pointed out by white arrows in Figs. 6b and c) as well as invasion of blood cells, the presence of elongated epithelioid cells in the inner surface of the follicle wall (indicated by black arrows in Fig. 6e), macrophages in the cystic fluid (showed by red arrows in Fig. 6f), and reduction of granulosa cells layers. DHEA significantly increased the occurrence of morphological cystic features in antral follicles with a diameter >300 μm per ovary (Fig. 6, lower panel); the oral administration of rhFSH in DHEA-treated mice was able to significantly decrease the percentage of atretic/cystic signs in large follicles, even if it is still higher than CTRL (P <0.05). Moreover in the 150–300 μm follicle

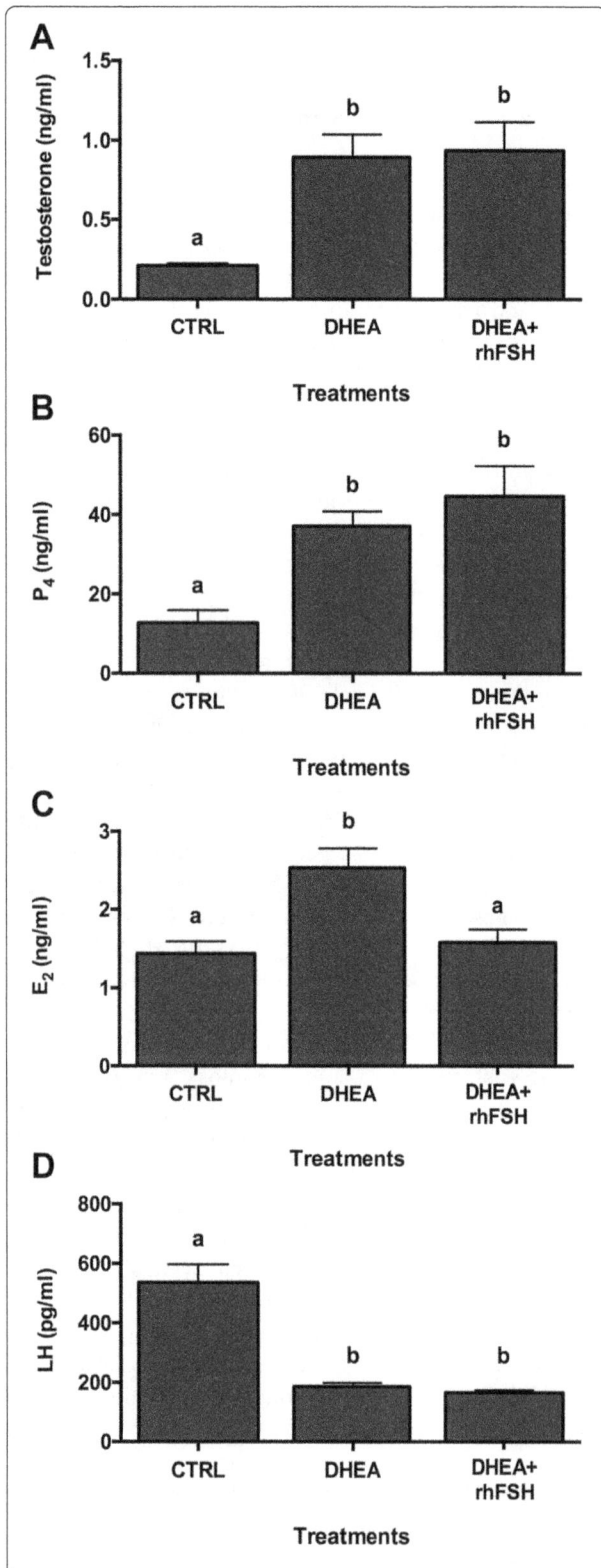

Fig. 3 Effect of different hormonal treatments on Testosterone, Progesterone, Estradiol, and Luteinizing Hormone serum concentration. **a** Testosterone; **b** Progesterone; **c** Estradiol; **d** Luteinizing hormone. Data were analyzed by one-way ANOVA, followed by Fisher's LSD multiple comparison test; in each graph, different letters indicate significant differences between groups (P <0.05)

population, rhFSH administration importantly reduced the percentage of atretic/cystic follicles on total follicular population compared to DHEA treatment alone (Fig. 7).

Localization of aromatase cytochrome P450

In all ovaries regardless the treatment, P450 aromatase protein was absent or weak in 150–300 μm early-small antral follicles (Fig. 8) while was localized in the cytoplasm of granulosa cells in >300 μm large antral follicles, with P450 arom concentrated inside the cytoplasm of

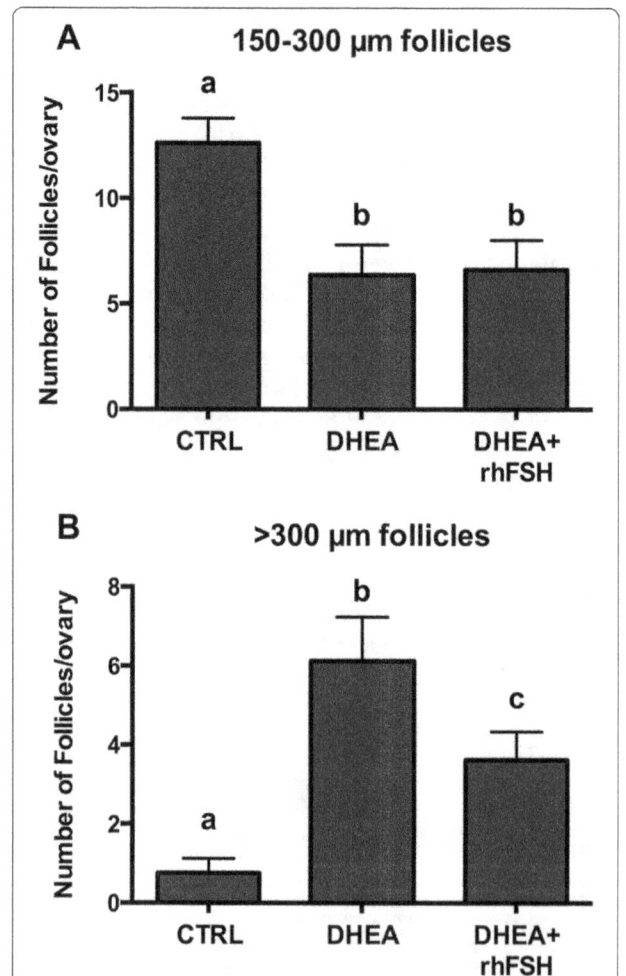

Fig. 4 Effect of hormonal treatments on the number of antral follicles per ovary. **a** antral follicles of 150–300 μm in diameter; **b** antral follicles >300 μm in diameter. Data were analyzed by one-way ANOVA, followed by Fisher's LSD multiple comparison test; in each graph, different letters indicate significant differences between groups (P <0.05)

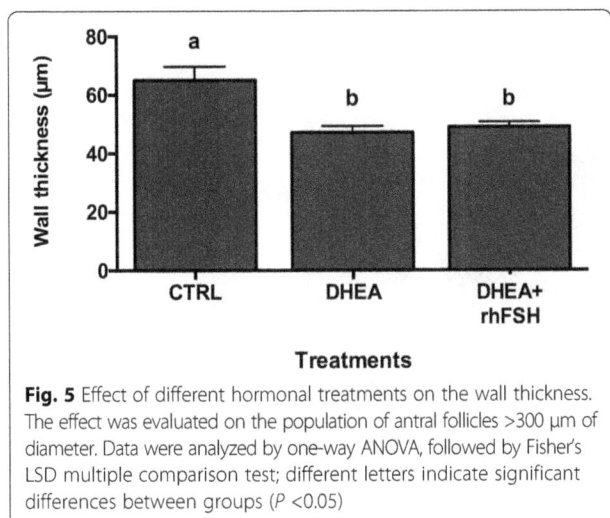

Fig. 5 Effect of different hormonal treatments on the wall thickness. The effect was evaluated on the population of antral follicles >300 µm of diameter. Data were analyzed by one-way ANOVA, followed by Fisher's LSD multiple comparison test; different letters indicate significant differences between groups (P <0.05)

mural cells, lying on the basal membrane (Fig. 8) with little or no staining in the cumulus cells. Control sections did not exhibit any positive staining.

Cumulus expansion and meiotic maturation rate evaluation

The biological effect of the peptide derived from in silico enzymatic digestion of FSH was analyzed on the cumulus expansion and on the maturation rate of bovine COCs. The peptide did not induce cumulus expansion (Fig. 9a), since the ratio between cumulus areas after culture and before culture was similar to that of COCs cultured in absence of FSH (P >0.05). Moreover the FSH peptide was not able to promote oocyte maturation (Fig. 9b), even when used at concentration 100, 1000 or 10000 times higher (data not shown). Moreover, treatment with the peptide concurrently to FSH did not affect the biological effects, since cumulus expansion index and maturation rate were comparable to that of FSH alone (data not shown).

Discussion

Most of the animal models used to understand the development of PCOS-related dysfunctions are based on induced hyperandrogenism [53]. DHEA, an androgen of mainly adrenal origin, is often increased in women with PCOS [54]. Therefore DHEA is utilized to induce PCOS in different rodent models. The dose commonly used (6 mg/100 g body weight) ensures a hyperandrogenized status equivalent to that found in women with PCOS [55]. The treatment that we utilized is commonly used in mice to induce the PCOS phenotype, characterized by infertility and ovaries containing more atretic follicles and follicular cysts [56–58]. Our data confirm the previous finding that DHEA treatment increased the number of large follicles (>300 µm of diameter) per ovary,

simultaneously reducing the small antral follicles population. In addition to the increase in follicles number, our results demonstrated that DHEA treatment induced an increase of the number of large follicles presenting morphological signs of atresia and/or cysts (from 0.0 % in the Control group to 67.26 % ± 3.5 in the DHEA group). Motta and colleagues found that mouse cysts had a thin theca layer and a packed stratum of granulosa cells [55]. These findings are confirmed by our results, since DHEA treated mice exhibit a reduced thickness of follicular wall (theca interna layer plus granulosa cell layer) in the large follicles. We observed also that both serum E2 and P4 levels were increased with induction of cysts formation. These findings are in agreement with other authors [26, 28, 59, 60] who observed increase in both cytochrome P450 17-hydroxylase and steroidogenic acute regulatory protein (StAR) activities in theca cells from women with PCOS, suggesting a global enhancement of steroidogenesis. This is also consistent with studies on cultures of human theca cells derived from follicles isolated from the ovaries of PCOS and normal women where it has been demonstrated that PCOS theca cells produce greater amounts of testosterone, 17-hydroxyprogesterone and P4 than normal theca cells [61]. Although the mechanism for LH hypersecretion described in human PCOS is not entirely clear, some data suggest that it involves impaired negative feedback on LH secretion mediated by either high E2 or P4 levels in women with PCOS [62]. Unexpectedly in our study, serum LH was decreased while LH over-production is commonly considered one of the peculiar trait of PCOS [63]. While in the rat data on the effect of postnatal treatment with DHEA on LH concentration are reported, although contrasting [28, 29, 64], to the best of our knowledge this is the first study showing the effect on LH concentration after 20 days of DHEA administration in the mouse model.

Moreover, our results reveal that DHEA increased animal weight at the end of the treatment. These observations are in agreement with both the wide distribution of obesity in PCOS-affected women [65] and with the characterization of the murine model reported in literature [66].

The therapy of PCOS is focused on ovulation induction in those desiring pregnancy. This may be achieved indirectly with clomiphene citrate (CC), which is an oral selective estrogen receptor modulator which action results in increases in circulating FSH [13], or directly by FSH administration. The first line of treatment, CC, restores ovulation in about 80 %, but will result in pregnancy in only 35 % of patients [67]. Additionally, about 25 % of PCOS women do not respond to CC and are considered to be "clomiphene resistant" [67]. Even though FSH treatment is more effective than CC,

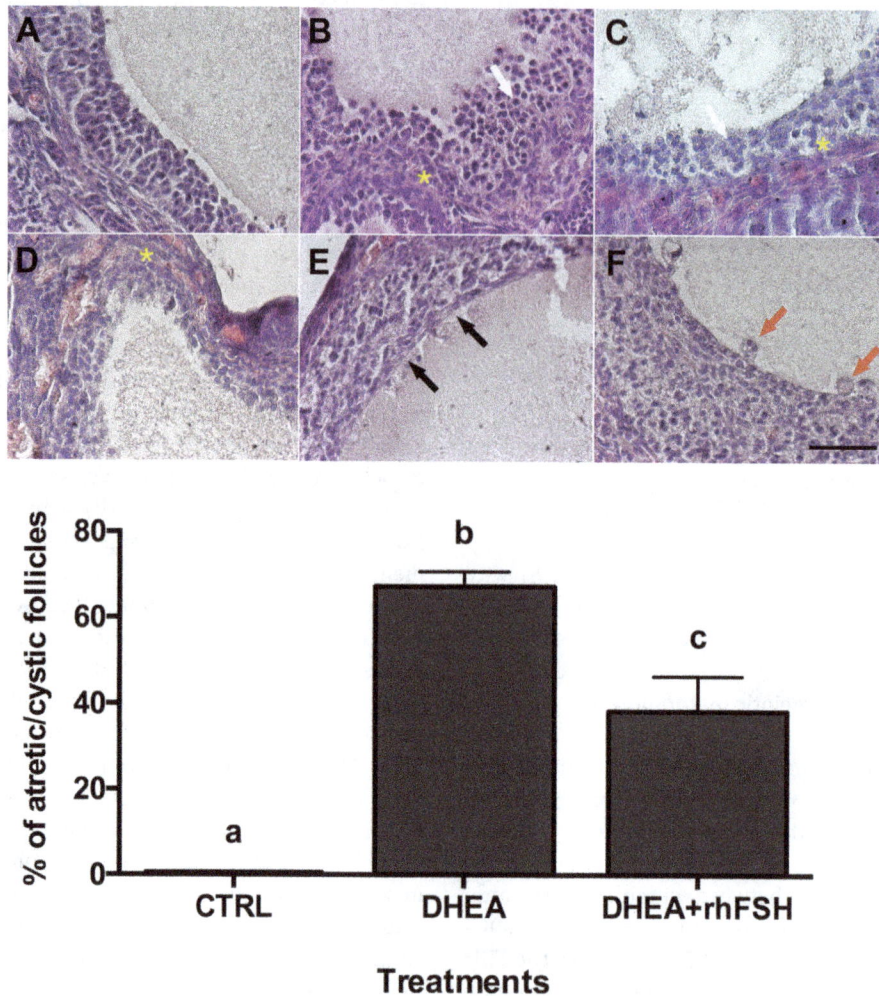

Fig. 6 Effect of different hormonal treatments on the percentage of follicles presenting atretic/cystic signs. *Upper panel* Representative images of typical morphological changes in antral follicle walls of ovaries isolated from controls (**a**) compared to DHEA-treated mice (**b, c, d, e, f**), stained with hematoxylin and eosin. In the control (**a**) theca externa, theca interna, basal membrane and granulosa cells layers appear normal. **b, c** and **d** represent progressive changes associated with follicular atresia (ie. pyknosis, disruption of the basement membrane (*asterisks*) and of granulosa layers (*white arrows*) and invasion of blood cells). Cystic features are described by thin and elongated epithelioid cells in the inner surface of the wall (**e**, *black arrows*) and macrophages in the cystic fluid (**f**, *red arrows*). Bar = 50 μm. *Lower panel* The effect of different hormonal treatment was evaluated on the population of antral follicles >300 μm of diameter. Data were analyzed by one-way ANOVA, followed by Fisher's LSD multiple comparison test; different letters indicate significant differences between groups ($P < 0.05$)

it is still considered a second line of treatment, mainly because of the lack of oral preparation and the risk of adverse effects [13, 14]. In order to reduce the risk of OHSS and multiple pregnancy, low-dose treatment programs have been successfully implemented [17, 18, 20]. The basic thinking behind this regiment is the "threshold theory", which demands the attainment and maintenance of follicular development with exogenous FSH without exceeding the threshold requirement of the ovary [67]. A low starting dose of FSH (usually 50–75 IU) is used for 7–14 days and, if necessary, a weekly 50 % increment of the initial or previous amount is administered until follicular development is initiated [17].

In our study we investigated the possibility of FSH oral administration. Gonadotropins, as most of the drugs constituted by protein formulations, are traditionally delivered via intramuscular, subcutaneous, or intravenous routes because of their reduced oral bioavailability. This is mainly due to the fact that peptides can be readily degraded and pass poorly through the intestinal mucosa [68, 69]. On the other hand, to the best of our knowledge this is the first study reporting that an oral administration of a low dose of rhFSH is able to ameliorate some peculiar features of PCOS in hyper-androgenized mice with treatment using higher doses potentially being more effective. However, this remains to be determined.

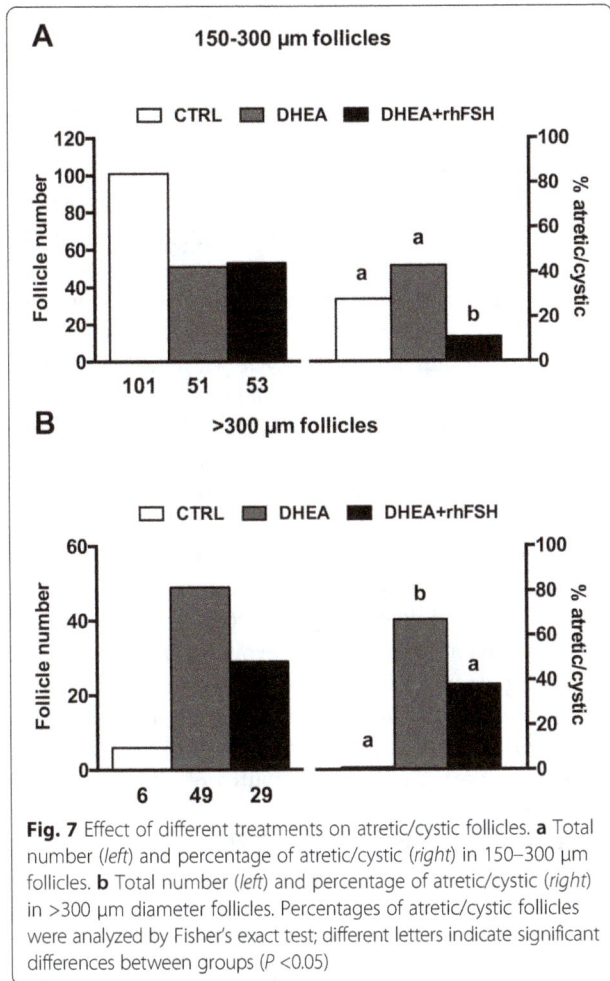

Fig. 7 Effect of different treatments on atretic/cystic follicles. **a** Total number (*left*) and percentage of atretic/cystic (*right*) in 150–300 μm follicles. **b** Total number (*left*) and percentage of atretic/cystic (*right*) in >300 μm diameter follicles. Percentages of atretic/cystic follicles were analyzed by Fisher's exact test; different letters indicate significant differences between groups (*P* <0.05)

During the first week, we orally administered 0.02 IU/die of rhFSH, which was derived from the dose of 50 IU in women and recalculated according to the average body weight in the mouse. The orally administered rhFSH was able both to reduce the number of large antral follicles and at the same time to maintain their viability, while reducing the percentage of atretic and cystic signs. The effect of FSH administration on cystic signs in ovarian follicles has not been extensively investigated, apart from a study in a Guinea pig model, which demonstrated that exogenous FSH treatment effectively reduced the ovarian cyst formation [70]. In our PCOS model, the oral administration of rhFSH normalized estradiol serum concentration. This phenomenon appears to reflect the follicular distribution after the oral administration of rhFSH, since rhFSH treated ovaries have a decrease in large antral follicles number (Fig. 4b) in favor of an increase in the new population of small growing healthy follicles (Fig. 7a). Compared to larger follicles, these smaller growing follicles synthetize and secrete less E2 than the larger follicles [71, 72], and this could account for the reduced E2 in the rhFSH treated mice. Further support from this concept is provided by the immunohistochemical detection of P450 aromatase in >300 μm large antral follicle and not in the smaller follicles. Thus the observed 50 % decrease in serum E2 observed in the rhFSH treated ovaries directly corresponds the 50 % decrease in the number of aromatase expressing follicles.

Thus rhFSH, even though orally administered, seemed to be able to partially restore the physiological status of ovarian follicles considering both morphological and functional aspects. During estrous cycle, FSH stimulates proliferation of granulosa cells in primary follicles, and

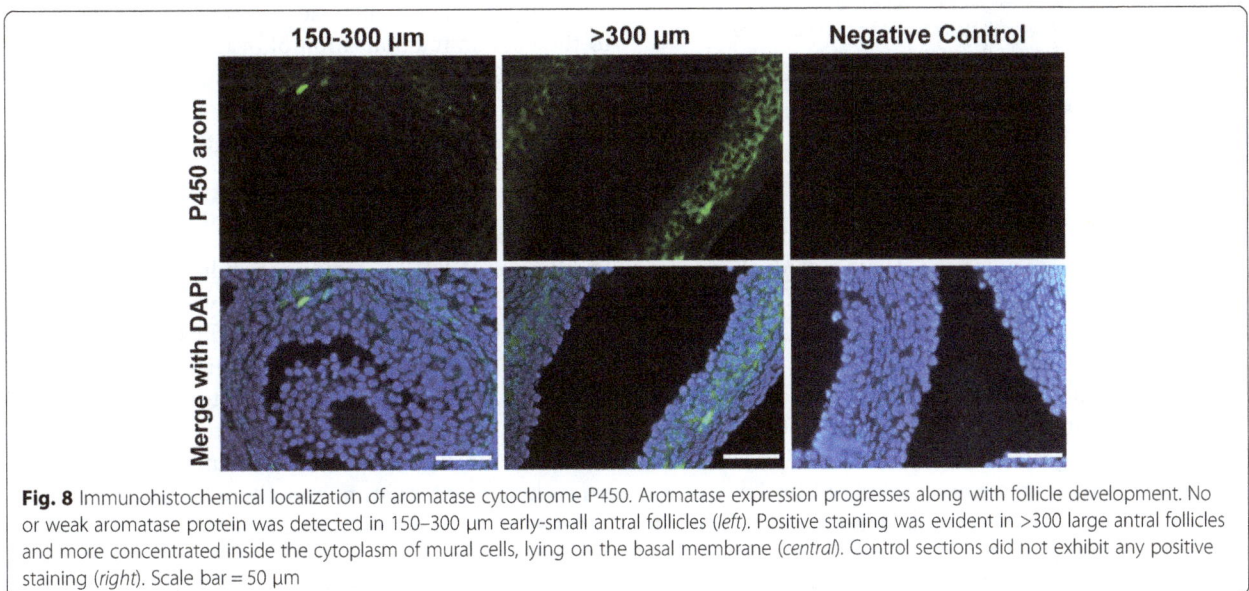

Fig. 8 Immunohistochemical localization of aromatase cytochrome P450. Aromatase expression progresses along with follicle development. No or weak aromatase protein was detected in 150–300 μm early-small antral follicles (*left*). Positive staining was evident in >300 large antral follicles and more concentrated inside the cytoplasm of mural cells, lying on the basal membrane (*central*). Control sections did not exhibit any positive staining (*right*). Scale bar = 50 μm

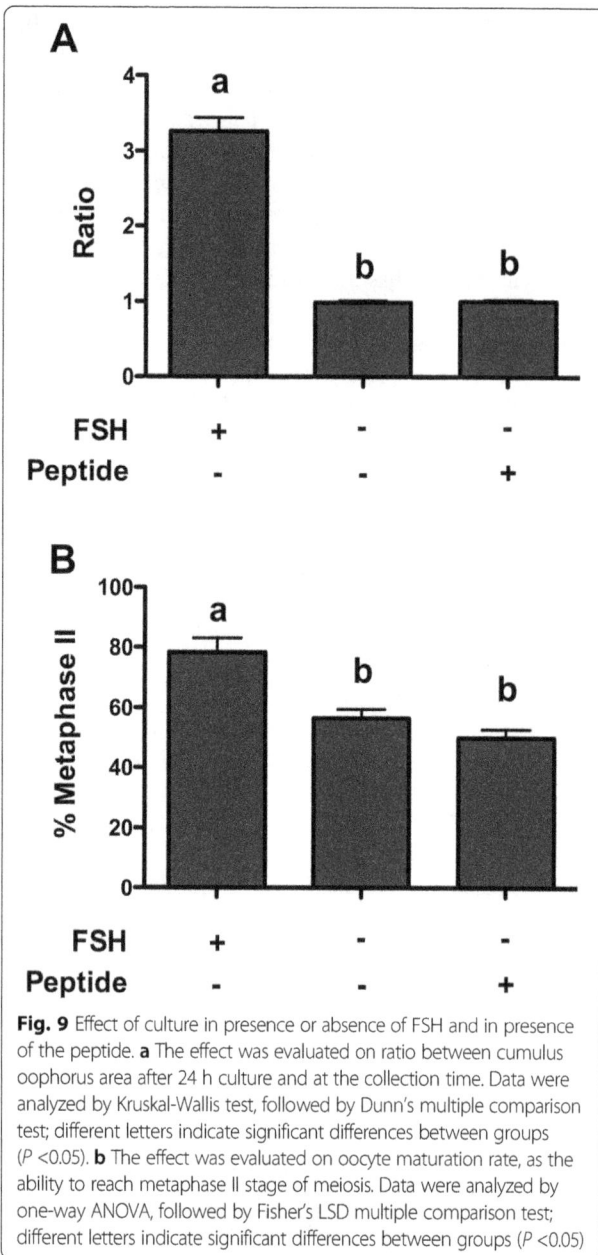

Fig. 9 Effect of culture in presence or absence of FSH and in presence of the peptide. **a** The effect was evaluated on ratio between cumulus oophorus area after 24 h culture and at the collection time. Data were analyzed by Kruskal-Wallis test, followed by Dunn's multiple comparison test; different letters indicate significant differences between groups ($P <0.05$). **b** The effect was evaluated on oocyte maturation rate, as the ability to reach metaphase II stage of meiosis. Data were analyzed by one-way ANOVA, followed by Fisher's LSD multiple comparison test; different letters indicate significant differences between groups ($P <0.05$)

FSH molecule digestion and containing amino acids responsible for specific receptor binding. Our results indicated that the selected peptide (from the amino acid 95–121 of β-chain) is not able to exert biological effects (i.e. cumulus expansion and oocyte maturation) in an *in vitro* model in the bovine species.

On the other hand World Health Organization has calculated that over 10 % of women are inflicted by infertility and subfertility (www.who.int). Assisted reproductive technologies (ART) are well-established treatments, representing substantial economic and healthcare implications for patients. Total number of ART cycle per annum will reach 2 million by the end of 2015 with a forecast cost for therapeutics market that is estimated in about 8 billion of euros. This valuation derived from the mean of direct cost of one fresh ART treatment cycle in several countries [75]. Considering that one treatment cycle is often not enough to achieve the childbirth, the amount is surely underestimated. This framework includes also the therapeutic market linked to PCOS considering also that the pharmaceutical market is evolving in a context of increasing economic pressure, it demands alternative approaches [76]. This situation has contributed to a revival of interest in peptides as potential drug candidates, considering alternative routes of administration. The peptide drug market is also growing twice as fast in the worldwide drug market [77]. Certainly peptides and proteins offer several advantages as compared to conventional drugs. These include high activity, high specificity, low toxicity, and minimal non-specific and drug-drug interactions [22], but the physiological, enzymatic and chemical barriers for oral administration route pose a significant challenge to the delivery of peptide and protein drugs [76]. Then oral delivery of peptides and proteins, and in particular of FSH [78], is currently a topic of intense research, which, together to the economic implication of ovarian stimulation not only in PCOS treatment [22, 78], strongly encourages further investigation in identifying FSH-derived peptides or a combination of peptides that have biologically activity.

Conclusions

In summary, DHEA treatment induced a global increase of Testosterone, E2 and P4 level confirming data from previous studies on DHEA-induced PCOS model in mouse where postnatal treatment of mice with DHEA for 20 consecutive days resulted in most females exhibiting follicular cysts with a thin granulosa cell layer and anovulation, increased numbers of atretic follicles, hyperandrogenism, and altered ovarian steroidogenesis with elevated serum levels of androgens, estrogens and progesterone [26, 55–57, 66, 79, 80]. Several evidences indicate that androgens modulate follicle

once a follicle reaches a diameter of approximately 150 μm, FSH induces antrum formation and aromatase activity within the granulosa cells with a gradual increase in estradiol synthesis [73, 74]. Moreover, our results demonstrate the feasibility of administering effective gonadotropin treatment orally.

However while oral administration is effective, we hypothesize that intact FSH is unlikely to be transferred from the gastrointestinal tract into the circulation, even though we cannot exclude it. In the present study we tested whether a bioactive peptide derived from FSH is functionally active. From this premise, we selected an amino acidic sequence derived from the development from the present and from other studies [81–83]. In particular, androgen-receptor KO mouse models have been used to establish that androgens actions through androgen-receptors are actually necessary for normal ovarian function and female fertility and recently has been demonstrated that androgens regulate ovarian follicular development by increasing follicle stimulating hormone receptors [83]. In the present study FSH treatment restored E2 to the control level and we hypothesize that this maybe due to FSH ability to suppress growth of large follicles >300, where aromatase is more expressed. However, how FSH affects DHEA-mediated follicle development in mouse model is unknown and to the best of our knowledge this is the first study showing FSH capability to modulate its activity. The mechanism involved in this interaction deserves certainly to be the subject of future research.

Finally, our results suggest that oral administration of FSH is able to attenuate some of the characteristic of PCOS in a hyperandrogenized mouse model. Although further investigation in identifying FSH-derived peptides potentially maintaining its proper biological activity are needed, this research could improve our understanding of the pathogenesis as well as lead to the development of innovative, more comfortable and cost effective treatments for PCOS infertility.

Competing interests
The authors declare that they have no competing interests.

Authors' contributions
IT and AML conceived the project, designed the experiments and wrote the manuscript. IT, SCM, VL, LT and FF carried out the experiments. IT and GS performed the morphometric analysis. IT, FF, SCM and AML accomplished statistical analysis and interpretation. All authors revised the manuscript and approved the final version to be published.

Acknowledgements
I.T. was funded by 'Dote Ricercatori' and 'Dote Ricerca Applicata' (FSE, Regione Lombardia, Italy). F.F. was supported by FP7-PEOPLE-2013-IOF Marie Curie Actions - International Outgoing Fellowships within the 7th European Community Framework Programme (Contract: 624874, "MateRNA"). V.L. was supported by - FP7-Marie Curie Actions-CIG - Career Integration Grants within the 7th European Community Framework Programme (Contract: 303640, "Pro-Ovum"). I.T. present address: Laboratory of Biomaterials and Tissue Engineering IRCCS Istituto Ortopedico Galeazzi, Milan, Italy
The authors thank Mrs. Patrizia Luchini for skillful assistance in conducting experiments. The authors greatly thank Dr. John J. Peluso of the Department of Cell Biology of the University of Connecticut Health Center, Farmington CT, USA, for critical reading and for valuable comments and suggestions.

References
1. Thessaloniki ESHRE/ASRM-Sponsored PCOS Consensus Workshop Group. Consensus on infertility treatment related to polycystic ovary syndrome. Fertil Steril. 2008;89(3):505–22.
2. The Amsterdam ESHRE/ASRM-Sponsored 3rd PCOS Consensus Workshop Group. Consensus on women's health aspects of polycystic ovary syndrome (PCOS). Hum Reprod. 2012;27(1):14–24.
3. Barthelmess EK, Naz RK. Polycystic ovary syndrome: current status and future perspective. Front Biosci (Elite Ed). 2014;6:104–19.
4. Sirmans SM, Pate KA. Epidemiology, diagnosis, and management of polycystic ovary syndrome. Clin Epidemiol. 2013;6:1–13.
5. Fauser BC, Tarlatzis BC, Rebar RW, Legro RS, Balen AH, Lobo R, et al. Consensus on women's health aspects of polycystic ovary syndrome (PCOS): the Amsterdam ESHRE/ASRM-Sponsored 3rd PCOS Consensus Workshop Group. Fertil Steril. 2012;97(1):28–38.e25.
6. Balen AH, Schachter ME, Montgomery D, Reid RW, Jacobs HS. Polycystic ovaries are a common finding in untreated female to male transsexuals. Clin Endocrinol (Oxf). 1993;38(3):325–9.
7. Imani B, Eijkemans MJ, te Velde ER, Habbema JD, Fauser BC. A nomogram to predict the probability of live birth after clomiphene citrate induction of ovulation in normogonadotropic oligoamenorrheic infertility. Fertil Steril. 2002;77(1):91–7.
8. Franks S, Stark J, Hardy K. Follicle dynamics and anovulation in polycystic ovary syndrome. Hum Reprod Update. 2008;14(4):367–78.
9. Webber LJ, Stubbs S, Stark J, Trew GH, Margara R, Hardy K, et al. Formation and early development of follicles in the polycystic ovary. Lancet. 2003;362(9389):1017–21.
10. Burt Solorzano CM, Beller JP, Abshire MY, Collins JS, McCartney CR, Marshall JC. Neuroendocrine dysfunction in polycystic ovary syndrome. Steroids. 2012;77(4):332–7.
11. Marshall JC, Dalkin AC, Haisenleder DJ, Paul SJ, Ortolano GA, Kelch RP. Gonadotropin-releasing hormone pulses: regulators of gonadotropin synthesis and ovulatory cycles. Recent Prog Horm Res. 1991;47:155–87. discussion 88–9.
12. McCartney CR, Eagleson CA, Marshall JC. Regulation of gonadotropin secretion: implications for polycystic ovary syndrome. Semin Reprod Med. 2002;20(4):317–26.
13. Perales-Puchalt A, Legro RS. Ovulation induction in women with polycystic ovary syndrome. Steroids. 2013;78(8):767–72.
14. Goodarzi MO, Dumesic DA, Chazenbalk G, Azziz R. Polycystic ovary syndrome: etiology, pathogenesis and diagnosis. Nat Rev Endocrinol. 2011;7(4):219–31.
15. Van Der Meer M, Hompes PG, De Boer JA, Schats R, Schoemaker J. Cohort size rather than follicle-stimulating hormone threshold level determines ovarian sensitivity in polycystic ovary syndrome. J Clin Endocrinol Metab. 1998;83(2):423–6.
16. Swanton A, Storey L, McVeigh E, Child T. IVF outcome in women with PCOS, PCO and normal ovarian morphology. Eur J Obstet Gynecol Reprod Biol. 2010;149(1):68–71.
17. Homburg R, Hendriks ML, Konig TE, Anderson RA, Balen AH, Brincat M, et al. Clomifene citrate or low-dose FSH for the first-line treatment of infertile women with anovulation associated with polycystic ovary syndrome: a prospective randomized multinational study. Hum Reprod. 2012;27(2):468–73.
18. Orvieto R, Homburg R. Chronic ultra-low dose follicle-stimulating hormone regimen for patients with polycystic ovary syndrome: one click, one follicle, one pregnancy. Fertil Steril. 2009;91(4 Suppl):1533–5.
19. Christin-Maitre S, Hugues JN. A comparative randomized multicentric study comparing the step-up versus step-down protocol in polycystic ovary syndrome. Hum Reprod. 2003;18(8):1626–31.
20. Leader A. Improved monofollicular ovulation in anovulatory or oligo-ovulatory women after a low-dose step-up protocol with weekly increments of 25 international units of follicle-stimulating hormone. Fertil Steril. 2006;85(6):1766–73.
21. Hamman JH, Enslin GM, Kotze AF. Oral delivery of peptide drugs: barriers and developments. BioDrugs. 2005;19(3):165–77.

22. Renukuntla J, Vadlapudi AD, Patel A, Boddu SH, Mitra AK. Approaches for enhancing oral bioavailability of peptides and proteins. Int J Pharm. 2013;447(1–2):75–93.

23. Walters KA, Allan CM, Handelsman DJ. Rodent models for human polycystic ovary syndrome. Biol Reprod. 2012;86(5):149. 1–12.

24. Shi D, Vine DF. Animal models of polycystic ovary syndrome: a focused review of rodent models in relationship to clinical phenotypes and cardiometabolic risk. Fertil Steril. 2012;98(1):185–93.

25. McNeilly AS, Duncan WC. Rodent models of polycystic ovary syndrome. Mol Cell Endocrinol. 2013;373(1–2):2–7.

26. Luchetti CG, Solano ME, Sander V, Arcos ML, Gonzalez C, Di Girolamo G, et al. Effects of dehydroepiandrosterone on ovarian cystogenesis and immune function. J Reprod Immunol. 2004;64(1–2):59–74.

27. Anderson E, Lee MT, Lee GY. Cystogenesis of the ovarian antral follicle of the rat: ultrastructural changes and hormonal profile following the administration of dehydroepiandrosterone. Anat Rec. 1992;234(3):359–82.

28. Lee MT, Anderson E, Lee GY. Changes in ovarian morphology and serum hormones in the rat after treatment with dehydroepiandrosterone. Anat Rec. 1991;231(2):185–92.

29. Ward RC, Costoff A, Mahesh VB. The induction of polycystic ovaries in mature cycling rats by the administration of dehydroepiandrosterone (DHA). Biol Reprod. 1978;18(4):614–23.

30. Gordon I. Laboratory production of cattle embryos. Biotechnology in Agriculture Series, No. 27. Dublin: CABI Publishing; 2003.

31. Assidi M, Richard FJ, Sirard MA. FSH in vitro versus LH in vivo: similar genomic effects on the cumulus. J Ovarian Res. 2013;6(1):68.

32. Wang X, Tsai T, Qiao J, Zhang Z, Feng HL. Impact of gonadotropins on oocyte maturation, fertilisation and developmental competence in vitro. Reprod Fertil Dev. 2014;26(5):752–7.

33. Calder MD, Caveney AN, Smith LC, Watson AJ. Responsiveness of bovine cumulus-oocyte-complexes (COC) to porcine and recombinant human FSH, and the effect of COC quality on gonadotropin receptor and Cx43 marker gene mRNAs during maturation in vitro. Reprod Biol Endocrinol. 2003;1:14.

34. Ali A, Sirard MA. Protein kinases influence bovine oocyte competence during short-term treatment with recombinant human follicle stimulating hormone. Reproduction. 2005;130(3):303–10.

35. Lazzari G, Tessaro I, Crotti G, Galli C, Hoffmann S, Bremer S, et al. Development of an in vitro test battery for assessing chemical effects on bovine germ cells under the ReProTect umbrella. Toxicol Appl Pharmacol. 2008;233(3):360–70.

36. Luciano AM, Franciosi F, Lodde V, Corbani D, Lazzari G, Crotti G, et al. Transferability and inter-laboratory variability assessment of the in vitro bovine oocyte maturation (IVM) test within ReProTect. Reprod Toxicol. 2010;30(1):81–8.

37. Lai H, Jia X, Yu Q, Zhang C, Qiao J, Guan Y, et al. High-fat diet induces significant metabolic disorders in a mouse model of polycystic ovary syndrome. Biol Reprod. 2014;91(5):127.

38. Modina SC, Tessaro I, Lodde V, Franciosi F, Corbani D, Luciano AM. Reductions in the number of mid-sized antral follicles are associated with markers of premature ovarian senescence in dairy cows. Reprod Fertil Dev. 2014;26(2):235–44.

39. Wang XN, Roy SK, Greenwald GS. In vitro DNA synthesis by isolated preantral to preovulatory follicles from the cyclic mouse. Biol Reprod. 1991;44(5):857–63.

40. Pedersen T, Peters H. Proposal for a classification of oocytes and follicles in the mouse ovary. J Reprod Fertil. 1968;17(3):555–7.

41. Griffin J, Emery BR, Huang I, Peterson CM, Carrell DT. Comparative analysis of follicle morphology and oocyte diameter in four mammalian species (mouse, hamster, pig, and human). J Exp Clin Assist Reprod. 2006;3:2.

42. Peluso JJ, England-Charlesworth C. Formation of ovarian cysts in aged irregularly cycling rats. Biol Reprod. 1981;24(5):1183–90.

43. Peluso JJ, England-Charlesworth C, Bolender DL, Steger RW. Ultrastructural alterations associated with the initiation of follicular atresia. Cell Tissue Res. 1980;211(1):105–15.

44. Manneras L, Cajander S, Holmang A, Seleskovic Z, Lystig T, Lonn M, et al. A new rat model exhibiting both ovarian and metabolic characteristics of polycystic ovary syndrome. Endocrinology. 2007;148(8):3781–91.

45. Gasteiger E, Hoogland C, Gattiker A, Duvaud S, Wilkins MR, Appel RD, et al. Protein identification and analysis tools on the ExPASy server. In: Walker JM, editor. The proteomics protocols handbook. Totowa: Humana Press; 2005. p. 571–607.

46. Fan QR, Hendrickson WA. Structure of human follicle-stimulating hormone in complex with its receptor. Nature. 2005;433(7023):269–77.

47. Jiang X, Dias JA, He X. Structural biology of glycoprotein hormones and their receptors: insights to signaling. Mol Cell Endocrinol. 2014;382(1):424–51.

48. Sonawani A, Niazi S, Idicula-Thomas S. In silico study on binding specificity of gonadotropins and their receptors: design of a novel and selective peptidomimetic for human follicle stimulating hormone receptor. PLoS One. 2013;8(5):e64475.

49. Luciano AM, Lodde V, Beretta MS, Colleoni S, Lauria A, Modina S. Developmental capability of denuded bovine oocyte in a co-culture system with intact cumulus-oocyte complexes: role of cumulus cells, cyclic adenosine 3′,5′-monophosphate, and glutathione. Mol Reprod Dev. 2005;71(3):389–97.

50. Lodde V, Modina S, Galbusera C, Franciosi F, Luciano AM. Large-scale chromatin remodeling in germinal vesicle bovine oocytes: interplay with gap junction functionality and developmental competence. Mol Reprod Dev. 2007;74(6):740–9.

51. Luciano AM, Franciosi F, Modina SC, Lodde V. Gap junction-mediated communications regulate chromatin remodeling during bovine oocyte growth and differentiation through cAMP-dependent mechanism(s). Biol Reprod. 2011;85(6):1252–9.

52. Schneider CA, Rasband WS, Eliceiri KW. NIH Image to ImageJ: 25 years of image analysis. Nat Methods. 2012;9(7):671–5.

53. Salilew-Wondim D, Wang Q, Tesfaye D, Schellander K, Hoelker M, Hossain MM, et al. Polycystic ovarian syndrome is accompanied by repression of gene signatures associated with biosynthesis and metabolism of steroids, cholesterol and lipids. J Ovarian Res. 2015;8(1):24.

54. Loughlin T, Cunningham S, Moore A, Culliton M, Smyth PP, McKenna TJ. Adrenal abnormalities in polycystic ovary syndrome. J Clin Endocrinol Metab. 1986;62(1):142–7.

55. Motta AB. Dehydroepiandrosterone to induce murine models for the study of polycystic ovary syndrome. J Steroid Biochem Mol Biol. 2010;119(3–5):105–11.

56. Elia E, Sander V, Luchetti CG, Solano ME, Di Girolamo G, Gonzalez C, et al. The mechanisms involved in the action of metformin in regulating ovarian function in hyperandrogenized mice. Mol Hum Reprod. 2006;12(8):475–81.

57. Sander V, Luchetti CG, Solano ME, Elia E, Di Girolamo G, Gonzalez C, et al. Role of the N, N′-dimethylbiguanide metformin in the treatment of female prepuberal BALB/c mice hyperandrogenized with dehydroepiandrosterone. Reproduction. 2006;131(3):591–602.

58. Solano ME, Sander VA, Ho H, Motta AB, Arck PC. Systemic inflammation, cellular influx and up-regulation of ovarian VCAM-1 expression in a mouse model of polycystic ovary syndrome (PCOS). J Reprod Immunol. 2011;92(1–2):33–44.

59. Fassnacht M, Schlenz N, Schneider SB, Wudy SA, Allolio B, Arlt W. Beyond adrenal and ovarian androgen generation: Increased peripheral 5 alpha-reductase activity in women with polycystic ovary syndrome. J Clin Endocrinol Metab. 2003;88(6):2760–6.

60. Wickenheisser JK, Quinn PG, Nelson VL, Legro RS, Strauss 3rd JF, McAllister JM. Differential activity of the cytochrome P450 17alpha-hydroxylase and steroidogenic acute regulatory protein gene promoters in normal and polycystic ovary syndrome theca cells. J Clin Endocrinol Metab. 2000;85(6):2304–11.

61. Strauss 3rd JF. Some new thoughts on the pathophysiology and genetics of polycystic ovary syndrome. Ann N Y Acad Sci. 2003;997:42–8.

62. Eagleson CA, Gingrich MB, Pastor CL, Arora TK, Burt CM, Evans WS, et al. Polycystic ovarian syndrome: evidence that flutamide restores sensitivity of the gonadotropin-releasing hormone pulse generator to inhibition by estradiol and progesterone. J Clin Endocrinol Metab. 2000;85(11):4047–52.

63. Blank SK, McCartney CR, Marshall JC. The origins and sequelae of abnormal neuroendocrine function in polycystic ovary syndrome. Hum Reprod Update. 2006;12(4):351–61.

64. Henmi H, Endo T, Nagasawa K, Hayashi T, Chida M, Akutagawa N, et al. Lysyl oxidase and MMP-2 expression in dehydroepiandrosterone-induced polycystic ovary in rats. Biol Reprod. 2001;64(1):157–62.

65. Chen X, Jia X, Qiao J, Guan Y, Kang J. Adipokines in reproductive function: a link between obesity and polycystic ovary syndrome. J Mol Endocrinol. 2013;50(2):R21–37.

66. Solano ME, Elia E, Luchetti CG, Sander V, Di Girolamo G, Gonzalez C, et al. Metformin prevents embryonic resorption induced by

hyperandrogenisation with dehydroepiandrosterone in mice. Reprod Fertil Dev. 2006;18(5):533–44.

67. Homburg R, Howles CM. Low-dose FSH therapy for anovulatory infertility associated with polycystic ovary syndrome: rationale, results, reflections and refinements. Hum Reprod Update. 1999;5(5):493–9.

68. Mahato RI, Narang AS, Thoma L, Miller DD. Emerging trends in oral delivery of peptide and protein drugs. Crit Rev Ther Drug Carrier Syst. 2003;20(2–3):153–214.

69. Sun L. Peptide-based drug development. Mod Chem Appl. 2013;1(1):1–2.

70. Campion CE, Trewin AL, Hutz RJ. Effects of follicle-stimulating hormone administration on oestradiol-induced cystic ovaries in guinea pigs. Zoolog Sci. 1996;13(1):137–42.

71. Roy SK, Greenwald GS. *In vitro* steroidogenesis by primary to antral follicles in the hamster during the periovulatory period: effects of follicle-stimulating hormone, luteinizing hormone, and prolactin. Biol Reprod. 1987;37(1):39–46.

72. Roy SK, Greenwald GS. *In vitro* effects of epidermal growth factor, insulin-like growth factor-I, fibroblast growth factor, and follicle-stimulating hormone on hamster follicular deoxyribonucleic acid synthesis and steroidogenesis. Biol Reprod. 1991;44(5):889–96.

73. Greenwald GS, Roy SK. Follicular development and its control. In: Knobil E, Neill JD, editors. Physiology of reproduction. Physiology of reproduction, Vols 1 and 2. 2nd ed. New York: Raven; 1994. p. 629–724.

74. Lederer KJ, Luciano AM, Pappalardo A, Peluso JJ. Proliferative and steroidogenic capabilities of rat granulosa cells of different sizes. J Reprod Fertil. 1995;103(1):47–54.

75. Connolly MP, Hoorens S, Chambers GM. The costs and consequences of assisted reproductive technology: an economic perspective. Hum Reprod Update. 2010;16(6):603–13.

76. Vlieghe P, Lisowski V, Martinez J, Khrestchatisky M. Synthetic therapeutic peptides: science and market. Drug Discov Today. 2010;15(1–2):40–56.

77. Bellmann-Sickert K, Beck-Sickinger AG. Peptide drugs to target G protein-coupled receptors. Trends Pharmacol Sci. 2010;31(9):434–41.

78. Low SC, Nunes SL, Bitonti AJ, Dumont JA. Oral and pulmonary delivery of FSH-Fc fusion proteins via neonatal Fc receptor-mediated transcytosis. Hum Reprod. 2005;20(7):1805–13.

79. Familiari G, Toscano V, Motta PM. Morphological studies of polycystic mouse ovaries induced by dehydroepiandrosterone. Cell Tissue Res. 1985;240(3):519–28.

80. Sander V, Solano ME, Elia E, Luchetti CG, Di Girolamo G, Gonzalez C, et al. The influence of dehydroepiandrosterone on early pregnancy in mice. Neuroimmunomodulation. 2005;12(5):285–92.

81. Sen A, Hammes SR. Granulosa cell-specific androgen receptors are critical regulators of ovarian development and function. Mol Endocrinol. 2010;24(7):1393–403.

82. Walters KA, Middleton LJ, Joseph SR, Hazra R, Jimenez M, Simanainen U, et al. Targeted loss of androgen receptor signaling in murine granulosa cells of preantral and antral follicles causes female subfertility. Biol Reprod. 2012;87(6):151.

83. Sen A, Prizant H, Light A, Biswas A, Hayes E, Lee HJ, et al. Androgens regulate ovarian follicular development by increasing follicle stimulating hormone receptor and microRNA-125b expression. Proc Natl Acad Sci U S A. 2014;111(8):3008–13.

12

The relationship between epicardial fat tissue thickness and visceral adipose tissue in lean patients with polycystic ovary syndrome

Dilek Arpaci[1*], Aysel Gurkan Tocoglu[2], Sabiye Yilmaz[3], Hasan Ergenc[2], Ali Tamer[2], Nurgul Keser[3] and Huseyin Gunduz[3]

Abstract

Background: Polycystic ovary syndrome (PCOS) is related to metabolic syndrome, insulin resistance, and cardiovascular metabolic syndromes. This is particularly true for individuals with central and abdominal obesity because visceral abdominal adipose tissue (VAAT) and epicardial adipose tissue (EAT) produce a large number of proinflammatory and proatherogenic cytokines. The present study aimed to determine whether there are changes in VAAT and EAT levels which were considered as indirect predictors for subclinical atherosclerosis in lean patients with PCOS.

Methods: The clinical and demographic characteristics of 35 patients with PCOS and 38 healthy control subjects were recorded for the present study. Additionally, the serum levels of various biochemical parameters were measured and EAT levels were assessed using 2D-transthoracic echocardiography.

Results: There were no significant differences in mean age ($p = 0.056$) or mean body mass index (BMI) ($p = 0.446$) between the patient and control groups. However, the body fat percentage, waist-to-hip ratio, amount of abdominal subcutaneous adipose tissue, and VAAT thickness were higher in the PCOS patient group than in the control group. The amounts of EAT in the patient and control groups were similar ($p = 0.384$). EAT was correlated with BMI, fat mass, waist circumference, and hip circumference but not with any biochemical metabolic parameters including the homeostasis model assessment of insulin resistance index or the levels of triglycerides, low-density lipoprotein cholesterol, and high-density lipoprotein (HDL) cholesterol. However, there was a small positive correlation between the amounts of VAAT and EAT. VAAT was directly correlated with body fat parameters such as BMI, fat mass, and abdominal subcutaneous adipose thickness and inversely correlated with the HDL cholesterol level.

Conclusions: The present study found that increased abdominal adipose tissue in patients with PCOS was associated with atherosclerosis. Additionally, EAT may aid in the determination of the risk of atherosclerosis in patients with PCOS because it is easily measured.

Keywords: Polycystic, Ovary, Epicardial, Adipose

* Correspondence: drarpaci@gmail.com
[1]Division of Endocrinology and Metabolism, Department of Internal Medicine, Faculty of Medicine, Bulent Ecevit University, Zonguldak, Turkey
Full list of author information is available at the end of the article

Background

Polycystic ovary syndrome (PCOS) is a heterogeneous disease that affects 5 to 10 % of women in the reproductive period [1]. Many studies have shown that PCOS is associated with various cardiovascular risk factors such as obesity, insulin resistance, hyperlipidemia, metabolic syndrome, and hypertension [1–3]. Additionally, patients with PCOS have a high incidence of central and abdominal obesity and marked increases in the waist circumference (WC) and waist-to-hip ratio (WHR) [4, 5].

Visceral abdominal adipose tissue (VAAT) surrounds the internal organs, and increased amounts of VAAT are more important than increased levels of subcutaneous fat in terms of the risks of metabolic syndrome, insulin resistance, and cardiovascular mortality [6]. Epicardial adipose tissue (EAT) and visceral adipose tissue (VAT), located between the myocardium and visceral epicardium, respectively, are derived from the same origin [7]. This is important because both of these body fat tissues produce large numbers of proinflammatory and proatherogenic cytokines [8, 9]. The reported findings regarding abdominal fat tissue and EAT in patients with PCOS are controversial [8–21]. For example, patients with PCOS have been shown to have increased [10–14], similar [15–17], or decreased [18] amounts of abdominal fat. Similarly, the amount of EAT in patients with PCOS has been reported to be increased and unchanged compared with healthy control groups [19–21]. However, not all patients with PCOS are obese; in fact, a 2001 study of 346 patients with PCOS found that 56 % of such patients are lean [22]; 56.0 % had a body mass index (BMI) of < 25 kg/m^2, 11.3 % had a BMI of 25 to 27 kg/m^2, and 32.7 % had a BMI of ≥ 27 kg/m^2 [22]. Thus, the present study aimed to determine whether there are changes in the amounts of VAAT and EAT in lean patients with PCOS compared with healthy control subjects.

Methods

Selection of subjects

The present study included 38 healthy control subjects and 35 patients with PCOS and concurrent hyperandrogenism and/or ovulatory dysfunction who were admitted to the Endocrinology and Metabolism Department of Sakarya Training and Research Hospital at Sakarya University from January 2013 to June 2014. Some of these patients were diagnosed by a gynecologist, and some were diagnosed by the present authors based on the presence of two of the three criteria from the Rotterdam European Society for Human Reproduction and Embryology/American Society for Reproductive Medicine (ESHRE/ASRM) for PCOS: a) oligomenorrhea, amenorrhea, or anovulation; b) the presence of clinical or biochemical hyperandrogenism; and/or c) the presence of polycystic ovaries as determined by a

pelvic ultrasound [22]. The control group comprised healthy secretaries, nurses, and doctors from our hospital who volunteered for the study and had regular menstrual cycles, normal androgen levels, the absence of hirsutism, and no polycystic ovary as determined by a pelvic ultrasound. The demographic data of the patient and control groups were recorded. The present study was approved by the Sakarya University Faculty of Medicine Ethics Committee (Date: 24.02.2014; No. 27), and all participants provided written informed consent.

Exclusion criteria

Subjects were excluded from the present study if they had history of smoking, diabetes, or hypertension; had been diagnosed with Cushing's syndrome (based on the 1-mg dexamethasone suppression test) or non-classic congenital adrenal hyperplasia (based on a 17-OH progesterone level of > 10 ng/dL after stimulation); exhibited cardiac disease; and/or had used antidiabetic, antihypertensive, antilipidemic, or oral contraceptive drugs within the past 3 months.

Measurements

The height and weight of all subjects were measured, and their BMI was calculated as the weight in kilograms divided by the square of height in meters. WC was measured from the narrowest part of the body between the iliac crest and the rib, and hip circumference (HC) was measured at the widest part of the hips. The WHR was calculated as the ratio of WC to HC [21].

Body composition analysis

The basal metabolic rate, body fat percentage, and total body water of each patient were evaluated with a Tanita Body Composition Analyzer (Model TBF-300; Tanita Corporation, Itabashi-ku, Tokyo, Japan) while the patient was in a standing position without shoes and with light clothing on after a ≥ 8-h fast with sufficient hydration. Abdominal subcutaneous fat tissue thickness and visceral abdominal fat tissue thickness were recorded using bioelectrical impedance with the Tanita Abdominal Fat Analyzer (AB-140 Viscan; Tanita Corporation, Tokyo, Japan). The blood pressure of each patient was assessed after at least 10 min of rest with a sphygmomanometer (ERKA; Bad Tölz, Germany); two measurements were performed, and the average of the blood pressure measurements was calculated [23].

Biochemical analysis

Blood samples were obtained from the patients in the morning after at least 8 h of fasting. The fasting plasma glucose (FPG) and fasting insulin levels of the patients were measured, and the homeostatic model assessment-insulin resistance (HOMA-IR) index was calculated using the following formula: (FPG [mg/dL] × fasting plasma insulin [µIU/mL] / 405). If the HOMA-IR index was > 2.7, insulin resistance was considered to be present [24]. Serum lipid levels of low-density lipoprotein (LDL) cholesterol, high-density lipoprotein (HDL) cholesterol, and triglycerides (TG) were measured using xylidine blue with an end-point colorimetric method (Roche Diagnostics GmbH; Mannheim, Germany). FPG levels were measured with a hexokinase method (Roche Diagnostics GmbH).

Echocardiography

All patients were directed to the Department of Cardiology at Sakarya Training and Research Hospital, and the EAT thickness was measured using 2D-transthoracic echocardiography by the same cardiologist. The parasternal long- and short-axis images of EAT, which allow for the most accurate measurement from the right ventricle, were obtained using a standard parasternal image in the left lateral decubitus position. EAT was defined as the echo-free space between the outer wall of the myocardium and the visceral layer of pericardium at endsystole in the right ventricle [25].

Statistical analysis

All statistical analyses were performed with SPSS software, version 15 (SPSS, Inc., Chicago, IL, USA). Nonparametric tests were utilized due to the prevalence of variables. The Mann–Whitney U test was applied to assess differences between groups, and Spearman's test was applied to assess correlations between the variables. A p value of < 0.05 was considered to indicate statistical significance, and a correlation was considered to be present if Spearman's value was ≥ 0.50. Continuous variables are expressed as either the mean ± standard deviation (SD) or the median (minimum–maximum), and categorical variables are expressed as either frequency or percentage. Continuous variables were compared with an independent-samples t-tests or the Mann–Whitney U test, and categorical variables were compared using Pearson's chi-square test. A p value of < 0.05 was considered to indicate statistical significance for all tests.

Results

The body fat distribution, total body water, WC, HC, WHR, amount of abdominal subcutaneous adipose tissue, VAAT thickness, blood pressure, and levels of LDL cholesterol, HDL cholesterol, are TG are provided in Table 1. There were no significant differences in the mean age ($p = 0.056$) or mean BMI ($p = 0.446$) between the patient and control groups, but the body fat percentage, WHR, amount of abdominal subcutaneous adipose tissue, and VAAT thickness were higher in the patient group. However, the patient and control groups had similar amounts of EAT ($p = 0.384$) (Table 1).

Table 1 Comparison of demographic, body analysis and laboratory parameters of the patient and the control group

Feature	Patients ($n = 35$)	Controls ($n = 38$)	P value
Age (years)	25.16 ± 4.12	27.44 ± 4.31	0.056
BMI (kg/m^2)	25.60 ± 5.22	23.67 ± 3.70	0.404
Fat mass (%)	31.74 ± 10.12	26.33 ± 7.61	**0.042**
Total body water (kg)	34.11 ± 4.48	32.72 ± 2.33	0.193
Waist circumference (cm)	91.76 ± 18.95	86.50 ± 9.71	0.677
Hip circumference (cm)	103.56 ± 15.27	100.55 ± 7.48	0.557
WHR	0.94 ± 0.06	0.89 ± 0.04	**0.007**
VAAT thickness	9.24 ± 4.67	6.77 ± 2.68	**0.042**
Abdominal subcutaneous adipose tissue thickness	40.48 ± 8.83	32.86 ± 9.48	**0.008**
Systolic blood pressure (mmHg)	120.10 ± 7.78	120.28 ± 7.28	0.979
Diastolic blood pressure (mmHg)	70.26 ± 7.40	72.76 ± 9.21	0.318
FPG (mg/dL)	89.16 ± 9.12	87.72 ± 7.92	0.565
Insulin (µIU/ mL)	9.77 ± 6.27	6.80 ± 3.45	0.073
HOMA-IR	2.13 ± 1.33	1.60 ± 0.67	0.082
TG (mg/dL)	11.52 ± 53.81	85.52 ± 31.49	0.058
LDL (mg/dL)	106.40 ± 35.57	96.38 ± 28.73	0.305
HDL (mg/dL)	55.69 ± 16.25	58.90 ± 11.96	0.300
EAT (mm)	4.72 ± 0.88	4.43 ± 1.31	0.384

BMI body mass index, *VAAT* visceral abdominal adipose tissue, *FPG* fasting plasma glucose, *HOMA-IR* Homeostatic Model Assessment-insulin resistance, *TG* triglyceride, *LDL* low density lipoprotein, *HDL* high density lipoprotein, *EAT* epicardial adipose tissue. Continuous variables were compared with an independent-samples t-tests or the Mann–Whitney *U* test, and categorical variables were compared using Pearson's chi-square test. A *p* value of <0.05 was considered to indicate statistical significance for all tests

EAT had a significantly positive correlation with BMI (r = 0.260, p = 0.034), fat mass (r = 0.250, p = 0.041), WC (r = 0.301, p = 0.016), and abdominal circumference (r = 0.254, p = 0.043), but it was not correlated with the HOMA-IR index or the levels of TG, LDL cholesterol, or HDL cholesterol (p > 0.05) (Table 2). There was a small positive correlation between VAAT and EAT (r = 0.248, p = 0.048). VAAT was also directly associated with BMI (r = 0.921, p < 0.01), fat mass (r = 0.941, p < 0.01), WC (r = 0.941, p < 0.01), HC (r = 0.876, p < 0.01), abdominal subcutaneous adipose thickness (r = 0.896, p < 0.01), the HOMA-IR index (r = 0.618, p < 0.01), and the levels of TG (r = 0.388, p < 0.01) and LDL cholesterol (r = 0.288, p = 0.016). Conversely, VAAT was inversely associated with the HDL cholesterol level (r = −0.488, p < 0.01) (Table 3).

Discussion

Although the patient and control groups in the present study had similar ages and BMIs, the lean patients with PCOS exhibited a higher WHR, VAAT, and abdominal subcutaneous fat tissue thickness than did the control group. In contrast, there were no significant differences in EAT. However, EAT was significantly correlated with VAAT, BMI, fat mass, WC, and HC.

Previous studies have shown a positive correlation between EAT thickness and VAAT thickness [26–28] independent of obesity [26, 27], and this correlation seems to be more important than WC [28]. Although there is an increased amount of EAT in obese patients with than without PCOS [19–21], EAT is not different between lean patients with PCOS and the normal population [21, 29]. Similarly, the present study found no differences in EAT between the two groups. Compared with normal individuals, patients with PCOS exhibit increases in total fat mass and organ-specific VAT [29]. Furthermore, these increases are positively correlated with both systolic and diastolic blood pressure and the levels of

Table 2 Correlation analysis between EAT and variables

Variable	r value	p value
BMI (kg/m^2)	0.260	**0.034**
Fat mass (%)	0.250	**0.041**
Waist circumference (cm)	0.301	**0.016**
Hip circumference (cm)	0.254	**0.043**
HOMA-IR	0.119	0.490
TG (mg/dL)	0.076	0.550
LDL (mg/dL)	0.158	0.209
HDL (mg/dL)	−0.185	0.141

BMI body mass index, *HOMA-IR* Homeostatic Model Assessment-insulin resistance, *TG* triglyceride, *LDL* low density lipoprotein, *HDL* high density lipoprotein, *EAT* epicardial adipose tissue. Continuous variables were compared with an independent-samples t-tests or the Mann–Whitney *U* test, and categorical variables were compared using Pearson's chi-square test. A *p* value of <0.05 was considered to indicate statistical significance for all tests

Table 3 Correlation analysis between VAAT and variables

Variable	r value	P value
EAT (mm)	0.248	**0.048**
BMI (kg/m^2)	0.921	<0.01
Fat mass (%)	0.941	<0.01
Waist circumference (cm)	0.941	<0.01
Hip circumference (cm)	0.876	<0.01
Abdominal subcutaneous adipose tissue thickness	0.896	<0.01
HOMA-IR	0.618	<0.01
TG (mg/dL)	0.388	<0.01
LDL (mg/dL)	0.288	**0.016**
HDL (mg/dL)	−0.488	<0.01

BMI body mass index, *HOMA-IR* Homeostatic Model Assessment-insulin resistance, *TG* triglyceride, *LDL* low density lipoprotein, *HDL* high density lipoprotein, *EAT* epicardial adipose tissue. Continuous variables were compared with an independent-samples t-tests or the Mann–Whitney *U* test, and categorical variables were compared using Pearson's chi-square test. A *p* value of <0.05 was considered to indicate statistical significance for all tests

fasting glucose, insulin, LDL cholesterol, TG, and transaminases but negatively correlated with the insulin sensitivity index and HDL cholesterol. Likewise, the present study found that fat mass, abdominal subcutaneous adipose tissue, and VAAT thickness were higher in the patient group than in the control group. Additionally, VAAT thickness was positively correlated with BMI, fat mass, WC, HC, abdominal subcutaneous adipose tissue thickness, and the levels of TG and LDL cholesterol but negatively correlated with HDL cholesterol.

Sahin et al. [21] reported that EAT is positively correlated with age, BMI, WC, the glucose level, the HOMA-IR index, and the TG level. Similarly, the present study found that EAT was positively correlated with BMI, WC, HC, and VAAT; however, in contrast to those previous findings, EAT was not correlated with fasting glucose, the HOMA-IR index, or the lipid parameters. This may be due to the fact that the patients with PCOS in the present study were lean rather than obese. Another study found that EAT is correlated with BMI, WC, VAT thickness, and insulin resistance [30]. In the present study, EAT was positively correlated with BMI, WC, and VAAT but not with the HOMA-IR index. EAT is reportedly more closely associated with VAT than with total body fat [28, 30].

In studies employing magnetic resonance imaging (MRI), the abdominal adipose tissue thicknesses of patients with PCOS and normal control subjects did not significantly differ [16, 31–33]. It has also been shown that VAAT thickness is increased only in mildly obese patients with PCOS relative to control subjects [15] and that obesity predicts insulin resistance independently of PCOS [31]. Furthermore, a study conducted using a bioimpedance device found that there was less VAT in lean patients with PCOS than in the control group [18].

In contrast, the present study found greater VAAT thickness in lean patients with PCOS than in the control group despite the fact that the EAT thickness did not change.

The gold standard tests for measuring VAT are MRI and computed tomography (CT) [34]. Thus, a limitation of the present study may be that the amounts of abdominal subcutaneous adipose tissue and VAT were assessed using bioelectrical impedance. However, it is difficult to measure adipose tissue using CT or MRI because of cost-effectiveness, the application of radiation, and the use of contrast media. Additionally, previous studies have shown that the results of bioelectrical impedance tests and CT scans when measuring VAT are closely correlated [35]. Consequently, given that the present study found a small positive correlation between EAT thickness and VAAT thickness, echocardiography would appear to be an easy, simple, noninvasive, reliable, and accessible method for the measurement of these parameters relative to the use of MRI scans [25]. EAT is important for the determination of both VAAT thickness and cardiovascular risk [26, 36], and increased abdominal adipose tissue is related to an increased risk of atherosclerosis [37] and mortality [38]. Because it can be difficult to measure abdominal adipose tissue, it may be more economical and efficient to determine these risk factors by measuring EAT.

Conclusions

The present study observed several associations between EAT thickness and cardiovascular risk in patients with PCOS. Because of the difficulties related to the measurement of abdominal adipose tissue thickness, the assessment of EAT may be a relatively easy-to-use but important tool for the determination of cardiovascular risk.

Abbreviations

PCOS: Polycystic ovary syndrome; VAAT: Visceral abdominal adipose tissue; EAT: Epicardial adipose tissue; BMI: Body mass index.

Competing interest

All authors declare that there were no conflict of interest or any funding source.

Authors' contributions

DA, AGT and SY contributed to conception and design, acquisition, analysis and interpretation of data and drafting the article. HE, AT, NK, HG carried out all the experiments described in the manuscripts. DA, SY, AT and HG contributed to conception, analysis and interpretation of data and reviewed the article critically for important intellectual content. All authors read and approved the final manuscript.

Author details

[1]Division of Endocrinology and Metabolism, Department of Internal Medicine, Faculty of Medicine, Bulent Ecevit University, Zonguldak, Turkey. [2]Department of Internal Medicine, Faculty of Medicine, Sakarya University Training and Research Hospital, Sakarya, Turkey. [3]Department of Cardiology, Sakarya University Training and Research Hospital, Sakarya, Turkey.

References

1. Diamanti-Kandarakis E. Role of obesity and adiposity in polycystic ovary syndrome. Int J Obes (Lond). 2007;31:8–13.
2. Schroder AK, Tauchert S, Ortmann O, Diedrich K, Weiss JM. Insulin resistance in patients with polycystic ovary syndrome. Ann Med. 2004;36:426–39.
3. Chen MJ, Yang WS, Yang JH, Chen CL, Ho HN, Yang YS. Relationship between androgen levels and blood pressure in young women with polycystic ovary syndrome. Hypertension. 2007;49:1442–7.
4. Escobar-Morreale HF, San Millan JL. Abdominal adiposity and the polycystic ovary syndrome. Trends Endocrinol Metab. 2007;18:266–72.
5. Pasquali R, Casimirri F, Cantobelli S, Labate AM, Venturoli S, Paradisi R, et al. Insulin and androgen relationships with abdominal body fat distribution in women with and without hyperandrogenism. Horm Res. 1993;39:179–87.
6. Goodpaster BH, Krishnaswami S, Harris TB, Katsiaras A, Kritchevsky SB, Simonsick EM, et al. Obesity, regional body fat distribution, and the metabolic syndrome in older men and women. Arch Intern Med. 2005;165:777–83.
7. Sacks HS, Fain JN. Human epicardial adipose tissue: a review. Am Heart J. 2007;153:907–17.
8. Iacobellis G, Barbaro G. The double role of epicardial adipose tissue as pro-and anti-inflammatory organ. Horm Metab Res. 2008;40:442–5.
9. Iacobellis G. Is obesity a risk factor for atrial fibrillation? Nat Clin Pract Cardiovasc. 2005;2:134–5.
10. Hutchison SK, Stepto NK, Harrison CL, Moran LJ, Strauss BJ, Teede HJ. Effects of exercise on insulin resistance and body composition in overweight and obese women with and without polycystic ovary syndrome. J Clin Endocrinol Metab. 2011;96:48–56.
11. Battaglia C, Battaglia B, Mancini F, Paradisi R, Fabbri R, Venturoli S. Ultrasonographic extended-view technique for evaluation of abdominal fat distribution in lean women with polycystic ovary syndrome. Acta Obstet Gynecol Scand. 2011;90:600–8.
12. Jones H, Sprung VS, Pugh CJ, Daousi C, Irwin A, Aziz N, et al. Polycystic ovary syndrome with hyperandrogenism is characterized by an increased risk of hepatic steatosis, compared to nonhyperandrogenic PCOS phenotypes and healthy controls, independent of obesity and insulin resistance. J Clin Endocrinol Metab. 2012;97:3709–16.
13. Cascella T, Palomba S, De Sio I, Manguso F, Giallauria F, De Simone B, et al. Visceral fat is associated with cardiovascular risk inwomenwith polycystic ovary syndrome. Hum Reprod. 2008;23:153–9.
14. Karabulut A, Yaylali GF, Demirlenk S, Sevket O, Acun A. Evaluation of body fat distribution inPCOSand its association with carotid atherosclerosis and insulin resistance. Gynecol Endocrinol. 2012;28:111–4.
15. Barber TM, Golding SJ, Alvey C, Wass JA, Karpe F, Franks S, et al. Global adiposity rather than abnormal regional fat distribution characterizes women with polycystic ovary syndrome. J Clin Endocrinol Metab. 2008;93:999–1004.
16. Mannerås-Holm L, Leonhardt H, Kullberg J, Jennische E, Odén A, Holm G, et al. Adipose tissue has aberrant morphology and function in PCOS: enlarged adipocytes and low serum adiponectin, but not circulating sex steroids, are strongly associated with insulin resistance. J Clin Endocrinol Metab. 2011;96:304–11.
17. Penaforte FR, Japur CC, Diez-Garcia RW, Chiarello PG. Upper trunk fat assessment and its relationship with metabolic and biochemical variables and body fat in polycystic ovary syndrome. J Hum Nutr Diet. 2011;24:39–46.
18. Dolfing JG, Stassen CM, van Haard PM, Wolffenbuttel BH, Schweitzer DH. Comparison of MRI-assessed body fat content between lean women with polycystic ovary syndrome (PCOS) and matched controls: less visceral fat with PCOS. Hum Reprod. 2011;26:1495–500.
19. Cakir E, Doğan M, Topaloglu O, Ozbek M, Cakal E, Vural MG, et al. Subclinical atherosclerosis and hyperandrogenemia are independent risk factors for increased epicardial fat thickness in patients with PCOS and idiopathic hirsutism. Atherosclerosis. 2013;226:291–5.
20. Aydogdu A, Uckaya G, Tasci I, Baysan O, Tapan S, Bugan B, et al. The relationship of epicardial adipose tissue thickness to clinical and biochemical features in women with polycystic ovary syndrome. Endocr J. 2012;59(6):509–16.
21. Sahin SB, Cure MC, Ugurlu Y, Ergul E, Gur EU, Alyildiz N, et al. Epicardial adipose tissue thickness and NGAL levels in women with polycystic ovary syndrome. J Ovarian Res. 2014;7:24.

22. Rotterdam ESHRE/ASRM-Sponsored PCOS Consensus Workshop Group. Revised 2003 consensus on diagnostic criteria and long-term health risks related to polycystic ovary syndrome. Fertil Steril. 2004;81:19–25.
23. Amariles P, Sabater-Hernández D, García-Jiménez E, Rodríguez-Chamorro MÁ, Prats-Más R, Marín-Magán F, et al. Effectiveness of Dader Method for pharmaceutical care on control of blood pressure and total cholesterol in outpatients with cardiovascular disease or cardiovascular risk: EMDADER-CV randomized controlled trial. J Manag Care Pharm. 2012;18(4):311–23.
24. Gokcel A, Ozsahin AK, Sezgin N, Karakose H, Ertorer ME, Akbaba M, et al. High prevalence of diabetes in Adana, a southern province of Turkey. Diabetes Care. 2003;26:3031–4.
25. Iacobellis G, Assael F, Ribaudo MC, Zappaterreno A, Alessi G, Di Mario U, et al. Epicardial fat from echocardiography: a new method for visceral adipose tissue prediction. Obes Res. 2003;11:304–10.
26. Iacobellis G, Ribaudo MC, Assael F, Vecci E, Tiberti C, Zappaterreno A, et al. Echocardiographic epicardial adipose tissue is related to anthropometric and clinical parameters of metabolic syndrome: a new indicator of cardiovascular risk. J Clin Endocrinol Metab. 2003;88:5163–8.
27. Iacobellis G, Leonetti F, Di Mario U. Images in cardiology: massive epicardial adipose tissue indicating severe visceral obesity. Clin Cardiol. 2003;26:237.
28. Singh N, Singh H, Khanijoun HK, Iacobellis G. Echocardiographic assessment of epicardial adipose tissue–a marker of visceral adiposity. McGill J Med. 2007;10:26–30.
29. Borruel S, Fernández-Durán E, Alpañés M, Martí D, Alvarez-Blasco F, Luque-Ramírez M, et al. Global adiposity and thickness of intraperitoneal and mesenteric adipose tissue depots are increased in women with polycystic ovary syndrome (PCOS). J Clin Endocrinol Metab. 2013;98(3):1254–63.
30. Fernández Muñoz MJ, Basurto Acevedo L, Córdova Pérez N, Vázquez Martínez AL, Tepach Gutiérrez N, Vega García S, et al. Epicardial adipose tissue is associated with visceral fat, metabolic syndrome, and insulin resistance in menopausal women. Rev Esp Cardiol (Engl Ed). 2014;67(6):436–41.
31. Morin-Papunen LC, Vauhkonen I, Koivunen RM, Ruokonen A, Tapanainen JS. Insulin sensitivity, insulin secretion, and metabolic and hormonal parameters in healthy women and women with polycystic ovarian syndrome. Hum Reprod. 2000;15:1266–74.
32. Dunaif A, Segal KR, Futterweit W, Dobrjansky A. Profound peripheral insulin resistance, independent of obesity, in polycystic ovary syndrome. Diabetes. 1989;38:1165–74.
33. Diamanti-Kandarakis E, Mitrakou A, Hennes MM, Platanissiotis D, Kaklas N, Spina J, et al. Insulin sensitivity and antiandrogenic therapy in women with polycystic ovary syndrome. Metabolism. 1995;44:525–31.
34. Iacobellis G, Sharma AM. Epicardial adipose tissue as new cardio-metabolic risk marker and poten tial therapeutic target in the metabolic syndrome. Curr Pharm Des. 2007;13:2180–4.
35. Nagai M, Komiya H, Mori Y, Ohta T, Kasahara Y, Ikeda Y. Estimating visceral fat area by multifrequency biolectrical impedance. Diabetes Care. 2010;33:1077–9.
36. Taguchi R, Takasu J, Itani Y, Yamamoto R, Yokoyama K, Watanabe S, et al. Pericardial fat accumulation in men as a risk factor for coronary artery disease. Atherosclerosis. 2001;157:203–9.
37. Gasteyger C, Tremblay A. Metabolic impact of body Fat distribution. J Endocrinol Invest. 2002;25:876–83.
38. Dagenais GR, Yi Q, Mann JF, Bosch J, Pogue J, Yusuf S. Prognostic impact of body weight and abdominal obesity in women and men with cardiovascular disease. Am Heart J. 2005;149:54–60.

13

Does metformin improve *in vitro* maturation and ultrastructure of oocytes retrieved from estradiol valerate polycystic ovary syndrome-induced rats

Fakhroddin Mesbah[1,2*], Mohsen Moslem[1], Zahra Vojdani[1,2] and Hossein Mirkhani[3,4]

Abstract

Background: Metformin decreases polycystic ovary syndrome (PCOS) symptoms, induces ovulation, and may improve developmental competence of *in vitro* oocyte maturation. This study was designed to define the effects of metformin on the characteristics of *in vitro* oocyte maturation in estradiol valerate (EV) PCOS-induced rats.

Methods: Forty-five adult female Sprague–Dawley rats were randomly divided into control; sham and PCOS-induced (treated by a single dose of estradiol valerate, 4 mg/rat, IM) groups. The body weight was measured weekly for 12 weeks. At the end of week 12, the serum levels of testosterone, estrogen, progesterone, LH, and FSH and blood glucose of all the rats were measured. About 380 cumulus oocyte complexes (control, 125; sham, 122; PCOS-induced rats, 133) were incubated in Ham's F10 in the absence and/or presence of metformin (M 5^{-10}) for 12, 24, 36, and 48 h. The cumulus cells expansion and nuclear and cytoplasmic maturation of the oocytes was evaluated using 1 % aceto-orcein staining, and transmission electron microscopy (TEM).

Results: No significant differences were observed in the body weight of the rats. The serum level of testosterone was reduced, and progesterone and LH were significantly increased in the PCOS-induced rats ($p < 0.05$). However, no significant differences were observed in the serum levels of estrogen and FSH among the groups. Blood glucose level was higher in the PCOS-induced rats than control, ($p < 0.01$). The expansion of cumulus cells was observed in the metformin-treated oocytes. The oocytes retrieved from PCOS-induced rats show a stage of meiotic division (GVBD, MI, A-T, and MII) in 57.12 % of metformin-untreated and fairly significantly increased to 64.28 % in metformin-treated oocytes, ($p < 0.05$), but no differences were observed in the MII stage within groups. The redistribution of some cytoplasmic organelles throughout the ooplasm, particularly the peripheral cortical granules, was defined in the metformin-treated oocytes.

Conclusions: Single dose of EV can creates a reversible PCO adult rat model. Metformin enhances the COCs to initiate meiotic resumption at the first 6 h of IVM. In our study the metformin inability to show all aspects of *in vitro* oocyte maturation and may be resulted from deficiency of EV to induce PCOS.

Keywords: Polycystic ovary syndrome, *In vitro* oocyte maturation, Metformin

* Correspondence: mesbahf@sums.ac.ir
[1]Department of Anatomical Sciences, Shiraz University of Medical Sciences, Shiraz 71348-53185, Iran
[2]Embryonic Stem Cell Lab, Shiraz University of Medical Sciences, Shiraz, Iran
Full list of author information is available at the end of the article

Background

Polycystic ovary syndrome is one of the major causes of anovulatory infertility in women. The etiology and pathology of PCOS are still questioned, but imbalances of testosterone, estrogen, progesterone, LH and FSH, obesity, insulin resistance, and hyperinsulinemia are crucial factors for ovarian hyperandrogenism and chronic anovulation [1]. In addition to infertility, patients with PCOS are at a risk of miscarriage [2], which has been reported during the first trimester of pregnancy in approximately 30 to 35 % of patients [3].

The protocols proposed for the treatment of PCOS include a diet plan, exercise and physical activity, drug treatments, and surgical procedures [4]. Drug treatments include the administration of metformin, glitazones, spironolactone, estrogen, and clomiphene citrate [5]. In recent years, metformin alone or in combination with other drugs is used to treat PCOS. Metformin, a biguanide antihyperglycemic drug, is utilized to treat type 2 diabetes. In women with PCOS associated with anovulation and resistance to clomiphene citrate, the administration of clomiphene citrate in combination with metformin satisfactorily increases the ovulation and pregnancy rate [6].

Many studies have reported that metformin can induce oocyte maturation and improve oocyte quality [7]. However, the role of metformin in promoting in vitro oocyte maturation remains unknown. The controversial effects of metformin on in vitro maturation (IVM) of oocytes have been demonstrated. Lee et al. demonstrated the effects of metformin on the in vitro developmental potential of porcine oocytes and embryos; further, they clearly asserted that metformin augments the actions of insulin as an insulin-sensitizing agent on the cytoplasmic aspect of oocyte maturation and the preimplantation embryonic development during in vitro production [8]. In addition, the administration of metformin in combination with oral contraceptives to women with PCOS can increase the probability of in vitro oocyte maturation in relation with miscarriage rate [9]. In contrast, Tosca et al. demonstrated that metformin activates adenosine monophosphate-activated protein kinase (AMPK), which inhibits the germinal vesicle breakdown (GVBD) in cumulus oocyte complexes (COCs) and most COCs arrested at the germinal vesicle (GV) stage, but not denuded bovine oocytes, [10]. Bilodeau-Goeseels et al. also reported that metformin, as an activator of AMPK, inhibited GVBD in bovine cumulus-enclosed oocytes and denuded oocytes and that AMPK might play contradictory roles in the regulation of bovine and murine oocyte maturation, [11].

Despite the ethical and technical restrictions on human experimentations, so far, the animal models that can display all features of human PCOS has not been well introduced. On the other hand, the effects of supplements on the in vitro oocyte maturation to be clearly determined, when all the main characteristics of PCOS are observed. Sabatini et al. revealed that metformin reduced the IVM of oocytes of the wild type and leptin deficient transgenic (ob/ob) mice models, but not in leptin receptor mutant mice (db/db) models, [12]. The in vitro maturation of oocytes consists of two principle features: nuclear and cytoplasmic maturation [8]. Thus far, the precise role of metformin in promoting all the aspects of oocyte maturation in animal models of PCOS has not been identified. The purpose of this study was that, despite the fact that EV PCOS-induced rat model lack some endocrine and metabolic features, whether metformin contributes to the quality of the in vitro maturation of oocytes? Therefore, the present study was designed to investigate the effects of metformin as an additive supplement on nuclear and cytoplasmic maturation as well as the expansion of cumulus cells as the third criterion of oocyte maturation in in EV PCOS-induced rats.

Methods

Experimental design

Forty-five adult female Sprague–Dawley rats (170–230 g) were randomly selected from the animal house of Shiraz University of Medical Sciences (SUMS). The animals were reared under standard conditions (12 h of darkness; 12 h of light; at 23 ± 2 °C), with ad libitum access to food and tap water. The SUMS Ethics Committee approved all the animal procedures. The animals were randomly classified into three groups: PCOS-induced, which received a single dose of EV, 4 mg/0.4 mL of olive oil/rat, IM, to induce PCOS; sham, received only olive oil, 0.4 mL/rat, IM; control, received no drug. This study was designed for a period of 12 weeks, and all the animal groups were kept under standard conditions in separate cages.

Measurement of weight, sex hormones and blood glucose

For defining the characteristics of the animal model of PCOS, the body weight of all the rats was measured once a week for 12 weeks on the same day at the same time; the serum levels of testosterone, estrogen, progesterone, LH, and FSH and blood glucose were also assessed (radioimmunoassay), at the end of week 12.

Histological study

To recognize the presence of cystic follicles in PCOS-induced rats, paraffinzed blocks of the ovaries were prepared. The blocks were cut into 5-μm-thick sections, stained with hematoxylin-eosin, and observed by a light microscope.

Oocyte collection and in vitro maturation

After 12 weeks, the rats were sacrificed and the ovaries excised to acquire COCs. The COCs with a homogeneous ooplasm and at least two layers of cumulus cells were selected for IVM. The COCs of each group were divided into two subgroups and incubated in Ham's F10 (Cat. No. T 071–01) supplemented with 2.1 mg of sodium bicarbonate/mL, 75 µg of penicillin G/mL, 75 µg of streptomycin/mL and 5 % human serum albumin, in the absence and/or presence of metformin (M 5^{-10}) for 12, 24, 36, and 48 h. The concentration of metformin (M 5^{-10}) was assigned based on the results of Lee et al. but not different concentration, because they have demonstrated that different concentrations of metformin alone does not affect the *in vitro* maturation of oocyte [8]. One of the subgroups of oocytes was stained with an aceto-orcein (1 %) solution to define nuclear maturation as the assortment of GV, GVBD, metaphase I (MI), anaphase-telophase (A-T), and MII, and as degenerated and non-detectable by using a light microscope [13, 14]. Cultured denuded oocytes were placed in the center of glass slide, covered and compressed gently with a cover slid which attached to the glass slid by a paraffin-vaseline wax bar on each corner of cover slid to hold and fixed them in acid acetic and methanol (1:3, v/v) for 24 h. Oocytes were stained with 1 % fresh aceto-orcein (1 % orcein in 45 % glacial acetic acid) by pushing aceto-orcein solution between glass slid and cover slid using insulin syringe, and immediately observed by light microscope. To prepare a 1 % aceto-orcein solution, 55 mL of glacial acetic acid was boiled and poured over 1 g of orcein powder. The solution was cooled, and 45 mL of distilled water was added to it.

Evaluation of the expansion of cumulus cells

In both subgroups of oocytes, the expansion of cumulus cells was evaluated using a modification of the method described by Nandi et al. [15] and was categorized as follows: complete expansion (almost all cumulus cells dispersed around the oocytes in a colloidal matrix), semi expansion (the cumulus investment had been initiated for the expansion and was partially dissociated), no expansion (none of the cumulus cells were expanded and they were adherent to the zona pellucida), and degeneration.

Oocyte preparation for transmission electron microscopy

The other subgroup of oocytes was fixed overnight in Karnovsky's solution (2.5 % glutaraldehyde and 2 % paraformaldehyde in 0.1-M sodium cacodylate buffer) and post-fixed in 1 % OsO_4 in 0.1-M sodium cacodylate buffer for 90 min. The samples were then dehydrated by passing them through an ethanol series, embedded in Epon 812 (TAAB, Aldermaston Berkshire, UK), and finally sectioned into semi-thin (1-µm-thick) slices. The sections were mounted on glass slides and stained with toluidine blue; they were examined using a light microscope. The tissue blocks were retrimmed and ultrathin (60–90 nm) sections were taken. These sections were

collected on copper grids, stained with uranyl acetate for 15 min and lead citrate for 12 min at room temperature, and examined using TEM (Philips CM10, Amsterdam, Netherlands).

Statistical analysis

To analyze the data related to the weight and the serum hormone levels, SPSS ver. 15 (SPSS Inc., Chicago, IL, USA) was used, and the weights of the rats were compared by mixed model analysis, and the serum level of hormones with one-way analysis of variance and post-hoc least significant difference. A chi-squared test was used to compare the rate of cumulus cell expansion and that of *in vitro* COCs maturation within the groups.

Results

Measurement of weight, sex hormones and blood glucose

The gain in body weight of the rats within the groups showed a growing trend, the mean (±SD) of the body weight of the rats from week 1 to week 12 increased from 186.20 ± 6.40 to 205.06 ± 3.50 g in the control group, from 186.60 ± 4.53 to 205.60 ± 2.10 g in the sham group, and from 170.26 ± 5.67 to 192.13 ± 2.10 g in the PCOS-induced group, although no significant differences were observed in the body weight of the rats.

The serum level of testosterone decreased, while the progesterone and LH significantly increased in the experimental rats ($p < 0.05$). No significant differences were observed in the estrogen and FSH levels in the three groups (Table 1). Blood glucose level was significantly increased the PCOS-induced (184.40 ± 11.03 mg/dL) vs control (154.40 ± 13.52 mg/dL) rats, ($p < 0.01$).

Histological observations

The histological features of the ovaries under the light microscope showed cystic and relatively degenerated follicles in the PCOS-induced rats (data not shown here and published previously as mention and cited in discussion section).

Table 1 Serum levels of testosterone, estrogen, progesterone, FSH, and LH in rats

a	Control (15 rats)	Sham (15 rats)	PCOS (15 rats)
Testosterone (ng/mL)	0.180 ± 0.068	0.180 ± 0.057	0.130 ± 0.031[a]
Estrogen (pg/mL)	11.120 ± 1.460	10.970 ± 0.470	11.570 ± 0.870
Progesterone (pg/mL)	50.990 ± 9.974	50.770 ± 6.678	56.700 ± 4.400[a]
FSH (ng/mL)	3.140 ± 0.350	3.790 ± 0.310	3.230 ± 0.470
LH (ng/mL)	0.160 ± 0.010	0.200 ± 0.030	0.760 ± 0.050[a]

PCOS polycystic ovary syndrome
[a] Significant differences from the control and sham groups ($p < 0.05$)

In vitro oocyte maturation

Out of the 380 COCs cultured in all groups for 12, 24, 36, and 48 h, the cumulus cells of 53.03 % and 32.83 % of the COCs in the PCOS-induced rats in the metformin-treated and-untreated groups had expanded completely (Fig. 1a), 30.30 % and 25.374 % had semi-expanded, 15.15 % and 34.32 % had not expanded (Fig. 1b), and 1.51 % and 7.46 % had degenerated, respectively (Table 2). The cumulus cells in 64.21 % of the COCs had completely expanded and/or semi-expanded in the absence of metformin, and had increased to 88.94 % in the presence of metformin in all the rats. In addition, in the PCOS-induced rats, the percentage of completely expanded and semi-expanded cumulus cells increased from 58.20 to 83.33 %. The total proportion of COCs with no expansion of the cumulus cells decreased from 30.00 % in the absence of metformin to 10.00 % in the presence of metformin. These results demonstrate that the rate of complete expansion and semi-expansion of the cumulus cells increased significantly, and the percantage of unexpanded cumulus cells decreased significantly in the presence of metformin ($p < 0.05$).

The nuclear maturation of oocytes was evaluated in the three groups: of 172 oocytes, 21 oocytes were in GV, 34 in GVBD (Fig. 2a), 37 in MI (Fig. 2b), 10 in A-T, 28 in MII, and 13 in degeneration; 29 were indistinguishable (Table 3). As mention in table 3, totally, 61.62 % of COCs show one of the stages of meiotic division (sum of GVBD, MI, A-T, and MII) in the absence of metformin (in total column of "without metformin") and significantly increased to 65.11 % in the presence of metformin (in total column of "with metformin"), while in PCOS-induced rats, a fairly significant increase from 57.12 % in metformin-untreated oocytes to 64.28 % in metformin-treated oocytes, ($p < 0.05$). No significant differences in the MII stage within the metformin-treated and -untreated COC groups were seen.

Light and electron microscope observations

The observation of semi-thin and ultrathin sections of COCs by a light (Fig. 3a, b, c) and a TEM (Fig. 4a, b, c, d, e, f) at different times in normal and PCOS-induced rats incubated with and without metformin, revealed the following features: a decrease in the number of connections between cumulus cells and each cell dispersed from the other; presence of many small and dark granulosa cells; decreased cytoplasmic projections of cumulus cells and oocytes in the zona pellucida; enlargement of the perivitelline space (PVS), particularly during 12–36 h of incubation; and redistribution of some cytoplasmic organelles, particularly cortical granules which close to the oolemma. However, polar bodies and Golgi complexes were not observed. Degenerated cells were observed in cumulus cell in metformin-treated group and non-uniform ZP, non-obvious oolemma and narrow PVS were noticed in the absence of metformin.

Discussion

Because of ethical and technical restrictions on human experimentation, researchers have used animal PCOS models. The animal models of PCOS have proven useful in determining the causes of PCOS, to perform preclinical trials, and to examine ovarian morphology, hormonal disorders, and the pathogenesis of anovulation in PCOS. Thus far, a persuasive animal model that can replicate all features of human PCOS has not been established. Among mammals, despite the fact that rhesus monkeys and sheep show major ovarian morphological changes [16], rodents are versatile and a more suitable and unique animal for PCOS models [17, 18]. Compare to rhesus monkeys and sheep, rats and mice are inexpensive, readily available, and

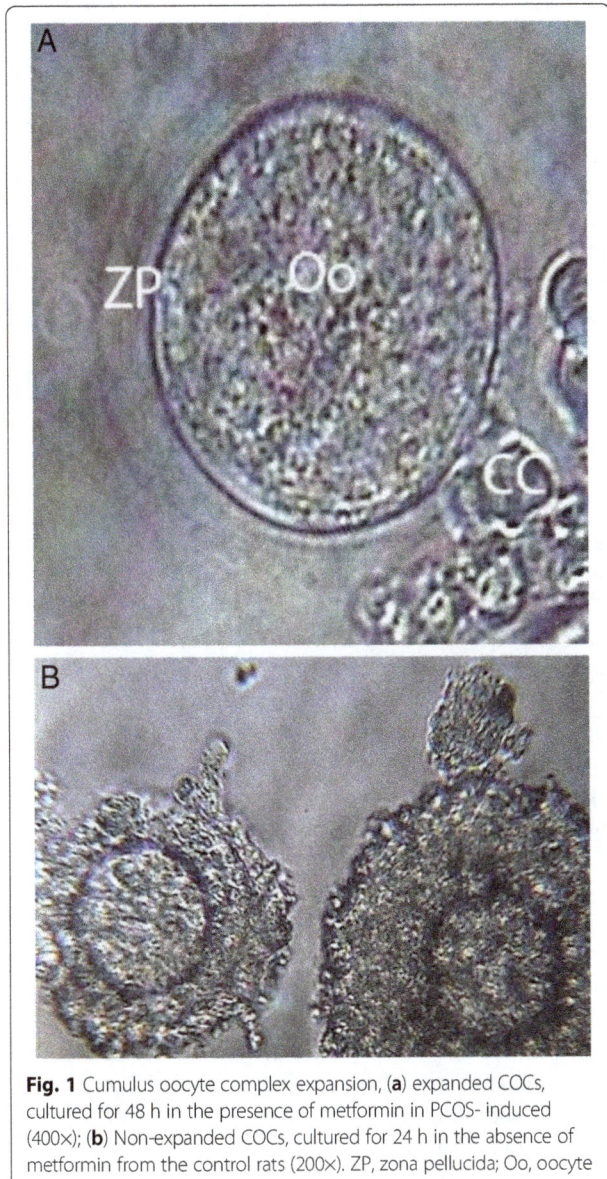

Fig. 1 Cumulus oocyte complex expansion, (**a**) expanded COCs, cultured for 48 h in the presence of metformin in PCOS- induced (400×); (**b**) Non-expanded COCs, cultured for 24 h in the absence of metformin from the control rats (200×). ZP, zona pellucida; Oo, oocyte

Table 2 Expansion of cumulus cells of rat cumulus oocyte complexes in control, sham, and PCOS groups in the absence or presence of metformin

Groups	Without metformin				With metformin				Total
	Control	Sham	PCOS	Total	Control	Sham	PCOS	Total	
	N (%)	N (%)	N (%)	N (%)	N (%)	N (%)	N (%)	N (%)	N (%)
Expansion	25 (40.32)	25 (40.98)	22 (32.83)	72 (37.98)	34 (53.96)	35 (57.37)	35 (53.03)[a]	104 (54.73)[a]	176 (46.31)
Semi expansion	16 (25.80)	17(27.86)	17 (25.37)	50 (26.31)	22 (34.92)	23 (37.70)	20 (30.30)	65 (34.21)[a]	115 (30.26)
No expansion	19 (30.65)	15 (24.59)	23 (34.32)	57 (30.00)	7 (11.11)	2 (3.27)	10 (15.15)[a]	19 (10.00)[a]	76 (20.00)
Degeneration	2 (3.23)	4 (6.55)	5 (7.46)	11 (5.78)	0 (00.00)	1 (1.63)	1 (1.51)[a]	2 (1.05)[a]	13 (3.43)
Total	62	61	67	190	63	61	66	190	380

PCOS polycystic ovary syndrome
[a]Significant differences from the absence of metformin ($p < 0.05$)

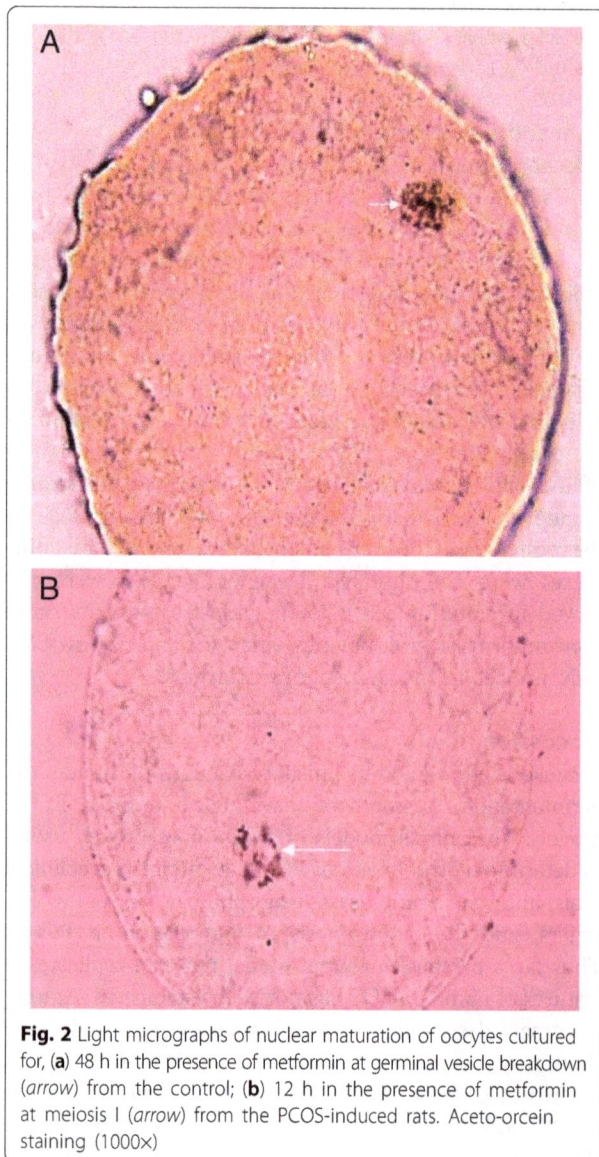

Fig. 2 Light micrographs of nuclear maturation of oocytes cultured for, (**a**) 48 h in the presence of metformin at germinal vesicle breakdown (*arrow*) from the control; (**b**) 12 h in the presence of metformin at meiosis I (*arrow*) from the PCOS-induced rats. Aceto-orcein staining (1000×)

easy to handle and maintain [16], they have a short reproductive cycle, short estrous cycles, and a short gestational period [17, 19]. Rodent models of PCOS have shown hyperandrogenism and hormonal alteration; ovarian morphological changes, including the presence of multi-cystic follicles; and metabolic disorders [17]. Rodent models of PCOS can be attained by a variety of methods, including constant exposure to light [20], genetic manipulation [17], and administration of hormones, such as testosterone (T) [17], dihydrotestosterone (DHT) [21], EV [22, 23], and letrozole (a non-steroidal aromatase inhibitor) [21, 24]. Among these hormones, T, DHT, and letrozole show many characteristics of human PCOS, including acyclicity, anovulation, polycystic ovaries, hyperandrogenism, and insulin resistance [17]. These features are dependent on the dose of hormones, menstrual cycle phase and duration of treatment, and the waiting time for induction of PCOS [25]. Several injections and/or gavages of T, DHT, and letrozole are likely to increase the possibility of stress and high mortality rates during the experiment and it is also a time-consuming method. However, after a single injection of the EV, it will take about 8–12 weeks to induce PCOS, therefor the stress of injection is reduced, it is well known that stress causes irregularities in the menstrual cycle. The EV-induced PCOS model displays characteristic morphological alterations in the ovary [26], particularly the multicystic follicle; as previously shown [27, 28], and mention shortly in results section, which is typically observed in human PCOS. In addition, the EV-induced PCOS model is used in many laboratories, develops hypertension and increases sympathetic activity [29]; these effects lead to increased blood glucose as in this study and it is utilized for autoimmune disorder responses in PCOS [30]. However, the major restrictions of the EV-induced PCOS model are a lack of exactly endocrine and metabolic features associated with human PCOS [17]. It seems that EV can creates a reversible PCO adult rat model, but not PCOS [16, 31, 32], Gonzalo Cruz et al. established an irreversible PCO model when neonatal rat exposure to EV [33]. Recently, Caldwell et al. have demonstrated that long-term DHT

Table 3 Nuclear maturation of rat oocytes in control, sham, and PCOS groups in the absence and presence of metformin

Groups	Without metformin				With metformin				Total
	Control	Sham	PCOS	Total	Control	Sham	PCOS	Total	
	N (%)	N (%)	N (%)	N (%)	N (%)	N (%)	N (%)	N (%)	N (%)
GV	4 (13.79)	3 (10.34)	4 (14.28)	11 (12.79)	3 (10.34)	4 (13.79)	3 (10.71)	10 (11.62)	21 (12.20)
GVBD	6 (20.68)	5 (17.24)	5 (17.85)	16 (18.60)	6 (20.68)	6 (20.68)	6 (21.42)[a]	18 (20.93)	34 (19.76)
MI	6 (20.68)	6 (20.68)	5 (17.85)	17 (19.76)	7 (24.13)	7 (24.13)	6 (21.42) [a]	20 (23.25)	37 (21.51)
A-T	1 (3.44)	3 (10.34)	2 (7.14)	6 (6.97)	1 (3.44)	1 (3.44)	2 (7.14)	4 (4.65)	10 (5.81)
MII	5 (17.24)	5 (17.24)	4 (14.28)	14 (16.27)	5 (17.24)	5 (17.24)	4 (14.28)	14 (16.27)	28 (16.27)
Deg	2 (6.89)	2 (6.89)	3 (10.71)	7 (8.13)	2 (6.89)	1 (3.44)	3 (10.71)	6 (6.97)	13 (7.55)
ND	5 (17.24)	5 (17.24)	5 (17.85	15 (17.44)	5 (17.24)	5 (17.24)	4 (14.28)	14 (16.27)	29 (16.86)
Total	29	29	28	86	29	29	28	86	172

PCOS polycystic ovary syndrome; *GV* germinal vesicle; *GVBD* germinal vesicle breakdown; *MI* metaphase I; *A-T* anaphase-telophase; *MII* metaphase II; *Deg.* degenerated; *ND* not-detectable
[a]Significant differences from without metformin, ($p < 0.05$)

administration in mice imitates an extensive of PCOS features [34].

The results of this present study show that a single intramuscular injection of EV induces experimental PCOS in rats, which can be identified by observing the cystic and atretic follicles as previously indicated in our laboratory [27, 28] and alterations in the serum levels of gonadotropins and increases blood glucose level. In our study, as in the study of Stener-Victorin et al. [29], EV may affect the hypothalamic–pituitary–adrenal axis and the ovary, following a hormonal disorder. Various PCOS animal models have shown dissimilar hormonal changes, but our findings confirm the results of studies by Singh [19], and Stener-Victorin et al. [29], who have reported alterations in the serum levels of gonadotropins.

Obesity is a subordinate symptom of PCOS in women [1]. In this study, weight gain in the PCOS-induced rats was lower than that in the control rats, which is comparable with the results of Stener-Victorin et al. [29]. The administration of EV increases adrenal glucocorticoid production, which enhances lipid metabolism, and leads to a decrease in the body weight [29]. However, the obesity is not always observed in women with PCOS [35, 36]. In addition, the amplification of sympathetic activities in women with PCOS was found to increase lipid metabolism and body activity, and consequently, decreases the body weight [31].

Metformin is an insulin-sensitizing drug [8, 37], usually prescribed in patients with PCOS, to induce ovulation, reduce the symptoms of hyperinsulinemia [8], and improve insulin sensitivity to decrease the serum levels of androgen [37]. It has been reported that metformin contributes to *in vitro* maturation of oocytes, which are collected from patients with PCOS [38], and associated with insulin, but not alone, have beneficial effects on oocyte maturation, oocyte quality and production of embryo [8]. Metformin improves the action of insulin on oocyte glutathione

(GSH) content, which knocks out the free radicals in the oocytes, resulting in enhanced oocyte competence [37]. These results suggest that metformin accompany with insulin may increase the cytoplasmic maturity of oocytes during IVM. Mansfield et al. demonstrated that metformin in the culture medium has a direct effect on cumulus and theca cells and mediates enzyme activities for the synthesis of steroid hormones. In addition, metformin has inhibitory effects on progesterone and estradiol production on the *in vitro* culture of granulosa cells; progesterone is the secreted end point in the steroid synthesis pathway in these cells [39]. Progesterone plays a role in bovine oocyte maturation, particularly in cytoplasmic maturation, but represents a different role and is dependent on cells (oocyte and/or cumulus cells) and the cell progesterone receptors [40]. In addition, progesterone induces meiosis resumption in cultured bovine COCs in a concentration-dependent manner [41]. Our data show that metformin does not affect all features of nuclear and/or cytoplasmic maturation. These controversial effects of metformin on nuclear and cytoplasmic maturation lead us to believe that the EV-induced PCOS animal model does not clearly present all the features of hyperandrogenism and hyperglycemia. It has been reported that metformin is more effective in a batch of transgenic PCOS-induced mice that categorized by hyperleptinemia and hyperinsulinemia [12]. The lacks of our study are that we have not measured leptin and insulin levels, but hyperglycemia was observed in the EV-induced PCOS animal model, which it may be due to the increase in sympathetic activity [29]. In the other hand it is believed that patients with the most obvious hyperandrogenism have most benefited from metformin treatment [42], therefore, in our study the metformin inability to show all aspects of *in vitro* oocyte maturation and may be resulted from deficiency of EV to induce PCOS.

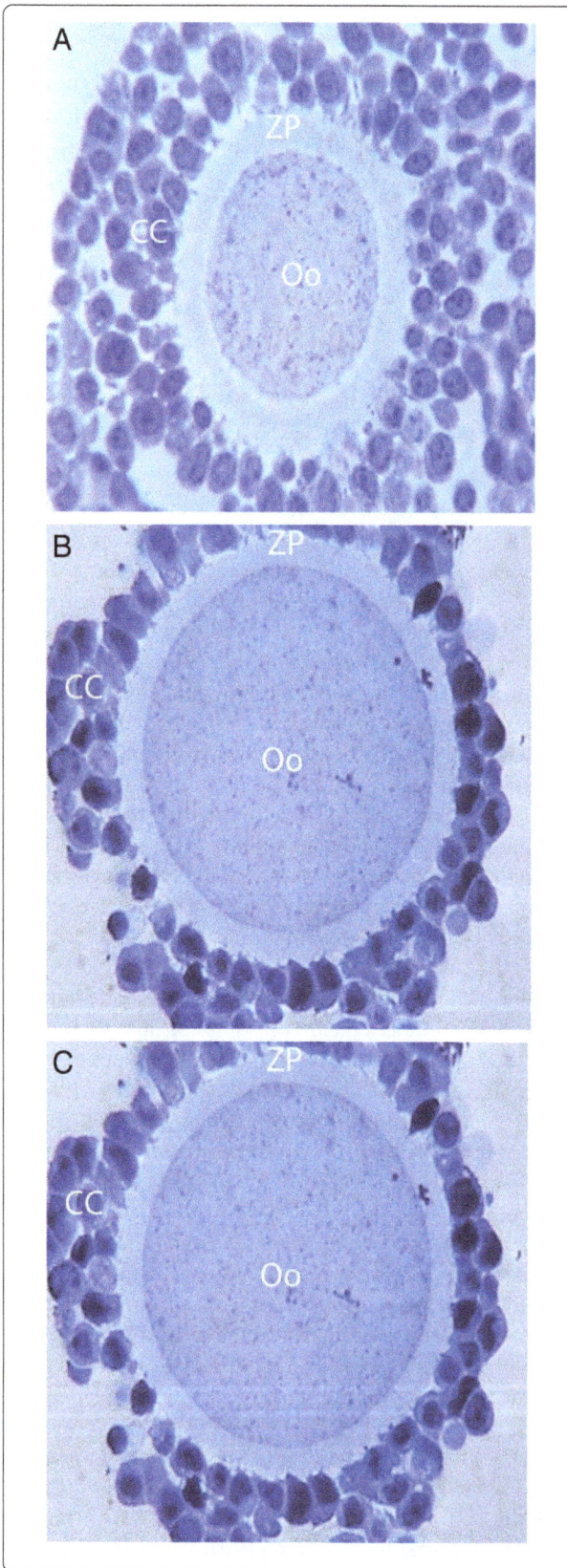

Fig. 3 Light micrographs of oocytes cultured for, (**a**) 12 h in the absence of metformin in the normal; (**b**) 24 h in the absence of metformin in the PCOS-induced; (**c**) 36 h in the presence of metformin in the PCOS-induced rats. Few atretic and dark small cumulus cells noticed in (**c**). Resinate 1 µm-sections, toluidine blue staining (400×). ZP, zona pellucida; Oo, oocyte; CC, cumulus cells

It is clearly known that the expansion of cumulus cells of COCs is a criterion for oocyte maturation. Nagyova reviewed the mechanisms involved in ovarian follicular processes, including the expansion of cumulus cells, the hyaluronan synthesis and progesterone production in COCs. The expansion of cumulus cells in mouse, porcine, bovine, and rat depends on a specific factor, "cumulus expansion enabling factor", which secreted by the oocytes and/or in some mammals, by cumulus cells [43]. It was concluded that optimal cumuli expansion promotes embryonic development in bovine oocytes. It is suggested that glutathione is needed for the expansion of cumulus cells and that hyaluronan accumulates in the expanded cumulus cells. Hyaluronan, which builds up within cumulus cells in porcine COCs during cumuli expansion, disrupts cell junctions of COCs and promotes meiotic resumption in oocytes [44]. Our findings concur with those of previous studies and show that in the presence of metformin in PCOS-induced rats, a higher number of cumulus cells of COCs (53.03 %) are completely expanded as compared to those in the absence of metformin (32.83 %). However, this contradicts the findings of Tosca et al. who concluded that metformin inhibits cumuli expansion and oocyte meiotic resumption in bovine COCs (not denuded oocytes), [45]. These results indicate that the presence of metformin in the culture medium may enhance the expansion of cumulus cells, but not in PCOS-induced rats, because metformin acts first on cumulus cell to dissociate around the oocyte [45]. Despite of metformin has a role on the resumption of meiotic division, a small percentage of oocytes reaches to MII stage. Bilodeau-Goeseels et al. reported that both metformin and aminoimidazole- carboxamide ribofuranoside (AICAR) (activators of AMPK) have inhibitory effects on cumulus cells expansion and nuclear maturation in bovine, but not mouse and are greater in COCs than in denuded oocytes due to the presence of cumulus-oocyte projections [11]. Also Nicolas reported that AMPK has same effects on cumulus cells expansion and nuclear maturation in porcine [46]. Metformin decreased progesterone and estradiol productions *in vitro* in human, rat and bovine granulosa cells [10, 39]. In relevant to the species, different mechanisms involved on estradiol production in granulosa cells and metformin may also reduce steroid levels in granulosa cells from follicular cysts. [10]. Increased estradiol and progesterone concentrations have been reported in the ovarian cyst [47].

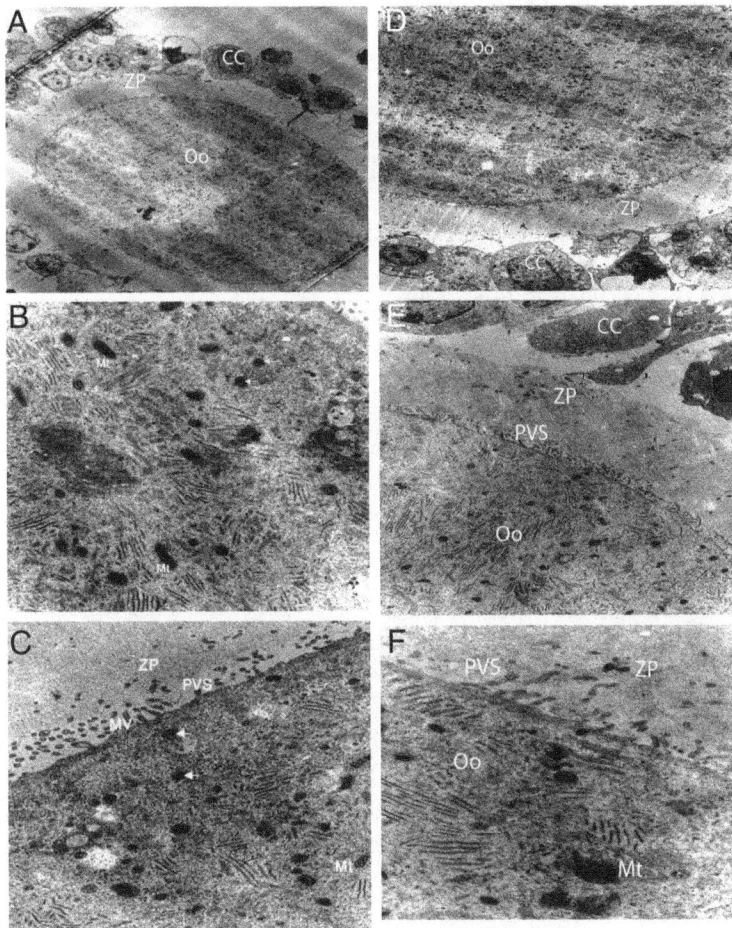

Fig. 4 Electron micrographs of oocytes cultured for, (**a**) 12 h in the absence of metformin from the PCOS-induced (1500×); (**b**) 12 h in the presence of metformin from the PCOS-induced, the arrows denote the cortical granules (8900×); (**c**) 24 h in the presence of metformin from the normal, the arrows denote the cortical granules (3200×); (**d**) 24 h in the presence of metformin from the PCOS-induced, degenerated cumulus cells were noticed. (1650×); (**e**) 36 h in the absence of metformin from the normal, degenerated cumulus cells were noticed. (3900×); (**f**) 36 h in the presence of metformin from the normal rats, PVS filled by microvilli. (1150×). ZP, zona pellucida; CC, cumulus cells; Oo, oocyte; Mt, mitochondria; PVS, perivitelline space; MV, microvilli

Resumption of meiotic division is the other principle of oocyte maturation and takes place largely in IVM. In our study, resumption of meiotic division was slightly increased in the presence of metformin, particularly in the PCOS-induced rats. Although the resumption of oocyte meiotic division is the first step of oocyte maturation, completion of oocyte maturation occurs when the oocyte reaches to the MII stage. In contrast to bovine [45] and porcine [48], which metformin arrested COCs at the GV stage, in our study 65.11 % of COCs were initiated meiotic resumption at the first 6 h of IVM in metformin supplemented medium. While, in PCOS-induced rats a fairly significant increase from 57.12 % in metformin-untreated oocytes to 64.28 % in metformin-treated oocytes. Our data show that, no differences were observed in the percentage of the MII stage between metformin-treated and –untreated oocytes, as reported in bovine

[45], these data clearly show that low percentage of oocytes reached to the MII of maturation. Thus, the nuclear maturation of oocytes in the PCOS-induced rats may be not affected by metformin. Tosca et al. reported that metformin decreases the number of cumulus and theca cells to generate steroid hormone genes, thus indirectly promoting the nuclear maturation of oocytes [10]. In contrast to our findings, Bilodeau-Goeseels et al. concluded that metformin activates AMPK, which inhibits GVBD in bovine COCs and denuded oocytes, but enhances oocyte meiotic resumption in mice, which is similar to that observed in the PCOS-induced rats in our study. Several studies also reported that AMPK may have contradictory roles in the management of bovine and murine oocyte maturation; it seems that a different mechanism is used to stimulate AMPK in rodents [11]. The difference between the rate of cumulus cell expansion

and nuclear maturation in PCOS-induced rat in presence and absence of metformin, may be as a result in a lack of orchestration between these phenomena.

Cytoplasmic maturation is a criterion for deducing the developmental competence of oocyte maturation *in vitro* and includes numerous morphological and biochemical features. The morphological changes include the reduction of the Golgi complex volume, increase in the number of lipid droplets and cortical granules, and enlargement of PVS [49]. The results of this study at the level of light and electron microscopy show that metformin influences few features of oocyte maturation. Cumulus cells around the oocytes in the metformin-treated group were dark, due to nuclear heterochromatin [50], and had lower cell density than the other groups. However, Nottola et al. [51] demonstrated that the presence of dark cumulus cells is related to the accumulation of lipid droplets in the ooplasm, which shows active steroidogenesis in healthy and mature granulosa cells. Our data show that the number of cell junctions between the other cumulus cells and oocytes were decreased, and these tended to expand. According to the findings of Tosca et al. [10], metformin reduces the production of steroids and enzymes in cumulus cells and consequently, causes a decrease in the number of connections between cumulus cells and oocytes; thus, cumulus cells initiate the expansion. Our findings on the effects of metformin, such as a declining trend of cellular links and redistribution of some cytoplasmic organelles, corroborate the findings of Suzuki et al. [52] with human oocytes and granulosa cells cultured in Ham's F-10. An increase in the number of apoptotic cells was observed in cumulus cell in the metformin-treated group. Note that a non-uniform zona pellucida, non-obvious oolemma, and narrow PVS were observed in the absence of metformin. It is well known that the enlargement of PVS is a morphological change in matured oocytes [49, 53]. As we have shown, the presence of cortical granules close to the inside of oolemma is a symptom of oocyte maturation, which is required to prevent polyspermy [54].

Conclusions

This study demonstrated that single dose of EV can creates a reversible PCO adult rat model, but not PCOS, it has no effect on the body weight of rats, but modifies sex hormones and blood glucose level. The results of this study revealed that, metformin enhances the COCs to initiate meiotic resumption at the first 6 h of IVM, but the most of the COCs have never completed meiotic division and the percentage of the MII stage is the same in metformin-treated and –untreated oocytes in EV PCOS-induced rats. In our study the metformin inability to show all aspects of *in vitro* oocyte maturation and may be resulted from deficiency of EV to induce PCOS. The results of this study suggest that further studies

including, assessment of glucose; insulin and leptin level; pre-treatment in vivo and deferent concentration of metformin; and spindle assembly detection are needed to evaluate the metabolic features and effects of metformin on oocyte at the molecular and cellular levels throughout the IVM of oocytes retrieved from EV PCOS-induced rat.

Abbreviations
AICAR: aminoimidazole- carboxamide ribofuranoside; AMPK: adenosine monophosphate-activated protein kinase; A-T: anaphase-telophase; COCs: cumulus oocyte complexes; DHT: dihydrotestosterone; EV: estradiol valerate; GSH: Glutathione; GV: Germinal vesicle; GVBD: Germinal vesicle breakdown; IVM: *in vitro* maturation; PCOS: polycystic ovary syndrome; PVS: perivitelline space; SUMS: Shiraz University of Medical Sciences; T: testosterone; TEM: transmission electron microscopy.

Competing interest
No potential conflict of interest relevant to this article was reported.

Authors' contributions
FM and MM were responsible for study design; ZV contributed to study design; FM and MM acquired, analyzed and interpreted the data; FM wrote the manuscript. HM commented on the administration of medication and the initial draft of manuscript. All authors read and approved the final manuscript.

Acknowledgments
This paper is the result of research project number 85–2824 of an MSc student thesis. The authors would like to thank the Vice Chancellery for Research of Shiraz University of Medical Sciences for financial support, and Mrs. Roohangeez Jafarpour for the electron microscopy technique and Mr. Izad Noori for performing the histological procedure.

Author details
[1]Department of Anatomical Sciences, Shiraz University of Medical Sciences, Shiraz 71348-53185, Iran. [2]Embryonic Stem Cell Lab, Shiraz University of Medical Sciences, Shiraz, Iran. [3]Department of Pharmacology, School of Medicine, Shiraz University of Medical Sciences, Shiraz, Iran. [4]Medicinal and Natural Products Chemistry Research Center, Shiraz University of Medical Sciences, Shiraz, Iran.

References
1. Szilagyi A, Szabo I. Endocrine characteristics of polycystic ovary syndrome (PCOS). Indian J Exp Biol. 2003;41:694–700.
2. Hart R. PCOS and infertility. Panminerva Med. 2008;50:305–14.
3. Jakubowicz DJ, Iuorno MJ, Jakubowicz S, Roberts KA, Nestler JE. Effects of metformin on early pregnancy loss in the polycystic ovary syndrome. J Clin Endocrinol Metab. 2002;87:524–9.
4. Salmi DJ, Zisser HC, Jovanovic L. Screening for and treatment of polycystic ovary syndrome in teenagers. Exp Biol Med (Maywood). 2004;229:369–77.
5. Badawy A, Elnashar A. Treatment options for polycystic ovary syndrome. Inter J of Women's Health. 2011;3:25–35.
6. Kocak I, Ustun C. Effects of metformin on insulin resistance, androgen concentration, ovulation and pregnancy rates in women with polycystic ovary syndrome following laparoscopic ovarian drilling. J Obstet Gynaecol Res. 2006;32:292–8.
7. Costello MF, Eden JA. A systematic review of the reproductive system effects of metformin in patients with polycystic ovary syndrome. Fertil Steril. 2003;79:1–13.
8. Lee MS, Kang SK, Lee BC, Hwang WS. The beneficial effects of insulin and metformin on *in vitro* developmental potential of porcine oocytes and embryos. Biol Reprod. 2005;73:1264–8.
9. Zhao JZ, Lin JJ, Yang HY, Zhang W, Huang XF, Huang YP. Effects of oral contraceptives and metformin on the outcome of *in vitro* maturation in infertile women with polycystic ovary syndrome. J Womens Health (Larchmt). 2010;19:261–5.

10. Tosca L, Chabrolle C, Uzbekova S, Dupont J. Effects of metformin on bovine granulosa cells steroidogenesis: possible involvement of adenosine 5' monophosphate-activated protein kinase (AMPK). Biol Reprod. 2007;76:368–78.

11. Bilodeau-Goeseels S, Sasseville M, Guillemette C, Richard FJ. Effects of adenosine monophosphate-activated kinase activators on bovine oocyte nuclear maturation in vitro. Mol Reprod Dev. 2007;74:1021–34.

12. Sabatini ME, Guo L, Lynch MP, Doyle JO, Lee H, Rueda BR, et al. Metformin therapy in a hyperandrogenic anovulatory mutant murine model with polycystic ovarian syndrome characteristics improves oocyte maturity during superovulation. J Ovarian Res. 2011;4:8.

13. Hewitt DA, England GC. The effect of oocyte size and bitch age upon oocyte nuclear maturation in vitro. Theriogenology. 1998;49:957–66.

14. Oliveira e Silva I, Vasconcelos RB, Caetano JV, Gulart LV, Camargo LS, Bao SN, et al. Induction of reversible meiosis arrest of bovine oocytes using a two-step procedure under defined and nondefined conditions. Theriogenology. 2011;75:1115–24.

15. Nandi S, Ravindranatha BM, Gupta PS, Sarma PV. Timing of sequential changes in cumulus cells and first polar body extrusion during in vitro maturation of buffalo oocytes. Theriogenology. 2002;57:1151–9.

16. Padmanabhan V, Veiga-Lopez A. Animal models of the polycystic ovary syndrome phenotype. Steroids. 2013;78(8):734–40. doi:10.1016/j.steroids.2013.05.004.

17. Walters KA, Allan CM, Handelsman DJ. Rodent models for human polycystic ovary syndrome. Biol Reprod. 2012;86:149.

18. Yanes LL, Romero DG, Moulana M, Lima R, Davis DD, et al. Cardiovascular-renal and metabolic characterization of a rat model of polycystic ovary syndrome. Gend Med. 2011;8(2):103–15. doi:10.1016/j.genm.2010.11.013.

19. Singh KB. Persistent estrus rat models of polycystic ovary disease: an update. Fertil Steril. 2005;84 Suppl 2:1228–34.

20. Lambert HH. Continuous red light induces persistent estrus without retinal degeneration in the albino rat. Endocrinology. 1975;97:208–10.

21. Manneras L, Cajander S, Holmang A, Seleskovic Z, Lystig T, Lonn M, et al. A new rat model exhibiting both ovarian and metabolic characteristics of polycystic ovary syndrome. Endocrinology. 2007;148:3781–91.

22. Shirwalkar H, Modi DN, Maitra A. Exposure of adult rats to estradiol valerate induces ovarian cyst with early senescence of follicles. Mol Cell Endocrinol. 2007;272:22–37.

23. Stener-Victorin E, Kobayashi R, Watanabe O, Lundeberg T, Kurosawa M. Effect of electro-acupuncture stimulation of different frequencies and intensities on ovarian blood flow in anaesthetized rats with steroid-induced polycystic ovaries. Reprod Biol Endocrinol. 2004;2:16.

24. Kafali H, Iriadam M, Ozardali I, Demir N. Letrozole-induced polycystic ovaries in the rat: a new model for cystic ovarian disease. Arch Med Res. 2004;35:103–8.

25. Tyndall V, Broyde M, Sharpe R, Welsh M, Drake AJ, McNeilly AS. Effect of androgen treatment during foetal and/or neonatal life on ovarian function in prepubertal and adult rats. Reproduction. 2012;143:21–33.

26. Dikmen A, Ergenoglu AM, Yeniel AO, Dilsiz OY, GulinnazErcan HY. Evaluation of glycemic and oxidative/antioxidative status in the estradiol valerate-induced PCOS model of rats. Eur J Obstet Gynecol Reprod Biol. 2012;160:55–9.

27. Mesbah F, Moslem M, Vojdani Z, Mirkhani H. Estradiol Valerate-induced Polycystic Ovary Syndrome: An Animal Model Study. Armeghan e Danesh. Winter. 2011;60:325–34. Article in Persian.

28. Noorafshan A, Ahmadi M, Mesbah SF, Karbalay-Doust S. Stereological study of the effects of letrozole and estradiol valerate treatment on the ovary of rats. CERM. 2013;40(3):115–21.

29. Stener-Victorin E, Ploj K, Larsson BM, Holmang A. Rats with steroid-induced polycystic ovaries develop hypertension and increased sympathetic nervous system activity. Reprod Biol Endocrinol. 2005;3:44.

30. Chapman JC, Min SH, Freeh SM, Michael SD. The estrogen-injected female mouse: new insight into the etiology of PCOS. Reprod Biol Endocrinol. 2009;7:47.

31. Shi D, Vine DF. Animal models of polycystic ovary syndrome: a focused review of rodent models in relationship to clinical phenotypes and cardiometabolic risk. Fertil Steril. 2012;98(1):185–93. doi:10.1016/j.fertnstert.2012.04.006.

32. McNeilly AS, Colin Duncan W. Rodent models of polycystic ovary syndrome. Mol and Cellul Endoc. 2013;373(1-2):2-7 http://dx.doi.org/10.1016/j.mce.2012.10.007.

33. Cruz G, Barra R, Gonzalez D, Sotomayor-Zarate R, Lara HE. Temporal window in which exposure to estradiol permanently modifies ovarian function causing polycystic ovary morphology in rats. Fertil Steril. 2012;98:1283–90.

34. Caldwell ASL, Middleton LJ, Jimenez M, Desai R, McMahon AC, Allan CM, et al. Characterization of Reproductive, Metabolic, and Endocrine Features of Polycystic Ovary Syndrome in Female Hyperandrogenic Mouse Models. Endocrinology. 2014;155:3146–59. http://dx.doi.org/10.1210/en.2014-1196.

35. Hart R, Hickey M, Franks S. Definitions, prevalence and symptoms of polycystic ovaries and polycystic ovary syndrome. Best Pract Res Clin Obstet Gynaecol. 2004;18:671–83.

36. Kushnir VA, Halevy N, Barad DH, Albertini DF, Gleicher N. Relative importance of AMH and androgens changes with aging among non-obese women with polycystic ovary syndrome. J of Ovarian Research. 2015;8:45. doi:10.1186/s13048-015-0175-x.

37. Motta AB. Dehydroepiandrosterone to induce murine models for the study of polycystic ovary syndrome. J Steroid Biochem Mol Biol. 2010;119:105–11.

38. Wei Z, Cao Y, Cong L, Zhou P, Zhang Z, Li J. Effect of metformin pretreatment on pregnancy outcome of in vitro matured oocytes retrieved from women with polycystic ovary syndrome. Fertil Steril. 2008;90:1149–54.

39. Mansfield R, Galea R, Brincat M, Hole D, Mason H. Metformin has direct effects on human ovarian steroidogenesis. Fertil Steril. 2003;79:956–62.

40. Aparicio IM, Garcia-Herreros M, O'Shea LC, Hensey C, Lonergan P, Fair T. Expression, regulation, and function of progesterone receptors in bovine cumulus oocyte complexes during in vitro maturation. Biol Reprod. 2011;84:910–21.

41. Siqueira LC, Barreta MH, Gasperin B, Bohrer R, Santos JT, Buratini Jr J, et al. Angiotensin II, progesterone, and prostaglandins are sequential steps in the pathway to bovine oocyte nuclear maturation. Theriogenology. 2012;77:1779–87.

42. Kolodziejczyk B, Duleba AJ, Spaczynski RZ, Pawelczyk L. Metformin therapy decreases hyperandrogenism and hyperinsulinemia in women with polycystic ovary syndrome. Fertil Steril. 2000;73:1149–54.

43. Nagyova E. Regulation of cumulus expansion and hyaluronan synthesis in porcine oocyte-cumulus complexes during in vitro maturation. Endocr Regul. 2012;46:225–35.

44. Yokoo M, Kimura N, Abe H, Sato E. Influence of hyaluronan accumulation during cumulus expansion on in vitro porcine oocyte maturation. Zygote. 2008;16:309–14.

45. Tosca L, Uzbekova S, Chabrolle C, Dupont J. Possible role of 5'AMP-activated protein kinase in the metformin-mediated arrest of bovine oocytes at the germinal vesicle stage during in vitro maturation. Biol Reprod. 2007;77:452–65.

46. Santiquet N, Sasseville M, Laforest M, Guillemette C, Gilchrist RB, Richard FJ. Activation of 5 Adenosine Monophosphate-Activated Protein Kinase Blocks Cumulus Cell Expansion through Inhibition of Protein Synthesis during In Vitro Maturation in Swine. Biol Reprod. 2014;91(2):51. doi:10.1095/biolreprod.113.116764.

47. Hatler TB, Hayes SH, Laranja da Fonseca LF, Silvia WJ. Relationship between endogenous progesterone and follicular dynamics in lactating dairy cows with ovarian follicular cysts. Biol Reprod. 2003;69:218–23.

48. LaRosa C, Downs SM. Stress stimulates AMP-activated protein kinase and meiotic resumption in mouse oocytes. Biol Reprod. 2006;74:585–92.

49. Hyttel P, Fair T, Callesen H, Greve T. Oocyte growth, capacitation and final maturation in cattle. Theriogenology. 1997;47:23–32.

50. Centurione L, Giampietro F, Sancilio S, Piccirilli M, Artese L, Tiboni GM, et al. Morphometric and ultrastructural analysis of human granulosa cells after gonadotrophin-releasing hormone agonist or antagonist. Reprod Biomed Online. 2010;20:625–33.

51. Nottola SA, Heyn R, Camboni A, Correr S, Macchiarelli G. Ultrastructural characteristics of human granulosa cells in a coculture system for in vitro fertilization. Microsc Res Tech. 2006;69:508–16.

52. Suzuki S, Kitai H, Tojo R, Seki K, Oba M, Fujiwara T, et al. Ultrastructure and some biologic properties of human oocytes and granulosa cells cultured in vitro. Fertil Steril. 1981;35:142–8.

53. Zamboni L, Mishell Jr DR, Bell JH, Baca M. Fine structure of the human ovum in the pronuclear stage. J Cell Biol. 1966;30:579–600.

54. Hyttel P, Xu KP, Smith S, Greve T. Ultrastructure of in-vitro oocyte maturation in cattle. J Reprod Fertil. 1986;78:615–25.

14

Circulating anti-mullerian hormone as predictor of ovarian response to clomiphene citrate in women with polycystic ovary syndrome

Wenyan Xi[1], Yongkang Yang[2], Hui Mao[1*], Xiuhua Zhao[1], Ming Liu[1] and Shengyu Fu[1]

Abstract

Background: To investigate the impact of high circulating AMH on the outcome of CC ovulation induction in women with PCOS.

Methods: This prospective cohort observational study included 81 anovulatory women with PCOS who underwent 213 cycles of CC ovarian stimulation. Serum AMH concentrations were measured on cycle day 3 before the commencement of CC in the first cycle, which were compared between responders and CC-resistant anovulation (CRA). Logistic regression analysis was applied to study the value of serum AMH for the prediction of ovarian responsiveness to CC stimulation. The receiver-operating characteristic (ROC) curve was used to evaluate the prognostic value of circulating AMH.

Main outcome measures: Serum AMH levels.

Results: Women who ovulated after CC therapy had a significantly lower AMH compared with the CRA (5.34 ± 1.97 vs.7.81 ± 3.49, $P < 0.001$). There was a significant gradient increase of serum AMH levels with the increasing dose of CC required to achieve ovulation ($P < 0.05$). In multivariate logistic regression analysis, AMH was an independent predictor of ovulation induction by CC in PCOS patients. ROC curve analysis showed AMH to be a useful predictor of ovulation induction by CC in PCOS patients, having 92 % specificity and 65 % sensitivity when the threshold AMH concentration was 7.77 ng/ml.

Conclusion: Serum AMH may be clinically useful to predict which PCOS women are more likely to respond to CC treatment and thus to direct the selection of protocols of ovulation induction.

Keywords: Anti-Müllerian hormone, Clomiphene citrate, Ovulation induction, Polycystic ovary syndrome

Background

Polycystic ovary syndrome (PCOS) is the most common endocrine disorder in women of reproductive age, with a prevalence of approximately 5–10 %. PCOS is the major cause of anovulatory infertility [1]. The recent studies suggest that anovulation results from ovarian follicle abnormalities in PCOS patitents are 2-fold [2, 3]. First, early follicular growth is excessive, thus women with PCOS are characterized by an excessive number of small antral follicles (2- to 3-fold that of normal ovaries). Secondly, the selection of one follicle from the increased pool of selectable follicles and its further maturation to a dominant follicle does not occur. This second abnormality in the folliculogenesis is named the follicular arrest (FA) and explains the ovulatory disorder of PCOS. Although the FA has not received yet a clear and unanimous explanation, Anti-Müllerian hormone (AMH) is considered as important contributors to this abnormality [4, 5].

AMH is produced specifically by granulose cells of early developing pre-antral and small antral follicles in

* Correspondence: xwyanzi@126.com
[1]Department of Obstetrics and Gynaecology, The Second Affiliated Hospital of Xi'an Jiaotong University, No. 157, Xiwu Road, Xi'an City 710004 Shaanxi Prov., China
Full list of author information is available at the end of the article

the ovary. Serum AMH levels in women with PCOS are 2- to 3-fold higher than in ovulatory women with normal ovaries [6, 7], which corresponds to the 2- to 3-fold increase in the number of small follicles seen in PCOS. The increased AMH has been hypothesized may reduce follicle sensitivity to FSH and oestradiol production, thus preventing follicle selection, resulting in follicle arrest at the small antral phase with the failure of dominance.

At present, the treatment of oligo- or anovulatory infertility is referred to as induction of ovulation. Clomiphene citrate (CC) is the treatment of first choice for ovulation induction in anovulatory women with PCOS. There are 20–25 % of women, however, remain anovulatory after receiving CC medication [8] and the exact cause of CC failure in some patients remain uncertain. Indentifying factors that determine the response of women with PCOS to CC will help selecting patients who are likely to benefit from this treatment, thus avoiding fruitless treatment and improving success rates.

Recently, AMH has been characterized as a promising novel clinical marker of ovarian reserve and predicting ovarian response to gonadotrophins during in vitro fertilization (IVF) in women without PCOS [9–11]. In PCOS women, we recent found AMH levels on day 3 of the IVF stimulation cycle still positively predict ovarian response to gonadotrophins [12]. However, different from our study, the predictive meaning of AMH was considered different between women with and without PCOS, for the authors found circulating AMH levels were negatively correlated with ovarian response to gonadotrophins during ovary induction in PCOS women [13]. Hence, the results of hitherto published studies are seemed not entirely in consensus. So we designed a study to investigate whether serum AMH has a role in predicting ovary response to CC treatment in a large cohort of infertile women with PCOS.

Methods

Patients

Subjects included 81 anovulatory women with PCOS who were referred to our department for ovulation induction between February 2012 and June 2014. The diagnosis of PCOS was based on the Rotterdam criteria, in which at least two of the following three criteria were met: oligomenorrhea or amenorrhea, hyperandrogenaemia, and sonographic appearance of polycystic ovaries [14]. Oligomenorrhoea was defined as cycles lasting longer than 35 days. Amenorrhea was defined as cycles lasting longer than 6 months. Hyperandrogenism was diagnosed either clinically (acne/hirsutism) and/or biochemically (testosterone >0.7 ng/ml). The ovary was considered polycystic on ultrasound scan if it contained ≥12 follicles (2–9 mm in diameter) and/or measured >10 ml in volume. All patients presented

with anovulatory cycles for at least 2 years. The inclusion criteria included: patients 35 years old or younger, BMI ≤30 kg/m without previous ovulation induction and partners with normal semen parameters. No PCOS patient had evidence of hyperprolactinemia, Cushing's syndrome, congenital adrenal hyperplasia or androgen-secreting tumors.

Ethical approval

This study was approved by the Ethics Committee of The Second Affiliated Hospital of Xi an Jiaotong University. All participants provided their informed consent before their involvement in this study.

Clomiphene citrate treatment

All women received an initial dose of 50 mg/d CC from cycle d3 until d7 after spontaneous or progestagen-induced withdrawal bleeding. In the case of an absent ovarian response, daily dosage was increased to 100 mg in the following cycles. If ovulation occurred, the dose remained unaltered during subsequent cycles. First ovulation was used as the end point. The duration of all patients included in the study was at least three treatment cycles. Ovulation was assessed by midluteal serum progesterone measurement (levels >10 ng/ml indicating ovulation) combined with transvaginal sonographic monitoring of follicle growth until the appearance of a preovulatory follicle (mean diameter ≥18 mm) and subsequent follicle rupture. Responders were defined as patients who ovulated during CC therapy, independent of the dose administered. Failure to ovulate in three CC cycles despite stimulation with the maximum dose (100 mg/d) was referred to as CC-resistant anovulation (CRA). Clinical pregnancy was defined as the presence of a gestational sac with cardiacactivity as detected by transvaginal ultrasound after 35 days of ovulation.

Hormone assays

Blood samples were collected on cycle day 3 before the commencement of CC in the first cycle of treatment to measure baseline serum concentrations of AMH. AMH was measured by using a second-generation enzyme-linked immunosorbent assay (ELISA) (Immunotech Beckman Coulter Laboratories, Villepinte, France). The analytical sensitivity of this assay is 0.14 ng/mL. Intra- and inter-assay coefficients of variation were ≤12.3 and ≤14.2 %, respectively.

Serum other hormonal concentrations including luteinizing hormone (LH), follicle stimulating hormone (FSH), testosterone (T), insulin and progesterone were measured using electrochemiluminescence immunoassay (Roche Diagnostics GmbH, Mannheim, Germany). Insulin resistance, defined by the homeostasis model assessment insulin resistance index (HOMA-IR), was calculated using the following equation: HOMA-IR = fasting insulin (IU/ml) × fasting glucose (mmol/L)/22.5 [15].

Transvaginal scan

In the same morning of the blood tests, a transvaginal ultrasound scan was performed to assess the ovarian volume (milliliters), and antral follicles count (AFC). The volume of each ovary was calculated by measuring the ovarian diameters (D) in three perpendicular directions and applying the formula for an ellipsoid: D1 × D2 × D3 × 0.5236. For the determination of the AFC, we calculated small follicles with a diameter between 2 and 9 mm, following the recommendations as described previously [16].

Statistical analysis

The Statistical Package for Social Sciences (SPSS 17.0, Chicago) was used for statistical analysis. Differences between responders and nonresponders were tested using the t-test, nonparametric test (Mann–Whitney U) and $\chi 2$-test as appropriate. Spearman's correlation coefficient was calculated to evaluate the relation of AMH to other characteristics of PCOS. Using the results of the ROC analysis, we defined an appropriate threshold level for AMH and determined the sensitivity and specificity of that threshold. Logistic regression analysis was applied to study the value of serum AMH and other study variables for the prediction of ovarian responsiveness to CC stimulation. $P < 0.05$ was considered statistically significant. Multiple logistic regression analysis with forward selection of parameters was applied with $P < 0.10$ for entry.

Results

The study included 81 anovulatory women with PCOS who received 213 cycles of CC ovulation induction. Patient characteristics are shown in Table 1. Of the 81 women included in the study, 43 (53.1 %) ovulated during ovulation induction with CC 50 mg/d. This number increased to 52 (64.2 %) after increasing CC dose up to the100 mg/d, 29(35.8 %) remaining anovulatory were considered CRA (Fig. 1). A total of 26(32.1 %) women conceived during up to three cycles of CC treatment. Of the 213 CC cycles, ovulation occurred in 114 cycles (53.5 %) and pregnancy in 26 cycles (12.2 %).

Women were divided into two groups based on their response to clomiphene citrate treatment: CC responders ($n = 52$) and CRA ($n = 29$). Patients who ovulated had a significantly lower serum AMH concentration compared with nonresponders (5.34 ± 1.97 vs.7.81 ± 3.49, $P < 0.001$). AFC and ovarian volume from responders group were statistically significantly lower than from the CRA group ($P < 0.05$). There were no significant differences between the groups in mean age, BMI, FSH, LH, LH/FSH, T and HOMA-IR (Table 1). In addition, patients who conceived had a significantly lower serum AMH concentrations compared with that of those who did not conceive (4.81 ± 2.06 vs. 6.89 ± 2.95 ng/ml, $P < 0.01$) (Table 2). When CC-resistant patients were excluded from analysis of pregnancy, serum AMH concentrations were comparable in women achieving pregnancy ($n = 26$) and those not conceiving ($n = 26$) (4.81 ± 2.06 ng/ml vs 5.67 ± 1.76 ng/ml, $P > 0.05$).

Spearman's correlations between serum AMH concentrations and other characteristics of PCOS showed AMH significantly correlated with serum LH ($r = 0.253$, $P < 0.05$), ovarian volume ($r = 0.297$, $P < 0.01$) and AFC ($r = 0.296$, $P < 0.01$). No statistically significant correlation between

Table 1 Baseline characteristics of 81 anovulatory women with PCOS who received CC ovulation induction, and separated for women who do (responders) or do not ovulate (CRA) after CC induction of ovulation

Variable	All participants	CC responders	CRA	P value
	$n = 81$	$n = 52$	$n = 29$	
Age (years)	26.62 ± 2.53	26.98 ± 2.48	25.97 ± 2.53	NS
BMI (kg/m2)	23.79 ± 2.78	23.53 ± 2.81	24.24 ± 2.71	NS
LH(IU/L)	8.29 ± 2.37	8.01 ± 2.29	8.77 ± 2.49	NS
FSH(IU/L)	5.73 ± 1.19	5.79 ± 1.28	5.62 ± 1.03	NS
LH/FSH	1.52 ± 0.59	1.46 ± 0.58	1.63 ± 0.62	NS
T(ng/ml)	0.56 ± 0.25	0.55 ± 0.23	0.58 ± 0.29	NS
HOMA-IR	3.18 ± 1.92	3.11 ± 2.16	3.31 ± 1.41	NS
Ovarian volume (ml)	10.43 ± 1.58	9.7 ± 1.32	10.49 ± 1.74	<0.05
AFC (n)	16.11 ± 3.71	15.44 ± 3.17	17.31 ± 4.33	<0.05
AMH	6.22 ± 2.8	5.34 ± 1.97	7.81 ± 3.49	<0.001

Note: Values are mean ± SD unless otherwise indicated

CRA CC-resistant anovulation, *BMI* body mass index, *LH* luteinizing hormone, *FSH* follicle stimulating hormone, *T* testosterone, *HOMA-IR* the homeostasis model assessment insulin resistance index, *AFC* antral follicles count, *AMH* antimüllerian hormone, *NS* Not statistially significant

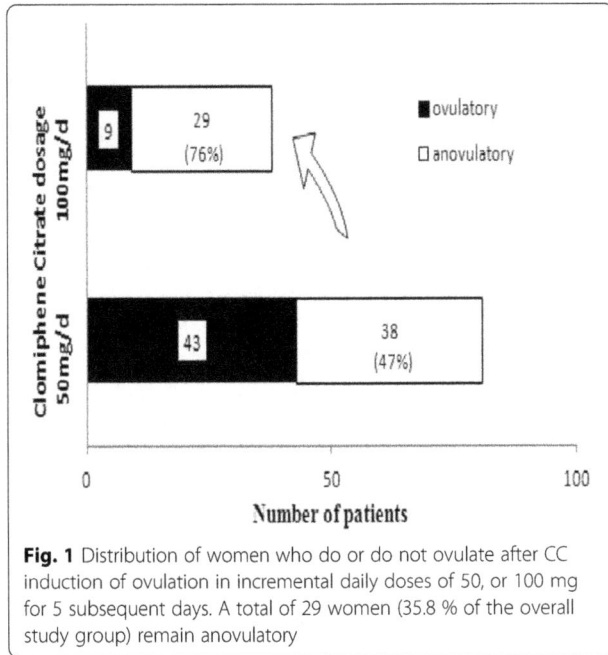

Fig. 1 Distribution of women who do or do not ovulate after CC induction of ovulation in incremental daily doses of 50, or 100 mg for 5 subsequent days. A total of 29 women (35.8 % of the overall study group) remain anovulatory

serum AMH and BMI, FSH, LH/FSH, T and HOMA-IR could be found (Table 3). Univariate logistic regression analysis showed that AMH, AFC and ovarian volume were significant predictors of ovarian response to CC stimulation. For the multivariate logistic regression analysis using stepwise forward selection on all variables, AMH was selected in the final model, while mean ovarian volume and AFC were not (date were not shown).

Figure 2 presents ROC for the sensitivity and specificity of the AMH at different levels in predicting no ovulation after CC therapy. The AMH shows a ROCAUC of 0.813 for no ovulation, indicating a useful potential for predicting CRA. Considering a serum AMH concentration of 7.77 ng/ml as cut-off,

Table 2 Comparison the characteristics of PCOS women who conceived on CC treatment (n = 26) and those who did not conceive (n = 55)

	Pregnant	Nonpregnant	P value
	n = 26	n = 55	
Age (years)	27.08 ± 2.23	26.40 ± 2.65	NS
BMI (kg/m2)	23.46 ± 2.83	23.94 ± 2.77	NS
LH(IU/L)	8.05 ± 2.12	8.40 ± 2.50	NS
FSH(IU/L)	5.55 ± 1.3	5.82 ± 1.14	NS
LH/FSH	1.55 ± 0.65	1.51 ± 0.57	NS
T(ng/ml)	0.55 ± 0.22	0.58 ± 0.27	NS
HOMA-IR	3.02 ± 1.35	3.27 ± 2.69	NS
Ovarian volume (ml)	9.52 ± 1.28	10.27 ± 1.48	<0.05
AFC (n)	15.04 ± 2.82	16.62 ± 3.98	NS
AMH	4.81 ± 2.06	6.89 ± 2.95	<0.01

Table 3 Spearman's correlations between plasma AMH and other factors in women with PCOS

Variable	r	P value
Age (years)	−0.012	NS
BMI (kg/m2)	0.027	NS
LH (IU/L)	0.253	<0.05
FSH(IU/L)	−0.06	NS
LH/FSH	0.207	NS
T(ng/ml)	0.065	NS
HOMA-IR	0.016	NS
Ovarian volume (ml)	0.297	<0.01
AFC (n)	0.296	<0.01

the sensitivity and specificity of predicting no ovulation were 92 and 65 % respectively. With this cut-off (7.77 ng/ml), the outcomes of CC ovarian stimulation were compared between cycles with high AMH vs. low AMH levels. Patients with AMH levels less than 7.77 ng/ml had significantly higher ovulation and pregnancy rates than those with AMH of 7.77 ng/ml or greater. In addition, patients with high AMH levels had significantly higher LH, ovarian volume and AFC (Table 4).

AMH and dose of CC

The mean serum concentration of AMH was compared between PCOS patients who responded to CC 50 mg (n = 43) vs those who responded to the higher dose 100 mg (n = 9). The results showed a significant

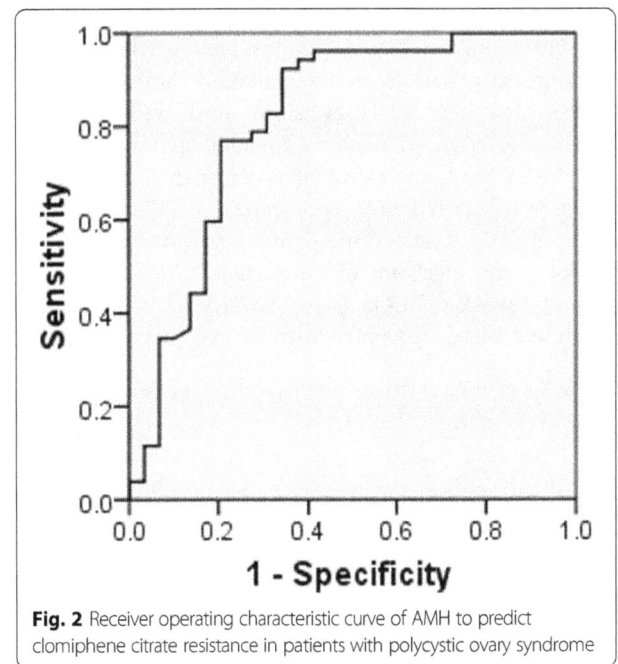

Fig. 2 Receiver operating characteristic curve of AMH to predict clomiphene citrate resistance in patients with polycystic ovary syndrome

Table 4 Comparison of PCOS women with high vs low AMH using a cutoff value of 7.77 ng/ml

	AMH <7.77 ng/ml $n = 59$	AMH ≥7.77 ng/ml $n = 22$	P value	PPV	NPV
Age (years)	26.68 ± 2.31	26.45 ± 3.08	NS		
BMI (kg/m2)	23.54 ± 2.80	24.45 ± 2.67	NS		
LH(IU/L)	7.92 ± 2.26	9.28 ± 2.43	<0.05		
FSH(IU/L)	5.73 ± 1.16	5.73 ± 1.29	NS		
LH/FSH	1.45 ± 0.55	1.72 ± 0.66	NS		
T(ng/ml)	0.56 ± 0.22	0.56 ± 0.33	NS		
HOMA-IR	3.12 ± 2.09	3.24 ± 1.39	NS		
Ovarian volume (ml)	9.72 ± 1.31	10.69 ± 1.82	<0.01		
AFC (n)	15.24 ± 3.06	18.45 ± 4.31	<0.01		
Ovulation/patient	46/81(57 %)	6/81(7 %)	<0.001	88.5	55.2
Pregnancy/patient	23/81(28 %)	3/81(4 %)	<0.01	88.4	34.5

$(P < 0.05)$ increase of serum AMH level with the increasing dose of CC (Table 5).

Discussion

Since the increased AMH would impair the action of FSH and contribute to the FA of PCOS, this evidence has led us to hypothesise that there is a subgroup of women with PCOS who have the higher levels of AMH and who are the more resistant to CC treatment. In this study, we really proved that patients with high AMH level are less likely to respond to CC treatment. Furthermore, we have identified a cut-off level of AMH (7.77 ng/ml), above which the chances of ovulation seem to be significantly reduced. These observations suggest that high AMH values reflect more impaired disruption in folliculogenesis and granulosa cell function.

However, it may seem paradoxical that serum AMH concentrations are known to positively predict ovarian response to gonadotrophin stimulation during IVF. For women with high AMH levels are considered to predict excessive ovarian response to gonadotropin. Meanwhile, low AMH levels indicative of a diminished ovarian reserve, is associated with poor response [17, 18]. Amer SA et al. [13] explained the contradiction may be due to the different spectrum of circulating AMH in women with and without PCOS. Since AMH levels were significantly increased in women with PCOS, they considered

levels above the optimum AMH values are associated with poor ovarian response to stimulation. It is interesting to note that, in contrast to Amer SA's opinion, Kaya et al. [19] and our previous study [12] found a positive association between serum AMH levels and ovarian responsiveness to gonadotrophins during IVF in women with PCOS. In that study as serum AMH levels increased, an increase in estrodiol levels on the day of hCG administration and the number of retrieved oocytes were observed, while the total dose of the gonadotrophins was significantly decreased. Thus, we suppose the predictive role of AMH is different in ovarian responsiveness to ovulation induction with CC and ovarian hyperstimulation with gonadotrophins for IVF treatment, because the goal of stimulation in women with anovulation is different than that in women undergoing IVF.

It is supposed that in anovulatory women with PCOS, increasing the serum FSH level may reduce the AMH excess, thus relieving its inhibition on the follicular growth, and allowing the emergence of a dominant follicle [20]. In ovulation induction the aim should be to achieve the ovulation of a single follicle, CC thus constitutes the first line treatment of choice in PCOS women. Chronic low-dose gonadotrophins (with a starting dose 37.5 or 50U daily) have been used to stimulate ovulation in women who fail to ovulate with CC. However, both CC and low-dose gonadotrophins make the serum FSH levels increased gently and may be not enough to reduce intra-ovarian AMH to a level consistent with resumption of ovulation in women with high AMH level. Therefore, as expected the patient with higher AMH were more deeply inhibited and more likely to remain anovulatory after ovulation induction. The aim of IVF treatment, however, is normally designed to promote multifollicular development and as such will usually employ higher doses of FSH (with a starting dose at least

Table 5 Serum AMH concentrations in PCOS patients achieving ovulation on different doses of CC

Dose (mg)	Clinical outcome		AMH levels achieving ovulation	P value
	Not ovulated, n (%)	Ovulated, n (%)		
50	38 (46.9)	43 (53.1)	5.07 ± 1.8	—
100	29 (76.3)	9 (23.7)	6.64 ± 2.34	<0.05*

Note: *The mean AMH levels was compared between PCOS patients who responded to CC 50 mg vs those who responded to the dose 100 mg

112.5U daily) than those used for ovulation induction. When the 'threshold' level of FSH for follicular growth is quickly exceeded and follicle arrest from AMH inhibition was relieved, resulting in an early visualization of multiple dominant follicles development.

Our findings are consistent with previous study by Mahran A and co-workers [21] who have evaluated the impact of circulating AMH on the success rates of CC ovulation induction in 60 women with anovulatory PCOS receiving 187 cycles of treatment, and found circulating AMH levels to be negatively correlated with the chances of ovulation. Simially, Amer SA et al. [13] have evaluated the impact of circulating AMH on the outcome of ovarian stimulation in 20 women with anovulatory PCOS undergoing 34 cycles of gonadotrophin treatment. They found circulating AMH levels to be negatively correlated with ovarian response to human menopausal gonadotrophin. On the other hand, our findings concur with those of El-Halawaty et al. [22], in that AMH levels were significantly higher in responders to CC therapy when compared to non-responder. However, their findings included a subgroup of obese PCOS women receiving a high dose of CC (150 mg/d). Only 25 % of participants in that study ovulated in response to the high CC in first cycle, which is much lower than the majority of publications reporting ovulation rates of 75–80 % after CC treatment [8].

AMH was reported to be one of the local inhibitors of FSH action by decreasing granulosa cell sensitivity to FSH [23, 24], since the antral follicles from AMH knockout mice are more sensitive to FSH than those from the wild type [25]. This effect of AMH was mainly the result of inhibited aromatase activity in granulosa cell. In keeping with this study, an inhibitory effect of AMH on FSH- induced aromatase mRNA expression and estradiol production has been shown in human GLCs [26]. Similarly, the inverse relationship between AMH and estradiol has also been found in PCOS women [6]. The fact that AMH is inhibitory to factors required for follicle growth and subsequently selection process of the dominant follicle [3], thus it is not surprising that AMH is a negatively predictive factor for ovarian response to CC therapy in PCOS women.

It is of note that AMH, LH, AFC and ovarian volume are closely related. Furthermore, AFC and ovarian volume were significantly higher in the CRA group compared with responder. These may therefore be confounding factors that could have an influence on responsiveness to CC. So we have used multiple logistic regression analysis to determine which of these factors is an independent predictor of ovulation. The analysis has shown that AMH serum level is the best overall predictor of ovarian response to CC treatment.

In current study, the AMH levels were significantly higher in non-pregnancy compared with pregnancy group. However, this difference was disappeared when CC-resistant women were excluded from the analyses. This may be due to the fact that most CC resistant patients in this study had relatively higher AMH were excluded from the non-pregnancy group.

In the present study, we found serum AMH levels with a threshold of 7.77 ng/ml had a sensitivity of 92 % and specificity of 65 % in predicting ovarian response to CC. This cut-off is greater than two times those of previously reported by Mahran A et al. [21] who reported that 3.4 ng/ml was an optimal cut-off for the prediction of CRA among 60 women with PCOS. It is possible that different kits for detecting AMH might result in substantial variation in the serum level of AMH. In addition, variations in PCOS manifestations and AMH across different racial/ethnic backgrounds may be ascribed to these differences. Therefore, it should be noted that our cutoff AMH level applies only to the AMH kit used in this study. More studies are needed to test which value would be most useful in clinical practice.

The main strength of this study is its prospective design with inclusion of anovulatory patients fulfilling the study inclusion. However, our study has certain limitations that should be noted. Definitions vary the dose required to define CC-resistance ranging from 100 mg to150 mg of CC [27, 28]. In the present study, we defined CC-resistance as failure to ovulate in three CC cycles with the maximum dose 100 mg of CC. The CC non-responder in our study may ovulate in response to 150 mg of CC administration. However, the doses in excess of 100 mg per day are not approved by Food and Drug Administration of United States. Therefore, we did not prescribe more than 100 mg per day of CC in this study.

Conclusions

In summary, this study demonstrates that the plasma AMH can predict ovarian response to CC treatment. Therefore, measurement of serum AMH concentration for anovulatory women with PCOS before treatment may be a useful tool in predicting the outcome of CC administration. This could help with counselling PCOS patients concerning the expected success of CC treatment and may render the ovulation-induction protocols more patient-tailored and more cost-effective.

Abbreviations
AFC: antral follicles count; AMH: Anti-Müllerian hormone; BMI: body mass index; CC: clomiphene citrate; CRA: CC-resistant anovulation; FA: follicular arrest; FSH: Follicle stimulating hormone; hCG: Human chorionic gonadotrophin; HOMA-IR: homeostasis model assessment insulin resistance index; IVF: In-vitro fertilisation; LH: Luteinizing hormone; PCOS: Polycystic ovarian syndrome; ROC: Receiver operating characteristic; T: testosterone.

Competing interests
The authors declare that they have no competing interests.

Authors' contributions
HM designed the study, carried out statistical analysis and drafted the manuscript. YY and XZ conceived of the study, obtained ethics approval and helped to draft the manuscript. SF recruited patients and collected blood samples. WX carried out AMH assays and collected data for analysis, reviewed the design and critically reviewed the manuscript. ML participated in the design of the study and critically reviewed the manuscript. All authors read and approved the final manuscript.

Acknowledgements
This study was funded by The Second Affiliation Hospital of Xi an JiaoTong University. We would like to express our gratitude to Shankun Liu for his help in statistical analysis and thank Xiaoning Lu for her invaluable help in the collection and storage of data.

Author details
[1]Department of Obstetrics and Gynaecology, The Second Affiliated Hospital of Xi'an Jiaotong University, No. 157, Xiwu Road, Xi'an City 710004 Shaanxi Prov., China. [2]Department of Obstetrics and Gynaecology, The Second Affiliated Hospital of Shaanxi University of Chinese Medicine, Xianyang City 712000 Shaanxi Prov., China.

References
1. Norman RJ, Dewailly D, Legro RS, Hickey TE. Polycystic ovary syndrome. Lancet. 2007;370:685–97.
2. Webber LJ, Stubbs S, Stark J, Trew GH, Margara R, Hardy K, et al. Formation and early development of follicles in the polycystic ovary. Lancet. 2003;27:1017–21.
3. Jonard S, Dewailly D. The follicular excess in polycystic ovaries due to intra-ovarian hyperandrogenism, may be the main culprit for the follicular arrest. Hum Reprzod Update. 2004;10:107–17.
4. Pigny P, Merlen E, Robert Y, Cortet-Rudelli C, Decanter C, Jonard S, et al. Elevated serum level of anti-Mullerian hormone in patients with polycystic ovary syndrome: relationship to the ovarian follicle excess and to the follicular arrest. J Clin Endocrinol Metab. 2003;88:5957–62.
5. Pigny P, Jonard S, Robert Y, Dewailly D. Serum anti-Mullerian hormone as a surrogate for antral follicle count for definition of the polycystic ovary syndrome. J Clin Endocrinol Metab. 2006;91:941–5.
6. Cook CL, Siow Y, Brenner AG, Fallat ME. Relationship between serum Mullerian-inhibiting substance and other reproductive hormones in untreated women with polycystic ovary syndrome and normal women. Fertil Steril. 2002;77:141–6.
7. Laven JS, Mulders AG, Visser JA, Themmen AP, Jong FH, Fauser BC. Anti-Mullerian hormone serum concentrations in normovulatory and anovulatory women of reproductive age. J Clin Endocrinol Metab. 2004;89:318–23.
8. Mitwally MF, Casper RF. Use of an aromatase inhibitor for induction of ovulation in patients with an inadequate response to clomiphene citrate. Fertil Steril. 2001;75:305–9.
9. Broer SL, Mol BW, Hendriks D, Broekmans FJ. The role of anti-Mullerian hormone in prediction of outcome after IVF: comparison with the antral follicle count. Fertil Steril. 2009;91:705–14.
10. Elgindy EA, El-Haieg DO, El-Sebaey A. Anti-Mullerian hormone: correlation of early follicular, ovulatory and midluteal levels with ovarian response and cycle outcome in intracytoplasmic sperm injection patients. Fertil Steril. 2008;89:1670–6.
11. Lekamge DN, Barry M, Kolo M, Lane M, Gilchrist RB, Tremellen KP. Anti-Mullerian hormone as a predictor of IVF outcome. Reprod Biomed Online. 2007;14:602–10.
12. Xi W, Gong F, Lu G. Correlation of serum Anti-Mullerian hormone concentrations on day 3 of the in vitro fertilization stimulation cycle with assisted reproduction outcome in polycystic ovary syndrome patients. J Assist Reprod Genet. 2012;29:397–402.
13. Amer SA, Mahran A, Abdelmaged A, El-Adawy AR, Eissa MK, Shaw RW. The influence of circulating anti-Müllerian hormone on ovarian responsiveness to ovulation induction with gonadotrophins in women with polycystic ovarian syndrome: a pilot study. Reprod Biol Endocrinol. 2013;11:115.
14. Rotterdam ESHRE/ASRM–Sponsored PCOS Consensus Workshop Group. Revised 2003 consensus on diagnostic criteria and long-term healthy risks related to polycystic ovary syndrome. Fertil Steril. 2004;81:19–25.
15. Matthews DR, Hosker JP, Rudenski AS, Naylor BA, Treacher DF, Turner RC. Homeostasis model assessment: insulin resistance and beta-cell function from fasting plasma glucose and insulin concentrations in man. Diabetologia. 1985;28:412–9.
16. Balen AH, Laven JS, Tan SL, Dewailly D. Ultrasound assessment of the polycystic ovary: international consensus definitions. Hum Reprod Update. 2003;9:505–14.
17. La Marca A, Sighinolfi G, Radi D, Argento C, Baraldi E, Artensio AC, et al. Anti-Mu llerian hormone (AMH) as a predictive marker in assisted reproductive technology (ART). Hum Reprod Update. 2010;16:113–30.
18. Nakhuda GS, Chu MC, Wang JG, Sauer MV, Lobo RA. Elevated serum müllerian-inhibiting substance may be a marker for ovarian hyperstimulation syndrome in normal women undergoing in vitro fertilization. Fertil Steril. 2006;85:1541–3.
19. Kaya C, Pabuccu R, Satlroglu H. Serum antimullerian hormone concentrations on day 3 of the in vitro fertilization stimulation cycle are predictive of the fertilization, implantation, and pregnancy in polycystic ovary syndrome patients undergoing assisted reproduction. Fertil Steril. 2010;94:2202–7.
20. Catteau-Jonard S, Pigny P, Reyss AC, Decanter C, Poncelet E, Dewailly D. Changes in serum anti-Mu llerian hormone level during low-dose recombinant follicular-stimulating hormone therapy for anovulation in polycystic ovary syndrome. J Clin Endocrinol Metab. 2007;92:4138–43.
21. Mahran A, Abdelmeged A, El-Adawy AR, Eissa MK, Shaw RW, Amer SA. The predictive value of circulating anti-müllerian hormone in women with polycystic ovarian syndrome receiving clomiphene citrate: A prospective observational study. J Clin Endocrinol Metab. 2013;98:4170–5.
22. El-Halawaty S, Rizk A, Kamal M, Aboulhassan M, Al-Sawah H, Noah O, et al. Clinical significance of serum concentration of anti-Müllerian hormone in obese women with polycystic ovary syndrome. Reprod Biomed Online. 2007;15:495–9.
23. Durlinger AL, Gruijters MJ, Kramer P, Karels B, Kumar TR, Matzuk MM, et al. Anti-Mullerian hormone attenuates the effects of FSH on follicle development in the mouse ovary. Endocrinology. 2001;142:4891–9.
24. Durlinger AL, Visser JA, Themmen AP. Regulation of ovarian function: the role of Anti-Mullerian hormone. Reproduction. 2002;124:601–9.
25. Durlinger AL, Kramer P, Karels B, de Jong FH, Uilenbroek JT, Grootegoed JA, et al. Control of primordial follicle recruitment by anti-Mullerian hormone in the mouse ovary. Endocrinology. 1999;140:5789–96.
26. Grossman MP, Nakajima ST, Fallat ME, Siow Y. Mullerian-inhibiting substance inhibits cytochrome P450 aromatase activity in human granulosa lutein cell culture. Fertil Steril. 2008;89:1364–70.
27. Verit FF, Erel O, Kocyigit A. Association of increased total antioxidant capacity and anovulation in nonobese infertile patients with clomiphene citrate-resistant polycystic ovary syndrome. Fertil Steril. 2007;88:418–24.
28. Ahmed MI, Duleba AJ, El Shahat O, Ibrahim ME, Salem A. Naltrexone treatment in clomiphene resistant women with polycystic ovary syndrome. Hum Reprod. 2008;23:2564–9.

15

Developmental programming: rescuing disruptions in preovulatory follicle growth and steroidogenesis from prenatal testosterone disruption

A Veiga-Lopez[1,2], J Moeller[1], D. H. Abbott[3] and V Padmanabhan[1*]

Abstract

Background: Prenatal testosterone (T) excess from days 30-90 of gestation disrupts gonadotropin surge and ovarian follicular dynamics and induces insulin resistance and functional hyperandrogenism in sheep. T treatment from days 60-90 of gestation produces a milder phenotype, albeit with reduced fecundity. Using this milder phenotype, the aim of this study was to understand the relative postnatal contributions of androgen and insulin in mediating the prenatal T induced disruptions in ovarian follicular dynamics.

Methods: Four experimental groups were generated: 1) control (vehicle treatment), 2) prenatal T-treated (100 mg i. m. administration of T propionate twice weekly from days 60-90 of gestation), 3) prenatal T plus postnatal anti-androgen treated (daily oral dose of 15 mg/kg/day of flutamide beginning at 8 weeks of age) and 4) prenatal T and postnatal insulin sensitizer-treated (daily oral dose of 8 mg/day rosiglitazone beginning at 8 weeks of age). Follicular response to a controlled ovarian stimulation protocol was tested during their third breeding season. Main outcome measures included the determination of number and size of ovarian follicles and intrafollicular concentrations of steroids.

Results: At the end of the controlled ovarian stimulation, the number of follicles approaching ovulatory size (≥6 mm) were ~35 % lower in prenatal T-treated (6.5 ± 1.8) compared to controls (9.8 ± 2.0). Postnatal anti-androgen (10.3 ± 1.9), but not insulin sensitizer (5.0 ± 0.9), treatment prevented this decrease. Preovulatory sized follicles in the T group had lower intrafollicular T, androstenedione, and progesterone compared to that of the control group. Intrafollicular steroid disruption was partially reversed solely by postnatal insulin sensitizer treatment.

Conclusions: These results demonstrate that the final preovulatory follicular growth and intrafollicular steroid milieu is impaired in prenatal T-treated females. The findings are consistent with the lower fertility rate reported earlier in these females. The finding that final follicle growth was fully rescued by postnatal anti-androgen treatment and intrafollicular steroid milieu partially by insulin sensitizer treatment suggest that both androgenic and insulin pathway disruptions contribute to the compromised follicular phenotype of prenatal T-treated females.

Keywords: Steroids, Testosterone, Androgen antagonist, Insulin sensitizer

* Correspondence: vasantha@umich.edu
[1]Department of Pediatrics, University of Michigan, 7641A Med Sci II, Ann Arbor, MI 48109-5622, USA
Full list of author information is available at the end of the article

Background

With well over 5 million U.S. women affected, women with polycystic ovary syndrome (PCOS) are frequent patients in infertility clinics, seeking assistance in becoming pregnant [1]. A PCOS diagnosis is reached when two of the following three criteria are met: hyperandrogenism, oligo- or anovulation, and/or polycystic ovaries [2–4]. The reduced pregnancy rate in PCOS patients has been attributed to the oligo-anovulatory condition of the syndrome; this, in part, stems from a disrupted intrafollicular milieu, which includes reductions in cortisone [5], insulin growth like factor (IGF) I and II [6], and progesterone (P4) [7], increases in anti-Mullerian hormone (AMH) [8], testosterone, androstenedione, and proteomic dysregulation [9]. The compromised intrafollicular steroidal milieu in PCOS women likely accounts for the poor quality of oocytes [10, 11]. A recent meta-analysis study found removal of oocytes from the disrupted endogenous steroidal environment of PCOS women and maturing them in vitro helps achieve better conception rates [12]. Understanding the dysregulation of the intrafollicular milieu is essential for developing strategies to overcome infertility in PCOS.

Increasing evidence from several species (rhesus monkeys, sheep, rats, and mice) has demonstrated a link between prenatal exposure to testosterone (T) and development of a PCOS-like phenotype [13, 14]. Specifically, prenatal T-treatment disrupts the intrafollicular steroidal balance in preovulatory follicles (5-7 mm) and reduces embryonic potential in rhesus monkeys [11]. In sheep, prenatal T excess from days 30 to 90 of gestation (T30-90) enhances follicular recruitment and persistence [13] and causes disruptions in several key mediators of folliculogenesis [15–18]. A milder PCOS-like phenotype with reduced fecundity was found in sheep treated prenatally from days 60-90 of gestation (T60-90), where only 40 % of such prenatal T-treated females became pregnant [19]. These T60-90 females also developed insulin resistance [13].

Using the milder T60-90 phenotype [19] and a controlled ovarian stimulation protocol that effectively stimulates follicular development [20], we tested the hypothesis that prenatal T excess compromises maturation of the preovulatory follicle and disrupts the intrafollicular milieu in sheep. Since *i*) prenatal T-treated sheep manifest functional hyperandrogenism and insulin resistance [13]; *ii*) treatment with an androgen antagonist or insulin sensitizer improves ovulatory function in women with PCOS [21], the reproductive phenotype of whom prenatal T-treated sheep recapitulate; and *iii*) postnatal insulin sensitizer-treatment prevents a progressive loss in cyclicity of prenatal T-treated sheep [22], this study aimed to parse out the relative postnatal contribution of androgen and insulin towards dysfunctional follicle responses of T60-90 prenatal T-treated sheep to controlled ovarian stimulation in adulthood.

Methods

Prenatal and postnatal treatments

All procedures used were approved by the Institutional Animal Care and Use Committee of the University of Michigan and conducted at the University of Michigan Sheep Research Facility. Animal husbandry details have been published previously [23]. Mature Suffolk ewes (2 to 3 years in age) maintained under a natural photoperiod were mated and date of mating confirmed based on rump paint marks left by a raddled ram. Pregnant ewes were blocked by weight and body score and randomly assigned to one of two treatment groups: 36 animals in the prenatal T treatment group received 100 mg T propionate (Sigma-Aldrich Corp., St. Louis, MO) twice weekly in 2 ml of corn oil, i.m. from days 60 to 90 of gestation, while 12 controls received an equal volume of vehicle. Before puberty beginning at 8 weeks of age, prenatal T-treated females received either androgen antagonist, flutamide (Sigma-Aldrich, Corp.) ($n = 11$), the insulin sensitizer, rosiglitazone (Avandia; GlaxoSmithKline, Durham, NC) ($n = 12$), or no treatment ($n = 13$). Flutamide was administered orally at a dose of 15 mg/kg/ewe/day and rosiglitazone orally at a dose of 0.11 mg/kg/ewe/day as previously described [24].

Controlled ovarian stimulation

During their third breeding season (~2.5 years of age), the follicular response to a controlled ovarian stimulation protocol modified from that previously described [25] was tested in all females (see Fig. 1a). All females received 2 ml of prostaglandin $F_{2\alpha}$ ($PGF_{2\alpha}$, 5 mg/ml; Lutalyse, Pfizer Animal Health, MI) and an intravaginal P4 control internal drug release device (CIDR; Eazi-Breed CIDR sheep inserts, Pfizer Animal Health, NY) on day 0 that was replaced on day 7. Beginning on day 1, 10 µg/kg body weight of acyline, a GnRH antagonist (GnRHa) procured from the National Hormone and Peptide Program, was administered every 12 h for 10 days. This was followed by administration of 8 decreasing doses (two doses at each concentration) of FSH (0.6, 0.4, 0.3, and 0.1 mg/kg; Folltropin-V, Bioniche Animal Health, GA) starting on day 11. The P4 CIDR was removed after the sixth FSH dose.

Follicular dynamics

To monitor changes in follicular dynamics, transrectal ultrasonography was performed as previously described [26] using a scanner (Aloka SSD-900 V, Aloka Co. Ltd., Wallington, CT) fitted to a 7.5 MHz linear array transducer. Number of follicles ≥ 2 mm and corpora lutea were determined prior to the start of GnRHa treatment,

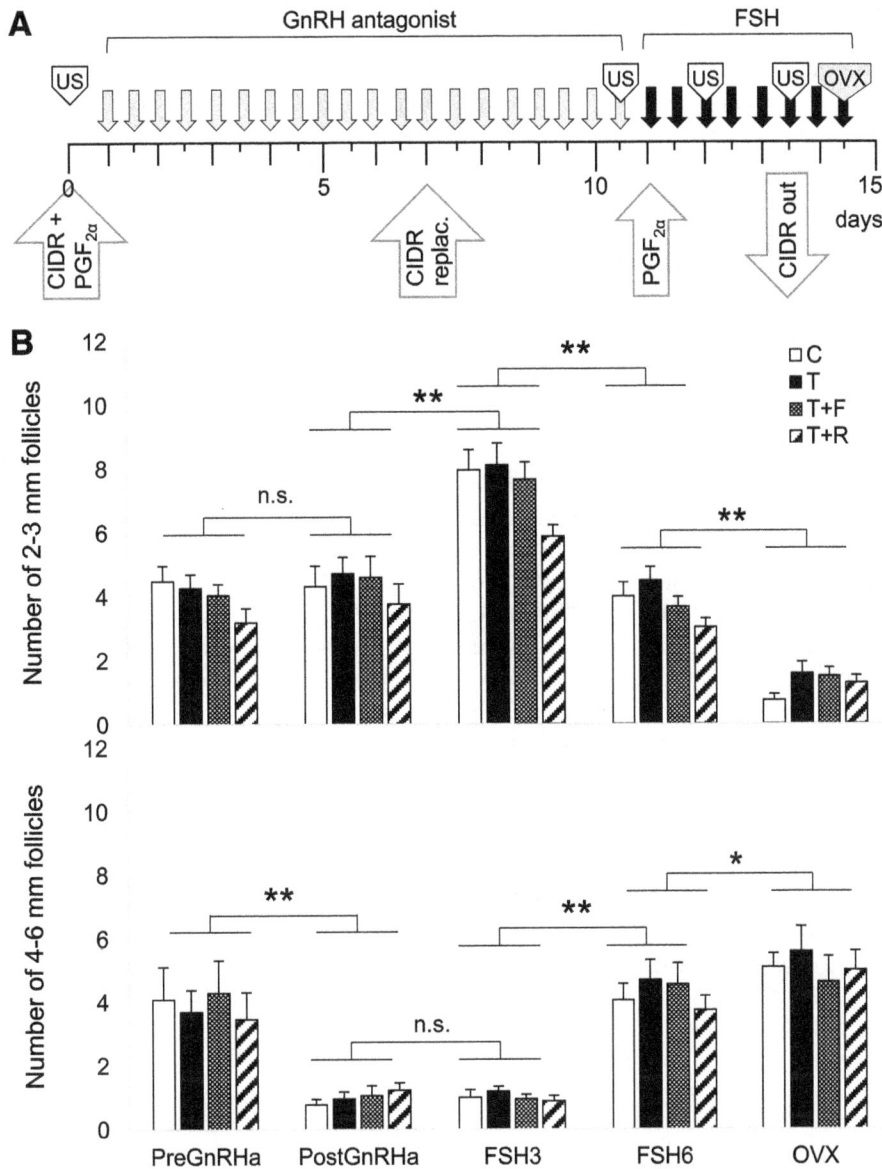

Fig. 1 a Scheme depicting synchronization and controlled ovarian stimulation protocol used in the study. See text for details. CIDR: intravaginal P4 control internal drug release device, $PGF_{2\alpha}$: prostaglandin $F_{2\alpha}$, FSH: follicle stimulating hormone, GnRH: gonadotropin releasing hormone, OVX: ovariectomy, replac.: replacement, US: transrectal ultrasonography. Grey and black arrows indicate time of GnRH antagonist and FSH administration, respectively. **b** Mean (± SEM) number of 2-3 mm (*top panel*) and 4-6 mm (*bottom panel*) before GnRH antagonist (PreGnRHa), after GnRH antagonist (PostGnRHa), before the 3rd and 6th FSH doses (FSH3 and FSH6, respectively), and ovariectomy (OVX) in control (*white bars*), T (*filled bars*), T + F (*dotted bars*), and T + R (*stripped dars*) females. See Fig. 1 for synchronization and controlled ovarian stimulation protocol and text for details of prenatal/postnatal treatment details. F: flutamide; R: rosiglitazone; n.s.: not significant; * $P < 0.01$, ** $P < 0.001$

after the last GnRHa dose, and after the 3rd and 6th FSH dose (Fig. 1a). Two hours after the 8th FSH dose, a subset (n = 6/group) of females were ovariectomized following procedures previously described [27], and all follicles ≥ 3 mm were dissected [20]. After recording their diameter, follicular fluid was aspirated and frozen at -20 °C. Prior to measurements, all follicular fluids were diluted 1:100 in 1x PBS supplemented with 1 % BSA. After follicular dissection and aspiration, the collapsed follicle was not useful to undertake histological studies.

Intrafollicular steroids

Follicular fluid concentrations of androstenedione (A4), estradiol (E_2), estrone, P4, and T were measured by quadruple linear ion trap mass spectrometer (LC-MS/MS) from one 3 mm, one 4 mm, and two 5-6 mm follicles that were randomly selected from each ovariectomized female. Samples (400 µl) were extracted after diluting with ultrapure water (500 µl). An internal deuterated standard and 1 ml of 2-methoxy-2-methylpropane was added to each sample, vortexed vigorously, and incubated for 5 min at room temperature. The steroid-containing organic phase was air-dried and re-suspended in 100 µl of ethanol and 500 µl of water. A second liquid-liquid extraction was performed with dichloromethane. The steroid-containing dichloromethane phase was air-dried and samples re-suspended in $NaHCO_3$ buffer (25 µl), and estrone and E_2 were derivitized with 50 µl of dansyl chloride (200 mg/ml in acetonitrile), heated to 40 °C for 4 min, and transferred into minivials.

A4, T, E_2, estrone, and P4 were assayed in the Assay Services Laboratories at the Wisconsin National Primate Research Center using a QTRAP 5500 LC-MS/MS (AB Sciex, USA) equipped with an atmospheric pressure chemical ionization source. The system included two Shimadzu LC20ADXR pumps and a Shimadzu SIL20ACXR autosampler. Thirty µl samples were injected onto a Phenomenex Kinetex 2.6u C18 100A, 100 × 2.1 mm column (Phenomenex) for separation. LC-MS/MS results were generated in positive-ion mode with optimized voltages. Calibration curve concentrations for estrogens were 1.56-0.003 ng/ml and 3.91-0.0076 ng/ml ng/ml for remaining steroids. Linearity was r > 0.9990 and curve fit was linear with 1/x weighting. Interassay coefficients of variation were determined by a pool of human serum and ranged from 6.09-19.47 % for all steroids. Assay sensitivities for A4, E_2, estrone, P4 and T were 0.015, 0.005, 0.0015, 0.015, and 0.0325 ng/ml, respectively.

Statistical analysis

For analyses of follicular dynamics, follicles were grouped as 2-3 mm, 4-6 mm, ≥2 mm, ≥4 mm, and ≥6 mm follicles. For intrafollicular steroid measurements, follicle classes included 3 mm, 4 mm, and 5-6 mm in diameter. Follicle size distribution among treatment groups and intrafollicular steroid concentrations among follicular classes within each treatment group and within a follicular class across treatment groups were analyzed by ANOVA and linear mixed effect model with Tukey posthoc tests. Percent change in intrafollicular steroid concentrations between 3 mm and 5-6 mm follicles was derived by subtracting concentration in 3 mm from that in larger follicles. Appropriate transformations were applied, as needed, to account for normality of data allowing analyses by parametric tests. All analyses were carried out using PASW Statistics for Windows release 18.0.1 and data presented as mean ± SEM. $P < 0.05$ was considered significant.

Results

Follicular size dynamics

GnRHa treatment decreased the number of 4-6 mm, but not 2-3 mm, follicles ($P < 0.001$; Fig. 1b). FSH administration increased number of 2-3 mm follicles ($P < 0.001$) by the third dose followed by a decline by the 6th FSH dose ($P < 0.001$). This decline in 2-3 mm was accompanied by a marked increase ($P < 0.001$) in the number of 4-6 mm follicles ($P < 0.001$). At ovariectomy, a further decline in 2-3 mm follicles and an increase in 4-6 mm follicles ($P < 0.001$) were found. GnRHa- and FSH-induced changes in 2-3 and 4-6 mm follicles in all treatment groups did not differ from the control group.

When all follicles ≥2 mm were considered, FSH increased the total number of follicles by the third FSH dose ($P < 0.001$; Fig. 2), increasing further until the sixth FSH dose ($P < 0.001$) but not beyond. In contrast, GnRHa administration significantly reduced ≥4 mm follicles ($P < 0.001$; Fig. 2). An increase in ≥4 mm follicles was observed following the third FSH dose and beyond ($P < 0.001$). There were no differences in follicular classes ≥2 mm and ≥4 mm between control and all treatment groups.

An increase was evident by the sixth FSH dose in ≥6 mm follicles ($P < 0.001$), culminating in a 3-fold increase at ovariectomy ($P < 0.001$; Fig. 2). Prenatal T treatment reduced ≥6 mm follicle number, with an initial decline evident by sixth FSH dose and achieving significance at ovariectomy (Fig. 2). Postnatal treatment with flutamide, but not rosiglitazone, prevented the prenatal T-induced reduction in ≥6 mm follicles.

Intrafollicular steroids

Figure 3a shows changes in intrafollicular concentrations of steroids. In control females, intrafollicular T concentrations were higher in 3 mm vs. larger follicles ($P < 0.05$), while the reverse was found for intrafollicular E_2 and P4, with higher concentrations found in 5-6 mm follicles ($P < 0.05$). Control females had an increase in E_2 with follicle size ($P < 0.05$) that was not seen in T and T + R females. T + F females had high E_2 concentrations regardless of follicle size. There was no follicle size effect on intrafollicular T and E_2 concentrations in T and T + F females, while an increase in P4 was evident in 5-6 mm follicles of T + R females.

No differences were found among treatment groups with intrafollicular T, A4, estrone, E_2, and P4 concentrations in the different follicular classes. When analysis was restricted only to control and T-treated females, T females had lower T and P4 ($P < 0.05$) and tended to have lower A4 ($P = 0.07$) in 5-6 mm follicles. Overall evaluation of change in steroids between the 3 and 5-6 mm sized follicles (Fig. 3b) revealed increases in A4, estrone, E_2, and P4 and a reduction in T in control

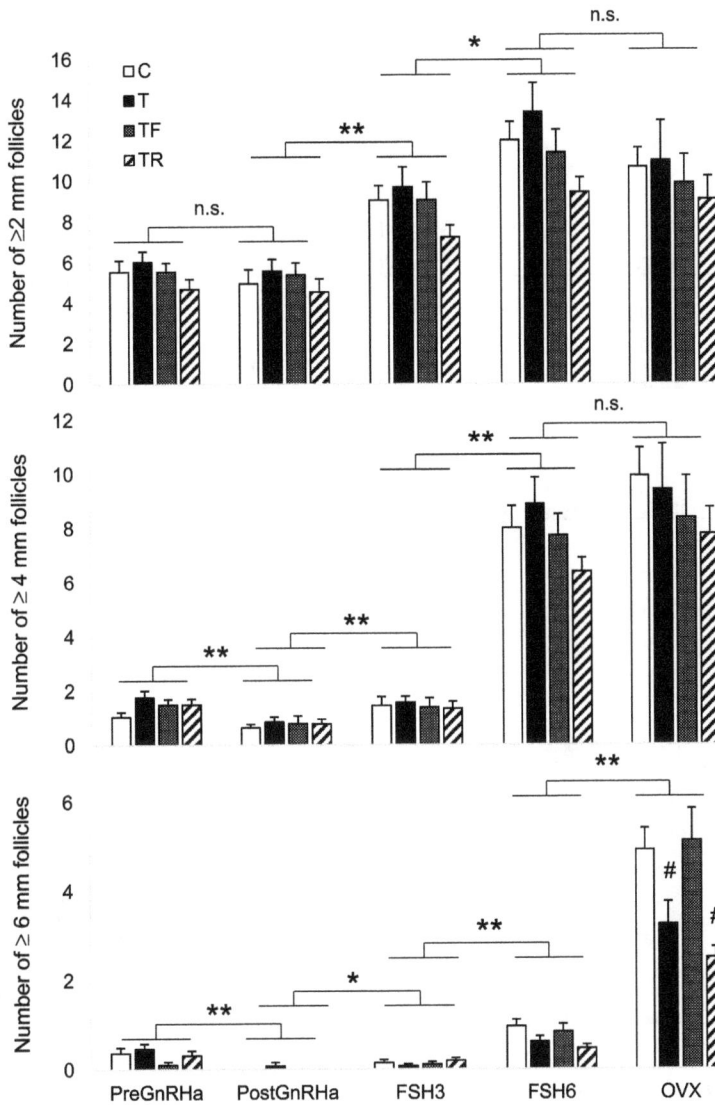

Fig. 2 Mean (± SEM) number of ≥2 mm (*top panel*), ≥ 4 mm (*middle panel*), and ≥ 6 mm (*bottom panel*) follicles before GnRH antagonist (PreGnRHa), after GnRH antagonist (PostGnRHa), before the 3rd and 6th FSH dose (FSH3 and FSH6, respectively), and ovariectomy (OVX) in control (C; *white bars*), T (*filled bars*), T + F (*dotted bars*), and T + R (*stripped bars*) females. See Fig. 1 for synchronization and controlled ovarian stimulation protocol and text for prenatal/postnatal treatment details. F: flutamide; R: rosiglitazone; n.s.: not significant; * $P < 0.01$, ** $P < 0.001$. # represents significant different ($P < 0.05$) compared to the control group

females, while reductions in A4, estrone, and P4 were observed in T females. The increase in E_2 from 3 to 5-6 mm was of a higher magnitude in control compared to T females. The changes in A4, estrone, and E_2 were more pronounced in T + F than T females. The directionality of changes in steroids between 3 and 5-6 mm in T + R females mirrored that of control females.

Comparison of steroid ratios across follicular stages found the follicular androgen to estrogen ratios (T:E_2, T + A4:E_2, T + A4:estrone + E_2, and T:estrone + E_2) in controls were lower in 5-6 mm compared 3 mm follicles ($P < 0.05$) (Fig. 4). The T:E_2 and T + A4:E_2 ratios were also lower in 5-6 mm vs. 3 mm follicles in T females. Intrafollicular

T:E_2, T + A4:E_2, T + A4:estrone + E_2, and T:estrone + E_2 ratios were all lower ($P < 0.05$) in 5-6 mm vs. 3 mm follicles within the T + R group. No treatment effect was found in steroid ratios. Data skewness prevented detection of differences in T:E_2 and T + A4:E_2 ratios in T + F females.

Discussion

This study is the first to demonstrate that prenatal T excess from days 60-90 of gestation impairs final preovulatory follicular growth (ovulatory size: ≥6 mm; [28]) and reduces intrafollicular concentrations of T, A4, and P4 in preovulatory sized follicles of sheep undergoing

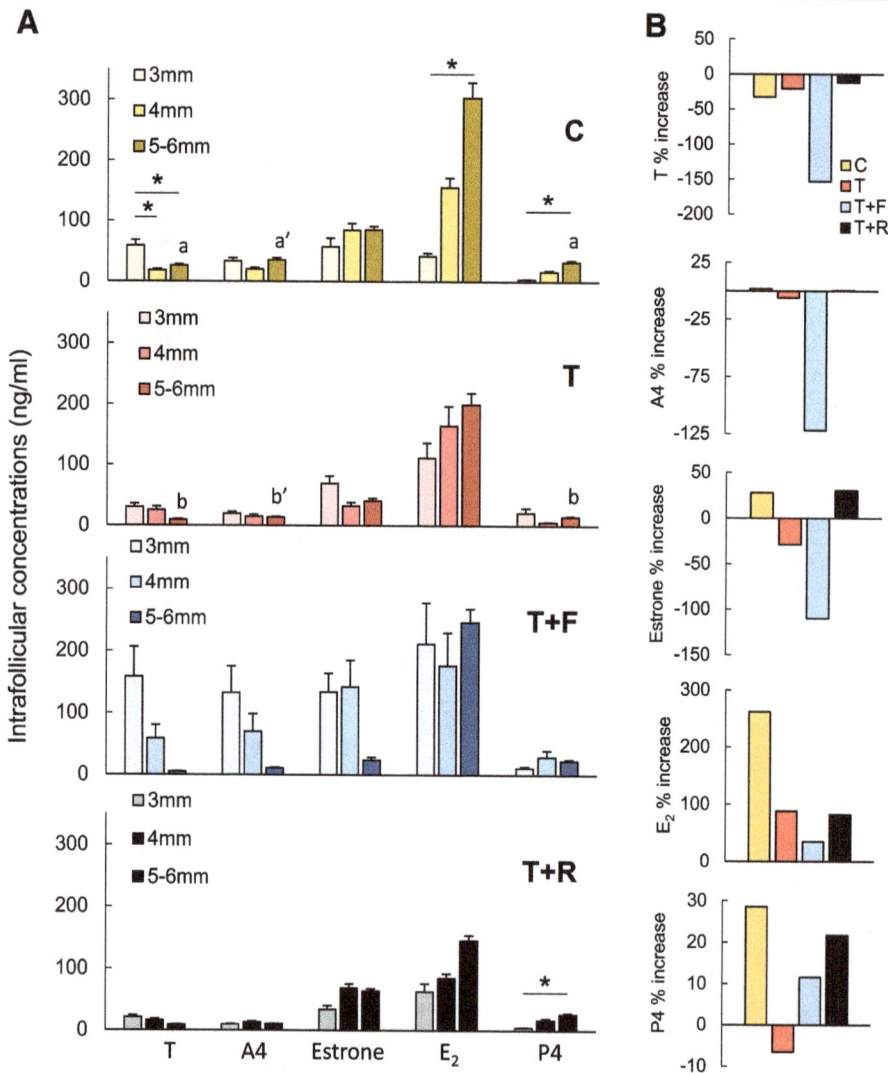

Fig. 3 a Mean (± SEM) intrafollicular concentrations (ng/ml) of testosterone (T), androstenedione (A4), estrone, estradiol (E$_2$), and progesterone (P4) at the time of ovariectomy and coincidentally with the 8th FSH dose in control (C; *yellow*), prenatal testosterone-treated (T; *red*), prenatal T plus postnatal flutamide (T + F; *blue*), and prenatal T plus postnatal rosiglitazone (T + R; *gray*) females. See Fig. 1 for synchronization and controlled ovarian stimulation protocol and text for prenatal/postnatal treatment details. Within group comparisons: asterisks represent differences within group within hormone and between follicular sizes. Posthoc analyses performed only when overall ANOVA among all three sizes was significant. Comparisons between C and T group are represented by a ≠ b if P < 0.05 and by a' ≠ b'if P = 0.07. F: flutamide; R: rosiglitazone. Data obtained from one 3 mm, one 4 mm, and two 5-6 mm follicles randomly selected from each female. **b** Percent change in intrafollicular steroids of T, A4, estrone, E$_2$, and P4 between 3 and 5-6 mm follicles in C (*yellow*), T (*red*), T + F (*blue*), T + R (*black*) groups. Percent change was calculated by subtracting the overall mean values between the 3 and 5-6 mm size within each group

controlled ovarian stimulation, a finding consistent with the lower fertility rates reported in these sheep [19]. The rescue of final growth by postnatal androgen antagonist, but not insulin sensitizer, administration suggests the impairment of prevoulatory follicle growth is mediated via androgenic action. This, in concert with the partial rescue of the intrafollicular steroid milieu with insulin sensitizer, suggests that both androgens and insulin contribute to reproductive disruption [29–31] and reduced fecundity [17] in adult prenatal T-treated sheep.

Prenatal T programming of follicular dynamics

The GnRHa treatment regimen used was effective in blocking follicular growth beyond the 3 mm stage in both the control and prenatal T-treated sheep, as was the case with T30-90 females exposed to a shorter GnRHa treatment [32]. The efficacy of pFSH to recruit follicular growth in controls was comparable to that achieved with oFSH or pFSH stimulation in other sheep breeds [25, 33]. pFSH used in this study was also as effective in stimulating follicular growth in the 3 treatment groups (T, T + F, and T + R) as the combined oFSH- LH

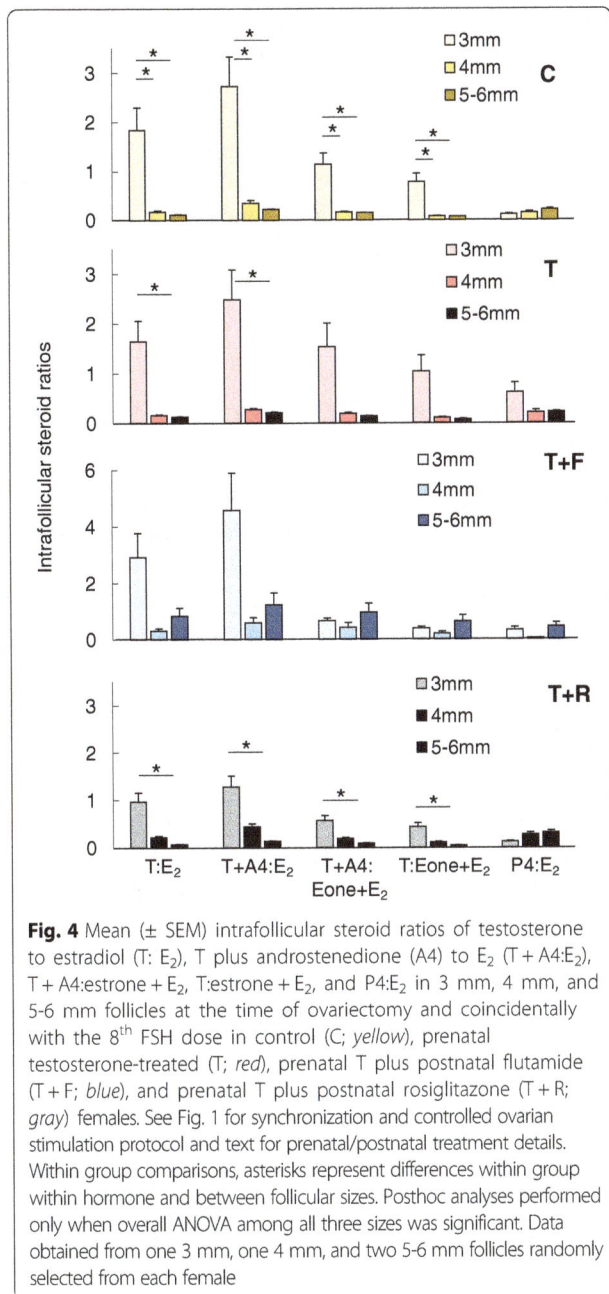

Fig. 4 Mean (± SEM) intrafollicular steroid ratios of testosterone to estradiol (T: E_2), T plus androstenedione (A4) to E_2 (T + A4:E_2), T + A4:estrone + E_2, T:estrone + E_2, and P4:E_2 in 3 mm, 4 mm, and 5-6 mm follicles at the time of ovariectomy and coincidentally with the 8th FSH dose in control (C; *yellow*), prenatal testosterone-treated (T; *red*), prenatal T plus postnatal flutamide (T + F; *blue*), and prenatal T plus postnatal rosiglitazone (T + R; *gray*) females. See Fig. 1 for synchronization and controlled ovarian stimulation protocol and text for prenatal/postnatal treatment details. Within group comparisons, asterisks represent differences within group within hormone and between follicular sizes. Posthoc analyses performed only when overall ANOVA among all three sizes was significant. Data obtained from one 3 mm, one 4 mm, and two 5-6 mm follicles randomly selected from each female

regimen used with T30-90 females [32]. These findings indicate responsiveness to exogenous FSH, and hence recruitment, was not impaired by prenatal T excess or postnatal treatment with androgen antagonist or insulin sensitizer. The finding that recruitment and growth of follicles up to 4 mm size was similar across groups is not surprising, because androgens increase FSH activity [34] and are not detrimental to follicular survival and growth of preantral and early antral follicles [35].

The reduced number of follicles ≥6 mm in T females suggests the final maturation of the preovulatory follicle is impaired. Given that *i)* the suppression was evident in

number of follicles ≥6 mm, but not in the number up to 4 mm, and *ii)* in sheep, follicles up to 4 mm size are considered FSH dependent and those beyond 4 mm as LH dependent [28], the shift from FSH to LH dependency appears to be impaired. One possibility is that this reduction in preovulatory sized follicles might be a function of advancement in LH dependency and hence a requirement for LH. Because LH was not co-administered with FSH, the final transition to preovulatory size might be compromised. This premise is supported by the lack of reduction in preovulatory sized follicles in the T30-90 females [32], when follicles were stimulated concomitantly with LH and FSH. Findings from both studies (this study and Steckler et al. [32]) suggest the compromised preovulatory follicular development might be rescued with exogenous LH supplementation. It is unclear if this impairment is a function of reduced number of LH receptors or altered LH signaling, both are aspects yet to be studied in this model but implicated in women with PCOS [36–38].

Importantly, the fact that postnatal androgen antagonist, not insulin sensitizer, treatment was able to rescue the number of preovulatory-sized follicles supports the notion that *i)* compromised androgen receptor expression/function in growing follicles or surrounding ovarian stroma is detrimental to progression beyond a critical size (4 mm in this case) and *ii)* that blockade of androgen action with an androgen antagonist would help overcome follicular growth arrest. In previous studies, we found prenatal T treatment from days 30-90 of gestation increases granulosa cell androgen receptor expression in antral follicles and is supportive of functional ovarian hyperandrogenism [15]. Although insulin plays a role in follicular development [39–41], failure of insulin sensitizer treatment to rescue this follicular growth defect suggests this dysfunction is driven primarily by the androgen signaling imbalance within the growing follicle.

Prenatal T programming of follicular steroid milieu

The opposing follicular size-related changes in intrafollicular T and estrogens in control females were similar to previous findings [20, 42]. A higher androgenic environment prevails in small follicles, with a shift towards a highly estrogenic milieu in preovulatory follicles; this is consistent with increased aromatase activity as follicles mature [42]. The transition from low E_2 in smaller follicles to high E_2 in larger follicles was the most striking change (4-fold increase) in the control group. Conversely, the E_2 increase was of much lower magnitude (< 1-fold) in the T group. Because androgens are the main substrate for estrogen production, the reduced magnitude of E_2 increase in T females may be driven by a reduced androgenic environment (T and A4) at earlier follicular stages. Androgen and estrogen receptors [17] and steroidogenic enzymes [43] are dysregulated in granulosa and theca cells of T30-90 sheep, and these disruptions remain to be determined in T60-90 females. It is also unclear whether the lower magnitude of E_2 increase in T females contributes to the delayed onset of LH surge that was reported earlier in these females [29].

Prenatal T-induced disruptions in intrafollicular steroid milieu were also reported in non-human primates [11]. Controlled ovarian stimulation studies in rhesus monkeys found 15-35 days of T treatment starting on gestational days 40-44, but not days 100-115, reduced intrafollicular A4 and E_2 concentrations in preovulatory sized follicles [11]. Although disruptions in intrafollicular A4 and E_2 parallel findings from the current study, timing and duration of T exposure differ between the sheep and monkey study. Our earlier findings of reduced granulosa cell CYP19A1 expression in antral follicles in the T30-90 model [43] agrees with the reduced intrafollicular E_2 in large antral follicles evidenced in the present study [43]. Considering the disrupted intrafollicular steroidal milieu of prenatal T-treated monkeys was accompanied by a reduction in oocyte competence [11], a similar intrafollicular disruption was evidenced in prenatal T-treated sheep is likely to be associated with compromised oocyte health. This, in fact, may explain the reduced fecundity in T60-90 females [19]. The strength of the present study is that the intrafollicular steroid milieu was identified in different size follicular classes as opposed to only the preovulatory follicular size in monkeys. Another strength is the parallel assessment of follicular growth at different time points during the ovarian stimulation protocol, which was helpful in dissecting out regulation of follicular growth from steroidogenesis.

Relative to interventions, postnatal flutamide treatment rescued follicular growth to where preovulatory follicle size was achieved, but treatment failed to ameliorate the disruptions in intrafollicular steroidal milieu. The steroidal transition from low E_2 to a high E_2 milieu between 3 to 6 mm size antral follicles seen in controls was not evident in T + F females. In addition, the directionality of change in intrafollicular concentrations of estrone and A4 in T + F animals, namely a reduction in both steroids in the 6 mm compared to 3 mm follicles as opposed to the increase in both steroids in the controls, point to an intrafollicular steroidal disruption that persists through antral follicle growth. The increase of T in the smaller 3 mm follicles of the T + F females may be a compensatory response to the blockade of androgen receptor signaling by flutamide treatment, which was present throughout the course of the study. Such a response would be analogous to the masculinizing effects of flutamide seen relative to other variables [44, 45]. To what extent the intrafollicular steroidal disruptions play a role in oocyte health and ultimately fertility remains unclear. Paradoxically, while flutamide treatment failed to ameliorate intrafollicular steroidal defects, the same treatment prevented pubertal advancement and enhanced preovulatory LH surge amplitude in the T30-90 females [24]. Considering T is an aromatizable androgen, the differing effects of flutamide in rescuing the various physiologic functions may be a function of whether androgen or estrogen (via aromatization) is the programming agent [31].

Despite the fact that T60-90 females are insulin resistant [13], the lack of rescue in the number of follicles that achieved a preovulatory size by rosiglitazone suggests the insulin pathway is not involved in growth of preovulatory follicles. In contrast, the intrafollicular steroid milieu of T + R follicles was more similar to that of the controls and is supportive of a role for insulin coupled with FSH as follicles mature in maintaining intrafollicular steroid balance [46]. The beneficial effects of insulin sensitizer therapies in enhancing insulin sensitivity and improving ovulatory function in women with PCOS [47, 48] may relate to normalization of intrafollicular steroidal milieu, as evidenced in the T + R animals.

In interpreting the impact of the interventions, it is important to recognize that GnRH antagonist treatment given prior to FSH stimulation to achieve a homogeneous follicular pool before FSH stimulation (as achieved in this study, Fig. 1) might have played a role in determining the impact of androgen antagonist and insulin sensitizer on follicular dynamics and the intra-follicular hormone milieu. However, considering that GnRH antagonist treatment is the same across treatments, any variability in the starting pool of follicles across treatment would suggest intrinsic ovarian differences originating from the T treatment and interventions respectively. It needs to be recognized that GnRH agonist and antagonist treatments are routinely used in standard IVF practices [49], and hence the approach taken with this study is consistent with this practice.

The outcomes achieved with the two interventions, namely the androgen antagonist helping rescue follicular growth and the insulin sensitizer partially rescuing intrafollicular steroidal milieu, suggest that both androgens and insulin may synergize in establishing optimal follicular growth and steroidogenesis. A combined intervention involving both may help compensate for any deficiency that one intervention has in order to achieve better success. While the finding in PCOS women is that combined treatment is more efficacious than monotherapies in treating anovulation [50] is supportive of this possibility, this remains to be tested.

Conclusions

Prenatal T excess from days 60-90 of gestation impairs final follicular growth and intrafollicular milieu under controlled ovarian stimulation protocols. This indicates an inherent ovarian defect that may contribute to the lower fertility seen in these females [19]. The differential benefit of postnatal androgen antagonist and insulin sensitizer treatment in rescuing follicular growth and steroidogenesis, respectively, raises the possibility that combined therapies during adolescence and early adulthood may be beneficial in enhancing fertility, a premise that remains to be tested.

Acknowledgements
We thank Douglas Doop for help with breeding, lambing, excellent animal care, and facility management, Gary McCalla for help with daily administration of androgen antagonist and insulin sensitizer treatments, Carol Herkimer for assistance with prenatal treatment and ovariectomies, and Kaitlyn Bates, Joe Majors, Shannon Lohman, Dr. Chunxia Lu, Sam Olson, Meg Ryan, and Rohit Shreedharan for help in various aspects of the animal experimentation. We are grateful to Dr. Fred Karsch for surgical help during ovariectomies.

Funding
This work was supported by NIH P01 HD44232 (VP). Effort spent by A.V-L. during the preparation of the manuscript was supported by AgBioResearch and the United States Department of Agriculture (USDA) National Institute of Food and Agriculture, Hatch project MICL02383.

Authors' contributions
AV-L participated in designing the experiment and generation of the animals, provided supervision in the performance of animal experiments, performed the ultrasonography and statistical analyses, and wrote the manuscript. JM participated in generating animals and in animal experiments, DHA provide oversight for the steroid measurements, VP paticipated in designing the experiment, provided oversight for integrating the study components, participated in data interpretation and writing of the manuscript. All authors read through the manuscript and provided input in finalizing the manuscript. All authors read and approved the final manuscript.

Competing interests
The authors declare that they have no competing interests.

Author details
[1]Department of Pediatrics, University of Michigan, 7641A Med Sci II, Ann Arbor, MI 48109-5622, USA. [2]Department of Animal Science, Michigan State University, East Lansing, MI 48824, USA. [3]Department of Obstetrics and Gynecology and Wisconsin National Primate Research Center, University of Wisconsin, Madison, WI 53715, USA.

References
1. Womeshealth.gov. Polycystic ovary syndrome (PCOS) fact sheet. http://www.womenshealth.gov/publications/our-publications/fact-sheet/polycystic-ovary-syndrome.html Last updated: December 23, 2014. Last accessed: January 29, 2016.
2. Rotterdam EA-SPCWG. Revised 2003 consensus on diagnostic criteria and long-term health risks related to polycystic ovary syndrome. Fertil Steril. 2004;81:19–25.
3. Zawadki J, Dunaif A. Diagnostic criteria for polycystic ovary syndrome: towards a rational approach. In: A D, JR G, FP H, GR M, eds. Polycystic ovary syndrome. Boston: Blackwell Scientific Publications; 1992. p. 377-84.
4. Azziz R, Carmina E, Dewailly D, Diamanti-Kandarakis E, Escobar-Morreale HF, Futterweit W, et al. Positions statement: criteria for defining polycystic ovary syndrome as a predominantly hyperandrogenic syndrome: an Androgen Excess Society guideline. J Clin Endocrinol Metab. 2006;91:4237–45.
5. Michael AE, Glenn C, Wood PJ, Webb RJ, Pellatt L, Mason HD. Ovarian 11beta-hydroxysteroid dehydrogenase (11betaHSD) activity is suppressed in women with anovulatory polycystic ovary syndrome (PCOS): apparent role for ovarian androgens. J Clin Endocrinol Metab. 2013;98:3375–83.
6. Barreca A, Del Monte P, Ponzani P, Artini PG, Genazzani AR, Minuto F. Intrafollicular insulin-like growth factor-II levels in normally ovulating women and in patients with polycystic ovary syndrome. Fertil Steril. 1996;65:739–45.
7. Lambert-Messerlian G, Taylor A, Leykin L, Isaacson K, Toth T, Chang Y, et al. Characterization of intrafollicular steroid hormones, inhibin, and follistatin in women with and without polycystic ovarian syndrome following gonadotropin hyperstimulation. Biol Reprod. 1997;57:1211–6.
8. Hossein G, Arabzadeh S, Hossein-Rashidi B, Hosseini MA. Relations between steroids and AMH: impact of basal and intrafollicular steroids to AMH ratios on oocyte yield and maturation rate in women with or without polycystic ovary undergoing in vitro fertilization. Gynecol Endocrinol. 2012;28:413–7.
9. Ambekar AS, Kelkar DS, Pinto SM, Sharma R, Hinduja I, Zaveri K, et al. Proteomics of follicular fluid from women with polycystic ovary syndrome suggests molecular defects in follicular development. J Clin Endocrinol Metab. 2015;100:744–53.
10. Homburg R, Berkowitz D, Levy T, Feldberg D, Ashkenazi J, Ben-Rafael Z. In vitro fertilization and embryo transfer for the treatment of infertility associated with polycystic ovary syndrome. Fertil Steril. 1993;60:858–63.
11. Dumesic DA, Schramm RD, Peterson E, Paprocki AM, Zhou R, Abbott DH. Impaired developmental competence of oocytes in adult prenatally androgenized female rhesus monkeys undergoing gonadotropin stimulation for in vitro fertilization. J Clin Endocrinol Metab. 2002;87:1111–9.
12. Siristatidis C, Sergentanis TN, Vogiatzi P, Kanavidis P, Chrelias C, Papantoniou N, et al. In Vitro Maturation in Women with vs. without Polycystic Ovarian Syndrome: A Systematic Review and Meta-Analysis. PLoS One. 2015;10:e0134696.
13. Padmanabhan V, Veiga-Lopez A. Animal models of the polycystic ovary syndrome phenotype. Steroids. 2013;78:734–40.
14. Abbott DH, Dumesic DA, Levine JE, Dunaif A, Padmanabhan V. Animal models and fetal programming of PCOS. In: Azziz JE, Nestler JE, Dewailly D, editors. Contemporary endocrinology: androgen excess disorders in women: polycystic ovary syndrome and other disorders. Totowa, NJ: Humana Press Inc; 2006. p. 259–72.
15. Ortega HH, Salvetti NR, Padmanabhan V. Developmental programming: prenatal androgen excess disrupts ovarian steroid receptor balance. Reproduction. 2009;137:865–77.
16. Salvetti NR, Ortega HH, Veiga-Lopez A, Padmanabhan V. Developmental programming: impact of prenatal testosterone excess on ovarian cell proliferation and apoptotic factors in sheep. Biol Reprod. 2012;87(22):1–10.
17. Ortega HH, Rey F, Velazquez MM, Padmanabhan V. Developmental programming: effect of prenatal steroid excess on intraovarian components of insulin signaling pathway and related proteins in sheep. Biol Reprod. 2010;82:1065–75.
18. Veiga-Lopez A, Ye W, Padmanabhan V. Developmental programming: prenatal testosterone excess disrupts anti-Mullerian hormone expression in preantral and antral follicles. Fertil Steril. 2012;97:748–56.
19. Steckler TL, Roberts EK, Doop DD, Lee TM, Padmanabhan V. Developmental programming in sheep: administration of testosterone during 60-90 days of pregnancy reduces breeding success and pregnancy outcome. Theriogenology. 2007;67:459–67.
20. Veiga-Lopez A, Dominguez V, Souza CJ, Garcia-Garcia RM, Ariznavarreta C, Tresguerres JA, et al. Features of follicle-stimulating hormone-stimulated follicles in a sheep model: keys to elucidate embryo failure in assisted reproductive technique cycles. Fertil Steril. 2008;89:1328–37.
21. Domecq JP, Prutsky G, Mullan RJ, Sundaresh V, Wang AT, Erwin PJ, et al. Adverse effects of the common treatments for polycystic ovary syndrome: a systematic review and meta-analysis. J Clin Endocrinol Metab. 2013;98:4646–54.

22. Veiga-Lopez A, Lee JS, Padmanabhan V. Developmental programming: insulin sensitizer treatment improves reproductive function in prenatal testosterone-treated female sheep. Endocrinology. 2010;151:4007–17.

23. Manikkam M, Crespi EJ, Doop DD, Herkimer C, Lee JS, Yu S, et al. Fetal programming: prenatal testosterone excess leads to fetal growth retardation and postnatal catch-up growth in sheep. Endocrinology. 2004;145:790–8.

24. Padmanabhan V, Veiga-Lopez A, Herkimer C, Abi Salloum B, Moeller J, Beckett E, et al. Developmental programming: prenatal and postnatal androgen antagonist and insulin sensitizer interventions prevent advancement of puberty and improve LH surge dynamics in prenatal testosterone-treated sheep. Endocrinology. 2015;156:2678–92.

25. Veiga-Lopez A, Gonzalez-Bulnes A, Garcia-Garcia RM, Dominguez V, Cocero MJ. The effects of previous ovarian status on ovulation rate and early embryo development in response to superovulatory FSH treatments in sheep. Theriogenology. 2005;63:1973–83.

26. Veiga-Lopez A, Wurst AK, Steckler TL, Ye W, Padmanabhan V. Developmental programming: postnatal estradiol amplifies ovarian follicular defects induced by fetal exposure to excess testosterone and dihydrotestosterone in sheep. Reprod Sci. 2014;21:444–55.

27. Jackson LM, Mytinger A, Roberts EK, Lee TM, Foster DL, Padmanabhan V, et al. Developmental programming: postnatal steroids complete prenatal steroid actions to differentially organize the GnRH surge mechanism and reproductive behavior in female sheep. Endocrinology. 2013;154:1612–23.

28. van den Hurk R, Zhao J. Formation of mammalian oocytes and their growth, differentiation and maturation within ovarian follicles. Theriogenology. 2005;63:1717–51.

29. Sharma TP, Herkimer C, West C, Ye W, Birch R, Robinson JE, et al. Fetal programming: prenatal androgen disrupts positive feedback actions of estradiol but does not affect timing of puberty in female sheep. Biol Reprod. 2002;66:924–33.

30. Savabieasfahani M, Lee JS, Herkimer C, Sharma TP, Foster DL, Padmanabhan V. Fetal programming: testosterone exposure of the female sheep during midgestation disrupts the dynamics of its adult gonadotropin secretion during the periovulatory period. Biol Reprod. 2005;72:221–9.

31. Padmanabhan V, Veiga-Lopez A. 2011 Developmental origin of reproductive and metabolic dysfunctions: androgenic versus estrogenic reprogramming. Semin Reprod Med. 2011;29:173–86.

32. Steckler TL, Lee JS, Ye W, Inskeep EK, Padmanabhan V. Developmental programming: exogenous gonadotropin treatment rescues ovulatory function but does not completely normalize ovarian function in sheep treated prenatally with testosterone. Biol Reprod. 2008;79:686–95.

33. Gonzalez-Bulnes A, Santiago-Moreno J, Cocero MJ, Lopez-Sebastian A. Effects of FSH commercial preparation and follicular status on follicular growth and superovulatory response in Spanish Merino ewes. Theriogenology. 2000;54:1055–64.

34. Gervásio CG, Bernuci MP, Silva-de-Sá MF, Rosa-E-Silva AC. The role of androgen hormones in early follicular development. ISRN Obstet Gynecol. 2014;2014:818010. doi:10.1155/2014/818010.

35. Vendola KA, Zhou J, Adesanya OO, Weil SJ, Bondy CA. Androgens stimulate early stages of follicular growth in the primate ovary. J Clin Invest. 1998;101:2622–9.

36. Liu N, Ma Y, Wang S, Zhang X, Zhang Q, Zhang X, et al. Association of the genetic variants of luteinizing hormone, luteinizing hormone receptor and polycystic ovary syndrome. Reprod Biol Endocrinol. 2012;30(10):36.

37. Comim FV, Teerds K, Hardy K, Franks S. Increased protein expression of LHCG receptor and 17α-hydroxylase/17-20-lyase in human polycystic ovaries. Hum Reprod. 2013;28:3086–92.

38. McAllister JM, Modi B, Miller BA, Biegler J, Bruggeman R, Legro RS, et al. Overexpression of a DENND1A isoform produces a polycystic ovary syndrome theca phenotype. Proc Natl Acad Sci USA. 2014;111:E1519–27.

39. Poretsky L, Bhargava G, Kalin MF, Wolf SA. Regulation of insulin receptors in the human ovary: in vitro studies. J Clin Endocrinol Metab. 1988;67:774–8.

40. Seto-Young D, Avtanski D, Strizhevsky M, Parikh G, Patel P, Kaplun J, et al. Interactions among peroxisome proliferator activated receptor-gamma, insulin signaling pathways, and steroidogenic acute regulatory protein in human ovarian cells. J Clin Endocrinol Metab. 2007;92:2232–9.

41. Kayampilly PP, Menon KM. Follicle-stimulating hormone increases tuberin phosphorylation and mammalian target of rapamycin signaling through an extracellular signal-regulated kinase-dependent pathway in rat granulosa cells. Endocrinology. 2007;148:3950–7.

42. Tsonis CG, Carson RS, Findlay JK. Relationships between aromatase activity, follicular fluid oestradiol-17 beta and testosterone concentrations, and diameter and atresia of individual ovine follicles. J Reprod Fertil. 1984;72:153–63.

43. Padmanabhan V, Salvetti NR, Matiller V, Ortega HH. Developmental programming: prenatal steroid excess disrupts key members of intraovarian steroidogenic pathway in sheep. Endocrinology. 2014;155:3649–60.

44. Mylchreest E, Sar M, Wallace DG, Foster PM. Fetal testosterone insufficiency and abnormal proliferation of Leydig cells and gonocytes in rats exposed to di(n-butyl) phthalate. Reprod Toxicol. 2002;16:19–28.

45. Herman RA, Measday MA, Wallen K. Sex differences in interest in infants in juvenile rhesus monkeys: relationship to prenatal androgen. Horm Behav. 2003;43:573–83.

46. Chaves RN, Duarte AB, Rodrigues GQ, Celestino JJ, Silva GM, Lopes CA, et al. The effects of insulin and follicle-simulating hormone (FSH) during in vitro development of ovarian goat preantral follicles and the relative mRNA expression for insulin and FSH receptors and cytochrome P450 aromatase in cultured follicles. Biol Reprod. 2012;87:69.

47. Pasquali R, Gambineri A. Insulin sensitizers in polycystic ovary syndrome. Front Horm Res. 2013;40:83–102.

48. Naderpoor N, Shorakae S, de Courten B, Misso ML, Moran LJ, Teede HJ. Metformin and lifestyle modification in polycystic ovary syndrome: systematic review and meta-analysis. Hum Reprod Update. 2015;21:560–74.

49. Garcia-Velasco JA, Fatemi HM. To pill or not to pill in GnRH antagonist cycles: that is the question! Reprod Biomed Online. 2015;30:39–42.

50. Ibáñez L, de Zegher F. Low-dose flutamide-metformin therapy for hyperinsulinemic hyperandrogenism in nonobese adolescents and women. Fertil Steril. 2006;86 Suppl 1:S24–5.

16

Application of receiver operating characteristic curve in the assessment of the value of body mass index, waist circumference and percentage of body fat in the Diagnosis of Polycystic Ovary Syndrome in childbearing women

Pan Dou[1], Huiyan Ju[2], Jing Shang[2], Xueying Li[3], Qing Xue[2], Yang Xu[2,5*] and Xiaohui Guo[4,5*]

Abstract

Background: There are various parameters to analyze obesity, however, no standard reference to predict, screen or diagnose PCOS with various obesity parameters has been established, and the accuracy of these parameters still needs to be studied.This study was to use the receiver operating characteristic (ROC) curve to explore the different values of three obesity parameters, body mass index (BMI), waist circumference (WC) and percentage of body fat (PBF) in the diagnosis of polycystic ovary syndrome (PCOS) in Chinese childbearing women.

Methods: Three hundred patients who were diagnosed with PCOS at Center of Reproductive Medicine and Genetics of Peking University First Hospital were enrolled in this study, and 110 healthy age-matched women were enrolled as controls. The characteristics of BMI, WC and PBF in PCOS patients were analyzed.

Results: Compared with the control group, all the three obesity parameters were significantly increased in PCOS group. In terms of ROC area under the curve, WC > PBF > BMI, and they were all significantly different from those of the control. At a cut-off point of 80.5 cm, WC has a sensitivity of 73.6 % and a specificity of 85 % in diagnosis of PCOS; At a cut-off point of 29 %, PBF has a sensitivity of 88.2 % and a specificity of 57.7 % in diagnosis of PCOS; and at a cut-off point of 26.6 kg/m^2, BMI has a sensitivity of 54.5 % and a specificity of 98 % in diagnosis of PCOS.

Conclusion: WC, BMI and PBF are valuable in screening and diagnosis of PCOS in Chinese childbearing women. PBF can be used to screen PCOS as it has a better sensitivity, while BMI can be used in the diagnosis of PCOS as it has a better specificity.

Keywords: Childbearing age, Polycystic ovary syndrome, Obesity, Body mass index, Waist circumference, percentage of body fat, Receiver operating characteristic, Area under the curve

Abbreviations: ROC, the receiver operating characteristic; BMI, body mass index; WC, waist circumference; PBF, percentage of body fat; PCOS, polycystic ovary syndrome; LH, luteinizing hormone; ASRM, the American Society for Reproductive Medicine; SHBG, sex hormone-binding globulin; WHO, World Health Organization; IDF, the International Diabetes Federation

* Correspondence: xuyangm@126.com; guoxh@medmail.com.cn
[2]Center of Reproduction and Genetics, Peking University First Hospital, Beijing, China
[4]Department of Endocrinology, Peking University First Hospital, Beijing, China
Full list of author information is available at the end of the article

Background

Polycystic ovary syndrome (PCOS) was first reported by Stein and Leventhal [1] in 1935, so it is also called Stein-Leventhal syndrome. It is the most common female endocrine and metabolic disorder, and its incidence rate is about 5.6 % among women aged 19–45 years old in China [2]. PCOS is a complex disease with high clinical heterogeneity, excess androgen production and elevated serum luteinizing hormone (LH) are its serological features. It is a major cause of infertility in women. Studies from different countries have shown that the comorbidity rate of obesity in patients with PCOS was 30–70 % [3, 4]. The reproductive, endocrinological and metabolic disorders (except hirsutism) in obese PCOS patients are more severe than non-obese patients, and the long-term risk of the incidence of metabolic syndrome, type 2 diabetes mellitus (DM), cardiovascular disease (CVD) as well as breast cancer, endometrial cancer and other complications was also increased exponentially [5]. There are various parameters to analyze obesity, however, no standard reference to predict, screen or diagnose PCOS with various obesity parameters has been established, and the accuracy of these parameters still needs to be studied. This study was designed based on the Rotterdam PCOS consensus criteria, to explore the accuracy and best cut-off points of three obesity parameter, i.e., body mass index (BMI), waist circumference (WC) and percentage of body fat (PBF), in PCOS diagnosis, as well as to compare their sensitivity and specificity to provide basis for rational application of obesity parameters in prediction, screen and diagnosis of PCOS among high-risk populations.

Methods

Study subjects

Three hundred study subjects who were diagnosed with PCOS at Reproduction and Genetic Center of Peking University First Hospital from June 2015 to January 2016 were selected. Patients were did not take any hormone medication within the past 3 months. 110 healthy women of childbearing age who have normal menstruation period and biphasic basal body temperature were selected as normal control. The ages of the two groups were matched to each other. This study was approved by the Ethics Committee of China Registered Clinical Trial and all the study subject have signed informed consent to voluntarily participate the study.

PCOS diagnostic criteria

Based on the American Society for Reproductive Medicine (ASRM) Rotterdam Revised Diagnostic Criteria, a patient can be with diagnosed as PCOS if two of the following three criteria are met: (1) no ovulation or irregular ovulation; (2) clinical (such as hirsutism, acne) or biochemical evidence associated with elevated androgen levels; (3)

enlarged ovaries, each side has 12 or more small follicles with a diameter of at least 2 ~ 9 mm; plus exclusion of hyperlactatemia and other metabolic diseases that produce high-level of androgen such as Cushing's syndrome, congenital adrenal hyperplasia, ovarian or adrenal tumors.

Anthropometric measurements

Measurements were carried out in the hospital's outpatient clinic, performed by the same observer in accordance with the provisions of WHO. For measurement of height (m), the examinee was required to be barefoot, the rear point of the feet, hip and the rear point of head were on the same vertical line, the measurement value was approximated to the nearest 0.5 cm; for measurement of body weight (kg), electronic scale was used, and the examinee was required to be fasted overnight and urine and stool were emptied, only underwear was allowed, the measurement values was approximated to the nearest 100 g, BMI was calculated with the formula: weight $(kg)/(height)^2$ (m^2); for measurement of waist circumference, the examinee was required to stand upright with two feet apart 25 ~ 30 cm, so that the weight is evenly distributed on both legs, the waist circumference was measured in a horizontal level through the midpoint that links the iliac crest and the lower margin of the 12th rib (the measurement tape was placed close to the skin, but cannot repress the soft tissue), the measurement values was approximated to the nearest 1 mm.

Body composition measurement

The body composition of the two groups was measured using bioelectrical impedance body composition analyzer (Multi-frequency bioelectrical impedance analyzer NQA-PI). On the test day, the examinee was asked to minimize eating and drinking, no tense activity was allowed within 6 h before the test to avoid its affection on body composition measurements. During measurement, the examinee was asked to take off socks, standing on the test bench with the body relaxed, with both feet on the foot electrodes and both hands holding firmly on the hand electrodes, then basal metabolic rate, total water, the amount of non-fat tissue, muscle mass, body fat mass, and percentage of body fat (PBF) were measured.

Statistical analysis

SAS 9.3 software was used in statistical analysis. 1). Measurement data were shown as $\bar{x} \pm s$, independent sample t test or Wilcoxon test was used to compare difference between the two groups, $P < 0.05$ was considered statistically significant; 2). Receiver operating characteristic curve (ROC curve) was drawn using Mann-Whitney method, and area under the ROC curve (area under curve, AUC) and Somers' D were used to determine the overall accuracy of each predictor (area under the curve ≥0.5 was considered to have diagnostic value, the larger the area, the larger the value); the optimal cut-off points for BMI, WC, PBF to predict PCOS was determined according to Youden index maximum points; 3). The cut-off point where the sensitivity reaches 90 % was determined as the reference standard for screening PCOS with BMI, WC and PBF; 4). The cut-off point where the specificity reaches 90 % was determined as the reference standard for diagnosis of PCOS with BMI, WC and PBF.

Results

Comparison of Age, BMI, WC and PBF between the two groups

Comparison was performed using independent samples t test or Wilcoxon test. The ages of the PCOS group were between 16 to 40 years with mean 28.55 ± 4.27 years; the ages of control group were between 23 to 38 years with mean 28.53 ± 3.26 years. There was no significant difference between the two groups (Table 1). As shown in Table 1 and Fig. 1, compared with the healthy control group, all three parameters, WC (89.67 ± 13.93 vs 75 ± 7.11), PBF (34.69 ± 5.72 vs 29.12 ± 5.05) and BMI (27.51 ± 5.37 vs 22.55 ± 2.9) in PCOS group were significantly increased ($P = 0.000$ for all comparisons), indicating that these three parameters are valuable in facilitating the screening or diagnosis of PCOS.

ROC curves of BMI, WC and PBF for diagnosing PCOS

The Rotterdam criteria was used as the gold standard when to evaluate the accuracy of BMI, WC and PBF to predict PCOS. Figure 2 is the ROC curve of the three obesity parameters for diagnosing PCOS, Table 2 is the area under the ROC curve of the three parameters for diagnosing PCOS. The results in Table 2 show that in general, the mean AUC for WC to diagnose PCOS is 0.814 with a standard error of 0.029 ($P < 0.001$ compared with 0.5 which was set as a standard comparison for

AUC, please refer to the Statistical Analysis section); the mean AUC for PBF to diagnose PCOS is 0.789 with a standard error of 0.025 ($P < 0.001$ compared with 0.5); the mean AUC for BMI to diagnose PCOS is 0.782 with a standard error of 0.028 ($P < 0.001$ compared with 0.5). Each of the two groups was further divided into three subgroups according to age: <26 y/o group, 26–31 y/o group and >31 y/o group, and the data were further analyzed according to age groups. It was shown that the AUCs of all the subgroups of the three obesity parameters were all significantly larger than 0.5 ($P < 0.001$). Comparisons were also performed among the three parameters and there is no significant difference between any of them, meaning that there is no better predictor for PCOS among them.

The cut-off points and other features of the three obesity parameters to diagnose PCOS

ROC curves as mentioned above was used to select the best cut-off points of each of the three parameters to diagnose PCOS. As mentioned in the Statistical Analysis section, the best cut-off points for each of the three parameters to diagnose PCOS was determined based on the maximum point of Youden index. In general, the best cut-off point for WC to diagnose PCOS is 80.5 cm, and at that point, its sensitivity to diagnose PCOS is 73.6 %, and specificity is 85.0 %; the best cut-off point for PBF to diagnose PCOS is 29 %, and at that point, its sensitivity to diagnose PCOS is 88.2 %, and specificity is 57.7 %; the best cut-off point for BMI to diagnose PCOS is 26.6 kg/m^2, and at that point, its sensitivity to diagnose PCOS is 54.5 %, specificity is 98.0 %. The results are shown in Table 3. In the age subgroups, the trend is similar: it seems that PBF has a better sensitivity and can be used to screen PCOS, while BMI can be used in the diagnosis of PCOS as it has a better specificity. The only

Table 1 Comparison of age, WC, PBF and BMI between control and PCOS groups

variables	Statistical parameters	Control group ($n = 300$)	PCOS group ($n = 110$)	P
Age (y/o)	$\bar{x} \pm s$	28.53 ± 3.26	28.55 ± 4.27	0.908
	Median	28.5 (27,30)	28 (26,31)	
	Range (Max, Min)	15 (23,38)	24 (16,40)	
WC (cm)	$\bar{x} \pm s$	75 ± 7.11	89.67 ± 13.93	0.000
	Median	75 (67,79)	89 (80,100)	
	Range (Max, Min)	28 (64,92)	60 (64,124)	
PBF (%)	$\bar{x} \pm s$	29.12 ± 5.05	34.69 ± 5.72	0.000
	Median	28.58 (26,32)	34.19 (30.98,38.27)	
	Range (Max, Min)	40.1 (6.55,46.65)	31.32 (16.11,47.43)	
BMI(kg/m^2)	$\bar{x} \pm s$	22.55 ± 2.9	27.51 ± 5.37	0.000
	Median	22.81 (20.39,24.01)	27.26 (23.36,31.61)	
	Range (Max, Min)	16.92 (17.46,34.37)	26.77 (17.46,44.23)	

Max Maximum, *Min* Minimum; *y/o* years old

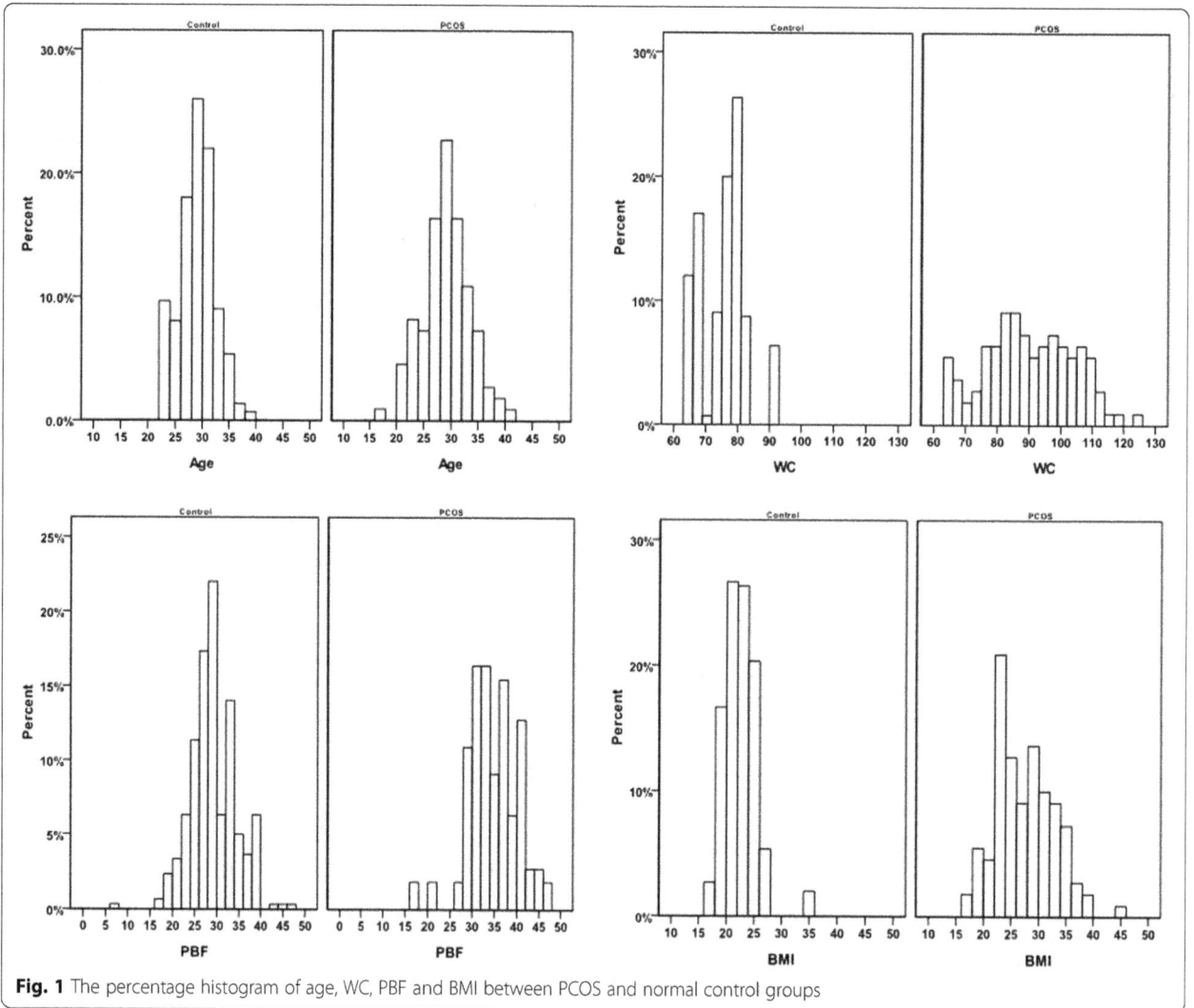

Fig. 1 The percentage histogram of age, WC, PBF and BMI between PCOS and normal control groups

exception is that in age subgroup of older than 31 y/o, WC has a better sensitivity than PBF (81.3 % vs 71.9 %).

Discussion

Studies from different countries have shown that the incidence rate of obesity in patients with PCOS was 30–70 % [3, 4]. Obese PCOS patients tend to have more severe endocrinological, reproductive and metabolic disorders (except hirsutism), manifested by increases of total testosterone level, fasting glucose level, fasting insulin level, insulin resistance and lipid lvel, and decrease of sex hormone-binding globulin (SHBG) level [6]. The current view of the main mechanism of PCOS is the accumulation of excessive visceral fat tissue which causes insulin resistance through secretion of factors such as leptin [7], adiponectin, interleukin-6. This was followed by promotion of androgen synthesis by theca cells and inhibition of hepatic synthesis of SHBG, which together lead to increase of free testosterone concentration in the blood , and subsequently exacerbation of hyperandrogenism further [8]. In addition

to affecting women's reproductive function and pregnancy outcomes, the risk of metabolic syndrome, type 2 DM, CVD and breast cancer, endometrial cancer and other long-term complications in obese PCOS patients are also exponentially increased [5]. The main causes of obesity in PCOS patients are excessive daily intake of carbohydrate-rich, high-glycemic and high saturated fat diet, and too little exercise [9]. Mild weight loss in overweight or obese PCOS patients (a decrease of 5–10 %) could lead to decline in serum testosterone levels, also lead to return of normal ovulation cycle, improve pregnancy success rate [10–13] , and improve hormone, glucose and lipid metabolism disorders [14] and decrease the risk for CVD [15]. Therefore, physicians should not only intervene against PCOS' clinical manifestations, but also should encourage weight loss in these PCOS patients to decrease long-term metabolic risk.

There are many parameters in analyzing obesity, among which, BMI, WC and PBF are the most widely used ones, but with different focus: BMI focus on evaluation of human density, WC focus on evaluation of human girth, PBF focus

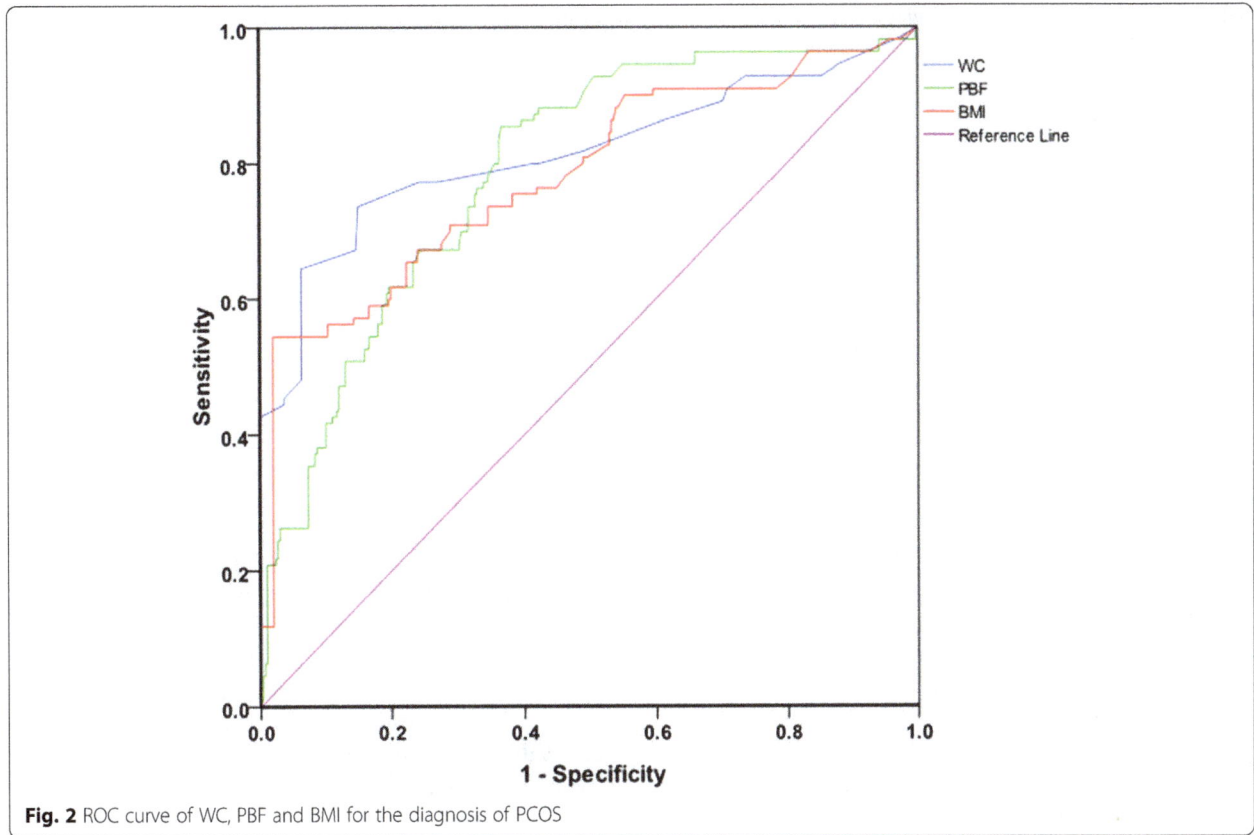

Fig. 2 ROC curve of WC, PBF and BMI for the diagnosis of PCOS

on evaluation of body fat [16]. The accuracy of using these three parameters to predict and diagnose obese PCOS still need to be assessed. In the meantime, due to the difference in race among different countries around the world, there is difference in detection rate of obesity when different cut-off points of obesity parameters were used, therefore, it is

necessary to study the cut-off points of BMI, WC and PBF unique to Chinese women of child-bearing age with PCOS. This study was based on the Rotterdam diagnosis criteria for PCOS [17], where we analyzed the BMI, WC and PBF of 300 women of child-bearing age with PCOS who visited the Reproduction and Genetic Center in Peking University

Table 2 AUC of ROC of WC, PBF and BMI to diagnose PCOS

Age (y/o)	Obesity parameter	AUC ± SE	95 % CI of AUC		Somers' D	P^a	P
			Lower limit	Upper limit			
<26	WC (cm)	0.798 ± 0.068	0.665	0.930	0.596	<0.001	0.558[b]
	PBF (%)	0.769 ± 0.060	0.650	0.887	0.537	<0.001	0.526[c]
	BMI (kg/m^2)	0.817 ± 0.059	0.701	0.933	0.634	<0.001	0.134[d]
26–31	WC (cm)	0.787 ± 0.0423	0.704	0.8700	0.574	<0.001	0.551[b]
	PBF (%)	0.765 ± 0.0361	0.694	0.8355	0.529	<0.001	0.544[c]
	BMI (kg/m^2)	0.768 ± 0.0403	0.689	0.8472	0.537	<0.001	0.898[d]
>31	WC (cm)	0.889 ± 0.043	0.806	0.973	0.779	<0.001	0.001[b]
	PBF (%)	0.838 ± 0.042	0.756	0.920	0.676	<0.001	0.090[c]
	BMI (kg/m^2)	0.773 ± 0.061	0.654	0.891	0.545	<0.001	0.138[d]
合计	WC (cm)	0.814 ± 0.029	0.758	0.870	0.629	<0.001	0.100[b]
	PBF (%)	0.789 ± 0.025	0.7397	0.838	0.577	<0.001	0.261[c]
	BMI (kg/m^2)	0.782 ± 0.028	0.7265	0.838	0.564	<0.001	0.724[d]

[a]AUC compared with 0.5
[b]compared with BMI
[c]compared with WC
[d]compared with PBF

Table 3 Cut-off points and other parameters of WC, PBF and BMI in diagnosis of PCOS

Age (y/o)	Obesity parameter	Cut-off point	Sensitivity (%)	Specificity (%)	Youden index	NPV (%)	PPV (%)
<26	WC (cm)	93.5	56.5	100	0.565	69.7	100
	PBF (%)	28.3	91.3	64.2	0.555	88.1	71.8
	BMI (kg/m^2)	26.6	56.5	100	0.565	69.7	100
26–31	WC (cm)	80.5	69.1	84.5	0.536	73.2	81.7
	PBF (%)	29.9	85.5	60.9	0.464	80.8	68.6
	BMI (kg/m^2)	26.5	45.5	98.9	0.444	64.5	97.6
>31	WC (cm)	81.0	81.3	93.2	0.745	83.3	92.3
	PBF (%)	33.0	71.9	83.6	0.555	74.8	81.4
	BMI (kg/m^2)	26.6	68.8	94.5	0.633	75.2	92.6
Total	WC (cm)	80.5	73.6	85.0	0.586	76.3	83.1
	PBF (%)	29.0	88.2	57.7	0.459	83.0	67.6
	BMI (kg/m^2)	26.6	54.5	98.0	0.525	68.3	96.5

First Hospital from June 2015 to January 2016, as well as 110 cases of age-matched healthy women as normal control. We compared the sensitivity and specificity of the three obesity parameters in diagnosing PCOS, trying to provide evidence for reasonable use of obesity parameters in facilitating the diagnosis of PCOS among high risk population.

The results of this study showed that compared with the healthy control group, all three parameters in PCOS group, BMI, WC and PBF were significantly increased, consistent with previous reports [18], indicating the severity of overweight and obesity in patients with PCOS which leads to exacerbation of endocrine and reproductive metabolic disorders [19].

Our results also showed that, the AUC features of the three obesity parameters were greater than 0.5. AUC reflects the sensitivity and specificity of a certain index in general in the diagnosis of diseases, and the overall diagnostic accuracy of this indicator: $0.5 < AUC \leq 0.7$ means a low diagnostic accuracy, $0.7 < AUC \leq 0.9$ means medium diagnostic accuracy, $0.9 < AUC < 1.0$ means a high diagnostic accuracy [20]. This study demonstrated that these three parameters are all valuable for predicting obesity PCOS, and there was no significant difference among them. Previous studies show that, WC is superior in the accuracy of BMI and other parameters in predicting metabolic syndrome in China [21, 22], metabolic syndrome in PCOS patients in South Korea [23] and Brazil [24]. The reason, mainly is that obesity and overweight are two different concepts. BMI represents body mass and represents a proportional relationship between weight and height, and it cannot reflect the body fat content [25–28], and therefore it is not appropriate to use BMI alone to assess the degree of obesity. WC is an indicator of central obesity and central obesity is not correlated with human mass index, it mainly refers to the accumulation of visceral fat, thus it is a

better predictor of risk of metabolic syndrome and cardiovascular disease [29], and WC is the simplest method of human body measurement. Results of this study suggest that at the time of the census of PCOS among childbearing women, it is recommended that the first choice is WC measurement since it is simple and has equal value in diagnosing PCOS.

Based on bioelectrical impedance principle, body composition analyzer can measure content of water in human body, as well as calculate PBF. It is an accurate, noninvasive and simple method to measure of the content and the proportion of human body fat [30]. Previous studies have shown that BMI showed high specificity and low sensitivity in the diagnosis of obesity, pointing out that BMI missed almost half of the obese population diagnosed by PBF [31–33]. Recent studies have shown that even with normal-weight, high PBF was also associated with insulin resistance [34], PBF is a better indicator to predict obesity [35], so more and more scholars began to study the value of measurement of body composition in obesity diagnosis [36–40]. The results of this study showed the AUC of PBF is not significantly different from the other two parameters, not consistent with previous findings [41]. Nevertheless, this study suggests that in the future, on the basis of PCOS sample, we can further dig into the value of body fat percentage measured using bioelectrical impedance method in the diagnosis of PCOS.

World Health Organization (WHO) [42] and the International Diabetes Federation (IDF) [43] have determined the cut-off point of BMI and WC in diagnosing obesity according to differences in the ethnic, race and morphology: For Chinese adult, $24 \text{ kg/m}^2 \leq BMI < 28 \text{ kg/m}^2$ is defined as overweight, the $BMI \geq 28 \text{ kg/m}^2$ is defined as obese; or female waist ≥ 80 cm is defined as overweight or central obesity; The normal range value of female PBF is 23 ± 5 % and $PBF \geq 30$ % is defined as obese. Korean studies

[23] showed that WC 80 cm was the best cut-off point for the best prediction of PCOS in Korean women; Brazilian studies [24] show WC 95 cm was the best cut-off point for the best prediction of PCOS in Brazilian women. The results of this study confirmed that, BMI 26.6 kg/m^2, WC 80.5 cm and PBF 29 %, were the best cut-off point for diagnosing PCOS. The results of this study is similar to the studies with South Korea, which may be related to ethnic characteristics.

The results of this study also showed that, the three obesity parameters have different sensitivity and specificity. For example, whether in general or in age subgroups, BMI always has the best specificity among the three. While with only one exception in one age subgroup, PBF always has the best sensitivity among the three. These results indicate that, to screen for high-risk PCOS patients in Chinese women of reproductive age, PBF is the first choice as it is more sensitive, except in patients over 31 y/o, WC can be used as an alternative. So the cut-off point of PBF at 29 % can be used as reference standard for epidemiological investigation and preliminary screening of PCOS in the community, then the gold standard of Rotterdam criteria was used for confirmatory diagnosis. In this case, not only the risk factor of PCOS can be prevented earlier, but also avoid causing excessive pressure to the public, it can also adapt to the manpower burden in disease prevention and control, is a reasonable strategy in saving health resources.

While in diagnosing PCOS, BMI has better value as it is more specific. So the cut-off point of BMI at 26.6 kg/m^2 can be used to facilitate the diagnosis of PCOS as it has a specificity of 98 %. It can be used as a relatively reliable diagnosis reference for PCOS when limited by equipment or economic situation, i.e., no ultrasound or sex hormones test available.

One disadvantage of this study is that the study subjects enrolled in this study were all from northern China, in the future, we still need to further expand the sample size, to summarize population data from multiple regions in China, and to establish a more accurate cut-off points in the prediction, screening and diagnosis of PCOS, as well as to administer weight loss treatment in obese PCOS patients to prevent long-term complications.

Conclusion

To summarize, endocrine, reproductive and metabolic disorders are more severe in obese PCOS patients. BMI, WC and PBF are three important parameters to measure obesity. This study shows that patients with PCOS have serious overweight or obesity problems. WC, PBF and BMI are valuable in screening or diagnosing PCOS. PBF has a better sensitivity and can be used to screen PCOS, while BMI can be used in the diagnosis of PCOS as it has a better specificity.

Acknowledgement
Not applicable.

Funding
The study was supported by the International Science & Technology Cooperation Program of China (2013DFA30910) and Research Foundation of Peking University First Hospital(2015QN021).

Authors' contributions
YX, XG and PD mainly participated in literature search, study design, writing and critical revision. HJ, JS, XL, QX mainly participated in data collection, data analysis and data interpretation. All authors read and approved the final manuscript.

Competing interests
The authors declare that there is no conflict of interest.

Author details
[1]Department of Clinical Nutrition, Peking University First Hospital, Beijing, China. [2]Center of Reproduction and Genetics, Peking University First Hospital, Beijing, China. [3]Department of Biostatistics, Peking University First Hospital, Beijing, China. [4]Department of Endocrinology, Peking University First Hospital, Beijing, China. [5]No.7, Xishiku Road, Xicheng District, Beijing 100034, People's Republic of China.

References
1. Stein, Irving F, Leventhal, and Michael L. Amenorrhea associated with bilateral polycystic ovaries. 1935. DOI: http://dx.doi.org/10.1016/S0002-9378(15)30642-6.
2. Li R, Zhang Q, Yang D, et al. Prevalence of polycystic ovary syndrome in women in China: a large community-based study. Hum Reprod. 2013;28: 2562–9. doi:10.1093/humrep/det262.
3. Azziz R, Woods KS, Reyna R, Key TJ, Knochenhauer ES, Yildiz BO. The prevalence and features of the polycystic ovary syndrome in an unselected population. J Clin Endocrinol Metab. 2004;89:2745–9. doi:10.1210/jc.2003-032046.
4. Ehrmann DA. Polycystic ovary syndrome. N Eng J Med. 2005;352:1223–36. doi:10.1056/NEJMra041536.
5. Martínezbermejo E, Luqueramírez M, Escobarmorreale HF. Obesity and the polycystic ovary syndrome. Minerva Endocrinol. 2007;32:129–40.
6. Lim SS, Norman RJ, Davies MJ, Moran LJ. The effect of obesity on polycystic ovary syndrome: a systematic review and meta-analysis. Obes Rev. 2013;14: 95–109. doi:10.1111/j.1467-789X.2012.01053.x.
7. Jalilian N, Haghnazari L, Rasolinia S. Leptin and body mass index in polycystic ovary syndrome. Indian J Endocrinol Metab. 2016;20:324–8. doi:10.4103/2230-8210.180005.
8. Ehrmann DA, Liljenquist DR, Kasza K, et al. Prevalence and predictors of the metabolic syndrome in women with polycystic ovary syndrome. J Clin Endocrinol Metab. 2006;91:48–53. doi:10.1210/jc.2005-1329.
9. Moran LJ, Ranasinha S, Zoungas S, Mcnaughton S, Brown W, Teede H. The contribution of diet, physical activity and sedentary behaviour to body mass index in women with and without polycystic ovary syndrome. Hum Reprod. 2013;28:2276–83. doi:10.1093/humrep/det256.
10. Huber-Buchholz MM, Carey DG, Norman RJ. Restoration of reproductive potential by lifestyle modification in obese polycystic ovary syndrome: role of insulin sensitivity and luteinizing hormone. J Clin Endocrinol Metab. 1999; 84:1470–4. doi:10.1210/jcem.84.4.5596.

11. Crosignani PG, Colombo M, Vegetti W, Somigliana E, Gessati A, Ragni G. Overweight and obese anovulatory patients with polycystic ovaries: parallel improvements in anthropometric indices, ovarian physiology and fertility rate induced by diet. Hum Reprod. 2003;18:1928–32.

12. Legro RS, Dodson WC, Kunselman AR, et al. Benefit of Delayed Fertility Therapy with Preconception Weight Loss over Immediate Therapy in Obese Women with PCOS. J Clin Endocrinol Metab. 2016: jc20161659. doi:10.1210/jc.2016-1659.

13. Bhandari S, Ganguly I, Bhandari M, et al. Effect of sleeve gastrectomy bariatric surgery-induced weight loss on serum AMH levels in reproductive aged women. Gynecol Endocrinol. 2016: 1-4. DOI:10.3109/09513590.2016.1169267.

14. Ha L, Li X. Effect of high protein diet and regular exercise in obese patients with polycystic ovary syndrome. Ningxia Med. 2013;35:3.

15. Soares NP, Santos AC, Costa EC, et al. Diet-induced weight loss reduces DNA damage and cardiometabolic risk factors in overweight/obese women with polycystic ovary syndrome. Ann Nutr Metab. 2016;68:220–7. doi:10.1159/000444130.

16. He X, Tao Q, Li X. Influence of gender and age on the diagnostic criteria of overweight and obesity in adult with BMI. Chin J Public Health. 2009;25:4.

17. Rotterdam EA-SPcwg. Revised 2003 consensus on diagnostic criteria and long-term health risks related to polycystic ovary syndrome (PCOS). Hum Reprod. 2004;19:41–7.

18. Wijeyaratne CN, Seneviratne Rde A, Dahanayake S, et al. Phenotype and metabolic profile of South Asian women with polycystic ovary syndrome (PCOS): results of a large database from a specialist Endocrine Clinic. Hum Reprod. 2011;26:202–13. doi:10.1093/humrep/deq310.

19. Sam S. Adiposity and metabolic dysfunction in polycystic ovary syndrome. Horm Mol Biol Clin Investig. 2015;21:107–16. doi:10.1515/hmbci-2015-0008.

20. Pan B, Zhang X, Liu S. Evaluation of the ROC analysis in SPSS in the test/diagnosis. Strait J Prev Med. 2003;9:5.

21. Chen L, Lan Z, Zhang D. The value of different obese criteria for the assessment of insulin resistance in women with polycystic ovary syndrome. Sichuan Da Xue Xue Bao Yi Xue Ban. 2013;44:5.

22. Zeng Q, He Y, Dong S, et al. Optimal cut-off values of BMI, waist circumference and waist:height ratio for defining obesity in Chinese adults. Br J Nutr. 2014;112:1735–44. doi:10.1017/S0007114514002657.

23. Oh JY, Sung YA, Lee HJ, Oh JY, Chung HW, Park H. Optimal waist circumference for prediction of metabolic syndrome in young Korean women with polycystic ovary syndrome. Obesity (Silver Spring). 2010;18: 593–7. doi:10.1038/oby.2009.297.

24. Costa EC, Sa JC, Soares EM, Lemos TM, Maranhao TM, Azevedo GD. Anthropometric indices of central obesity how discriminators of metabolic syndrome in Brazilian women with polycystic ovary syndrome. Gynecol Endocrinol. 2012;28:12–5. doi:10.3109/09513590.2011.583956.

25. Lavie CJ, Milani RV, Ventura HO. Obesity and cardiovascular disease: risk factor, paradox, and impact of weight loss. J Am Coll Cardiol. 2009;53: 1925–32. doi:10.1016/j.jacc.2008.12.068.

26. Lavie CJ, De Schutter A, Patel D, Artham SM, Milani RV. Body composition and coronary heart disease mortality–an obesity or a lean paradox? Mayo Clin Proc. 2011;86:857–64. doi:10.4065/mcp.2011.0092.

27. Lavie CJ, Milani RV, Ventura HO, Romero-Corral A. Body composition and heart failure prevalence and prognosis: getting to the fat of the matter in the "obesity paradox". Mayo Clin Proc. 2010;85:605–8. doi:10.4065/mcp.2010.0333.

28. Romero-Corral A, Montori VM, Somers VK, et al. Association of bodyweight with total mortality and with cardiovascular events in coronary artery disease: a systematic review of cohort studies. Lancet. 2006;368:666–78. doi:10.1016/S0140-6736(06)69251-9.

29. Zhu S, Wang Z, Heshka S, Heo M, Faith MS, Heymsfield SB. Waist circumference and obesity-associated risk factors among whites in the third National Health and Nutrition Examination Survey: clinical action thresholds. Am J Clin Nutr. 2002;76:743–9.

30. Wattanapenpaiboon N, Lukito W, Strauss BJ, Hsu-Hage BH, Wahlqvist ML, Stroud DB. Agreement of skinfold measurement and bioelectrical impedance analysis (BIA) methods with dual energy X-ray absorptiometry (DEXA) in estimating total body fat in Anglo-Celtic Australians. Int J Obes Relat Metab Disord. 1998;22:854–60.

31. Habib SS. Body mass index and body fat percentage in assessment of obesity prevalence in saudi adults. Biomed Environ Sci. 2013;26:94–9. doi:10.3967/0895-3988.2013.02.003.

32. Okorodudu DO, Jumean MF, Montori VM, et al. Diagnostic performance of body mass index to identify obesity as defined by body adiposity: a systematic review and meta-analysis. Int J Obes (Lond). 2010;34:791–9. doi:10.1038/ijo.2010.5.

33. Carpenter CL, Yan E, Chen S, et al. Body fat and body-mass index among a multiethnic sample of college-age men and women. J Obes. 2013;2013: 790654. doi:10.1155/2013/790654.

34. Madeira FB, Silva AA, Veloso HF, et al. Normal weight obesity is associated with metabolic syndrome and insulin resistance in young adults from a middle-income country. PLoS One. 2013;8:e60673. doi:10.1371/journal.pone.0060673.

35. Lavie CJ, De Schutter A, Patel DA, Romero-Corral A, Artham SM, Milani RV. Body composition and survival in stable coronary heart disease: impact of lean mass index and body fat in the "obesity paradox". J Am Coll Cardiol. 2012;60:1374–80. doi:10.1016/j.jacc.2012.05.037.

36. Thibault R, Pichard C. The evaluation of body composition: a useful tool for clinical practice. Ann Nutr Metab. 2012;60:6–16. doi:10.1159/000334879.

37. Deurenberg-Yap M, Chew SK, Deurenberg P. Elevated body fat percentage and cardiovascular risks at low body mass index levels among Singaporean Chinese, Malays and Indians. Obes Rev. 2002;3:209–15.

38. Cruz P, Johnson BD, Karpinski SC, et al. Validity of weight loss to estimate improvement in body composition in individuals attending a wellness center. Obesity (Silver Spring). 2011;19:2274–9. doi:10.1038/oby.2011.102.

39. Wright CM, Sherriff A, Ward SC, McColl JH, Reilly JJ, Ness AR. Development of bioelectrical impedance-derived indices of fat and fat-free mass for assessment of nutritional status in childhood. Eur J Clin Nutr. 2008;62:210–7. doi:10.1038/sj.ejcn.1602714.

40. Bintvihok W, Chaikittisilpa S, Panyakamlerd K, Jaisamrarn U, Taechakraichana N. Cut-off value of body fat in association with metabolic syndrome in Thai peri- and postmenopausal women. Climacteric. 2013;16:393–7. doi:10.3109/13697137.2012.762762.

41. Zabuliene L, Tutkuviene J. Body composition and polycystic ovary syndrome. Medicina (Kaunas). 2010;46:142–57.

42. Consultation WHOE. Appropriate body-mass index for Asian populations and its implications for policy and intervention strategies. Lancet. 2004;363: 157–63. doi:10.1016/S0140-6736(03)15268-3.

43. Alberti KG, Zimmet P, Shaw J. Metabolic syndrome–a new world-wide definition. A consensus statement from the International Diabetes Federation. Diabet Med. 2006;23:469–80. doi:10.1111/j.1464-5491.2006.01858.x.

17

Expression pattern of circadian genes and steroidogenesis-related genes after testosterone stimulation in the human ovary

Minghui Chen[1,2], Yanwen Xu[1,2], Benyu Miao[1,2], Hui Zhao[4], Lu Luo[1,2], Huijuan Shi[3] and Canquan Zhou[1,2]*

Abstract

Background: Previous studies have shown that circadian genes might be involved in the development of polycystic ovarian syndrome (PCOS). Hyperandrogenism is a hallmark feature of PCOS. However, the effect of hyperandrogenism on circadian gene expression in human granulosa cells is unknown, and the general expression pattern of circadian genes in the human ovary is unclear.

Methods: Expression of the circadian proteins CLOCK and PER2 in human ovaries was observed by immunohistochemistry. The mRNA expression patterns of the circadian genes *CLOCK*, *PER2*, and *BMAL1*, and the steroidogenesis-related genes *STAR*, *CYP11A1*, *HSD3B2*, and *CYP19A1* in cultured human luteinized granulosa cells were analyzed over the course of 48 h after testosterone treatment by quantitative polymerase chain reaction.

Results: Immunostaining of CLOCK and PER2 protein was detected in the granulosa cells of dominant antral follicles but was absent in the primordial, primary, or preantral follicles of human ovaries. After testosterone stimulation, expression of *PER2* showed an oscillating pattern, with two peaks occurring at the 24th and 44th hours; expression of *CLOCK* increased significantly to the peak at the 24th hour, whereas expression of *BMAL1* did not change significantly over time in human luteinized granulosa cells. Among the four steroidogenesis-related genes evaluated, only *STAR* displayed an oscillating expression pattern with two peaks occurring at the 24th and 40th hours after testosterone stimulation.

Conclusions: Circadian genes are expressed in the dominant antral follicles of the human ovary. Oscillating expression of the circadian gene *PER2* can be induced by testosterone in human granulosa cells in vitro. Expression of *STAR* also displayed an oscillating pattern after testosterone stimulation. Our results indicate a potential relationship between the circadian clock and steroidogenesis in the human ovary, and demonstrate the effect of testosterone on circadian gene expression in granulosa cells.

Keywords: Circadian rhythm, Testosterone, Granulosa cells, Ovary, Human

Abbreviations: BMAL1, Brain and muscle arnt-like protein 1; CLOCK, Circadian locomotor output cycles kaput; CYP11A1, Cholesterol side-chain cleavage cytochrome P450; CYP19A1, Cytochrome P450; HSD3B2, 3-β-hydroxysteroid dehydrogenase type II; PER, Period; qRT-PCR, Quantitative reverse transcription-polymerase chain reaction; STAR, Steroidal acute regulatory protein

* Correspondence: zhoucanquan@hotmail.com
[1]Reproductive Medicine Center, The First Affiliated Hospital of Sun Yat-sen University, 58 2nd Zhongshan Road, Guangzhou GD510080, People's Republic of China
[2]Guangdong Provincial Key Laboratory of Reproductive Medicine, The First Affiliated Hospital of Sun Yat-sen University, 58 2nd Zhongshan Road, Guangzhou GD510080, People's Republic of China
Full list of author information is available at the end of the article

Background

A circadian clock is a biochemical mechanism that oscillates with a period of 24 h and is coordinated with the day–night cycle. In mammals, light signals perceived by the retina are transmitted via the retino-hypothalamic tract to the suprachiasmatic nuclei (SCN), which contain the master pacemaker for the generation of circadian rhythms [1]. The SCN synchronize countless subsidiary oscillators existing in the peripheral tissues throughout the body [2]. The basis for maintaining the circadian rhythm is a molecular clock consisting of interlocked transcriptional/translational feedback loops. The proteins encoded by the genes circadian locomotor output cycles kaput (*Clock*) and brain and muscle arnt-like protein 1 (*Bmal1*) heterodimerize and promote the rhythmic transcription of the period (*Per1*, *Per2*) and cryptochrome (*Cry1*, *Cry2*) gene families, whereas modified PER–CRY complexes repress the activity of the CLOCK–BMAL1 complex. Over several hours, PER–CRY complexes are degraded, and the CLOCK–BMAL1 complex is eventually released from feedback inhibition [3–6].

Quantitative reverse transcription-polymerase chain reaction (qRT-PCR) analysis revealed that transcripts for the core oscillator elements (*Arntl*, *Clock*, *Per1*, *Per2*, and *Cry1*) were present in the rat ovary [7]. Expression of *Arntl* and *Per2* was detected in the granulosa and theca layers of growing and antral follicles, as well as in the corpora lutea and stromal fibroblasts of the rat ovary [7]. *Per1* and *Per2* mRNAs in the rat ovary display rhythmic oscillation with a 24-h period [8]. Moreover, such rhythmic expression of a circadian gene can be induced in cultured ovarian cells. When cultured without any treatment, no rhythmic pattern in the expression of either *Per1* or *Bmal1* transcripts was observed in chicken granulosa cells; however, both serum shock and luteinizing hormone (LH) treatment could induce a rhythm of both *Per1* and *Bmal1* in these cells [9].

Polycystic ovarian syndrome (PCOS) is the most common endocrine disorder of reproductive-age women. A recent study highlighted the important role of circadian genes in the development of PCOS. This study showed that the level of *BMAL1* expression in granulosa cells in the PCOS group of women was lower than that of the group without PCOS. Estrogen synthesis and aromatase expression were downregulated after *BMAL1* knockdown and, conversely, were upregulated in KGN cells (a granulosa cell line) overexpressing *BMAL1* [10]. Hyperandrogenism is a hallmark feature of PCOS and is strongly implicated in the genesis of the disorder [11]. A high testosterone level reflects a type of androgen excess, which is one of the primary symptoms of PCOS. In the present study, we selected testosterone as a stimulator for cultured human granulosa cells and observed the temporal expression patterns of circadian genes and

steroidogenesis-related genes in human luteinized granulosa cells after testosterone stimulation. In addition, we evaluated the distribution of circadian protein expression in human ovaries by immunohistochemistry.

Methods

Immunohistochemistry

Paraffin sections of normal ovarian tissue were obtained from five women aged 29–35 years. All women had undergone bilateral salpingo-oophorectomy with or without hysterectomy for a uterine or unilateral ovarian malignant tumor before chemotherapy or radiotherapy. Informed consent was obtained from all patients. After deparaffinization, antigen retrieval, and blocking in normal goat serum (for CLOCK) or bovine serum (for PER2), the slides were incubated overnight at 4 °C in rabbit anti-human CLOCK polyclonal antibody diluted to 20 μg/mL (catalogue no. ab 65033,Abcam) or goat anti-human PER2 polyclonal antibody diluted to 7.5 μg/mL (catalogue no. ab118489, Abcam), respectively. Slides were washed and incubated with biotin-labeled goat anti-rabbit secondary antibody for CLOCK (CWBIO) or bovine anti-goat secondary antibody for PER2 (Santa Cruz Biotechnology) for 30 min, then washed and incubated with horseradish peroxidase-labeled streptavidin for 10 min. The peroxidase–antibody complex was visualized using 3, 3′-diaminobenzidine (CWBIO). Control experiments included samples treated in the same manner but with omission of the primary antibody. The sections were counterstained with hematoxylin.

Cell culture

For each experiment, human luteinized granulosa cells were obtained from the follicle fluid collected during ovum aspiration of 10 patients undergoing in vitro fertilization. All patients underwent the long protocol of gonadotropin-releasing hormone agonist treatment (1.0 mg tiptorelin acetate; Ipsen Pharma Biotech, France) with human chorionic gonadotropin as the trigger. The follicle fluid was pooled and centrifuged for 5 min at 2500 rpm. Granulosa cells were purified using 50 % Percoll (Sigma) through gradient centrifugation for 10 min at 2000 rpm. Ovarian tissue fragments were then removed from the granulosa cell suspension with a 40-μm cell strainer (Becton-Dickinson). Purified granulosa cells were plated on a 12-well plate (3.0×10^5/well) and cultured in Dulbecco's modified Eagle medium/Ham's F12 supplemented with penicillin (100 U/mL), streptomycin (100 μg/mL), and 10 % fetal bovine serum (Gibco) in a 37 °C incubator with 5 % CO_2. Cells were cultured for 9 days to reach confluence prior to any treatment. Cells were exposed to 100 ng/mL testosterone (Sigma) dissolved in serum-free medium for 2 h, washed with serum-free medium once, and then cultured further in serum-free medium until harvested. Cells in the control group were cultured in serum-free medium without testosterone treatment. Samples were harvested every 4 h starting at the beginning of treatment and continuing until 48 h.

RNA extraction and quantification

RNA was extracted with High Pure RNA Isolation Kit (Roche) according to the manufacturer's instructions, and quantitated by 260/280 UV spectrophotometry (NanoDrop ND-1000, Wilmington, DE, USA). Five hundred nanograms of RNA were subjected to reverse transcription with oligo-dT primers using Roche Transcriptor First-strand cDNA Synthesis Kit. The differential expression of target gene mRNA in granulosa cells was quantified using the following TaqMan® Gene Expression Assays (Applied Biosystems): *CLOCK* (Hs00231857_m1), *PER2* (Hs00256143_m1), *BMAL1* (Hs00154147_m1), steroidogenic acute regulatory protein (*STAR*; Hs00986559_g1), 3-β-hydroxysteroid dehydrogenase type II (*HSD3B2*; Hs00605123-m1), cholesterol side-chain cleavage cytochrome P450 (*CYP11A1*; Hs00167984_m1), and cytochrome P450 (*CYP19A1*; Hs00903413_m1). Quantification was accomplished with an Applied Biosystems 7500 real-time RT-PCR machine using TaqMan® Fast Advanced Master Mix (Invitrogen). The relative mRNA levels were calculated using the comparative cycle threshold method, using *ACTB* (Hs99999903_m1; Applied Biosystems) as a reference gene.

Statistical analysis

Data are presented as the least squares mean ± standard error of the mean from three replicate experiments. Least-squares analysis of variance (ANOVA) implemented by SPSS 13.0 was used to analyze all data. Tukey's multiple-comparison post-hoc test was used if equal variances were validated, or Dunnett's T3 post-hoc test was used if equal variances were not assumed, when ANOVA returned a value of $P \leq 0.05$. $P \leq 0.05$ was considered a statistically significant difference.

Results

Expression of circadian proteins in the human ovary

Immunohistochemistry results showed positive expression of CLOCK in the cumulus and mural granulosa cells in dominant antral follicles and in interstitial cells, but no CLOCK expression was observed in the primordial follicles, primary follicles, and preantral follicles, and in the theca cells of antral follicles. Expression of PER2 was observed in the cumulus cells and mural granulosa cells in the dominant antral follicles and in interstitial cells, was weak in the theca cells of the dominant antral follicle, but was absent in the primordial follicle, primary follicles, and preantral follicles (Fig. 1).

Expression patterns of circadian genes in human granulosa cells stimulated by testosterone

Treatment of testosterone induced oscillations in *PER2* expression, with the first peak and bottom occurring at the 24th and 32nd hours, respectively, and the second peak occurring at the 44th hour ($P_{4 \text{ vs. } 24} = 0.028$, $P_{24 \text{ vs. } 32} = 0.041$, $P_{24 \text{ vs. } 48} = 0.039$, $P_{4 \text{ vs. } 44} = 0.024$). Expression of *CLOCK* increased significantly at the 24th hour ($P_{4 \text{ vs. } 24} = 0.04$), whereas expression of *BMAL1* did not change significantly after testosterone stimulation. In the control group, after changing to serum-free medium, the expression levels of both *PER2* ($P_{4 \text{ vs. } 16} = 0.016$) and *CLOCK* ($P_{4 \text{ vs. } 12} = 0.022$, $P_{4 \text{ vs. } 16} = 0.031$, $P_{4 \text{ vs. } 20} = 0.006$, $P_{4 \text{ vs. } 36} = 0.011$) increased significantly; however, they did not display an oscillating pattern. The expression of *BMAL1* did not change significantly over time (Fig. 2).

Expression patterns of steroidogenesis-related genes in human granulosa cells stimulated by testosterone

Treatment of testosterone induced oscillations in *STAR* expression, with the first and second peaks occurring at the 24th and 40th hours, respectively ($P_{4 \text{ vs. } 24} < 0.001$, $P_{24 \text{ vs. } 32} < 0.001$, $P_{4 \text{ vs. } 40} = 0.001$). Expression of *CYP19A1* in granulosa cells was significantly repressed at the 12th hour ($P_{4 \text{ vs. } 12} = 0.003$), whereas the expression levels of *HSD3B2* and *CYP11A1* did not change significantly after testosterone stimulation. In the control group, changing to serum-free medium significantly stimulated *STAR* expression ($P_{4 \text{ vs. } 24} = 0.028$, $P_{4 \text{ vs. } 36} = 0.001$, $P_{4 \text{ vs. } 40} = 0.021$), but had no significant effects on the expression levels of *CYP11A1*, *HSD3B2*, and *CYP19A1* (Fig. 3).

Discussion

In this study, we detected the presence of both PER2 and CLOCK proteins in human dominant antral follicles, which were absent in the primordial, primary, and preantral follicles. Moreover, *CLOCK*, *PER2*, and *BMAL1* mRNAs were present in human luteinized granulosa cells. These distribution patterns of circadian genes in the human ovary are similar to those reported for the rat ovary. In the rat ovary, expression of *Per2* and *Bmal1* was detected in growing and antral follicles, as well as in the corpora lutea and stromal fibroblasts [7]. Circadian genes have previously been found to be involved in steroidogenesis in granulosa cells. BMAL1 knock-down can lead to downregulation of estrogen synthesis and aromatase expression; conversely, overexpression of BMAL1 resulted in upregulation of estrogen synthesis and aromatase expression in KGN cells [10]. In addition, inhibition of the expression of Per2 with Per2-specific small interfering RNA stimulated the expression of *Star* in granulosa cells from cows [12]. Both dominant antral follicle and corpora lutea can produce steroids hormone. Expression of circadian genes in dominant antral follicle

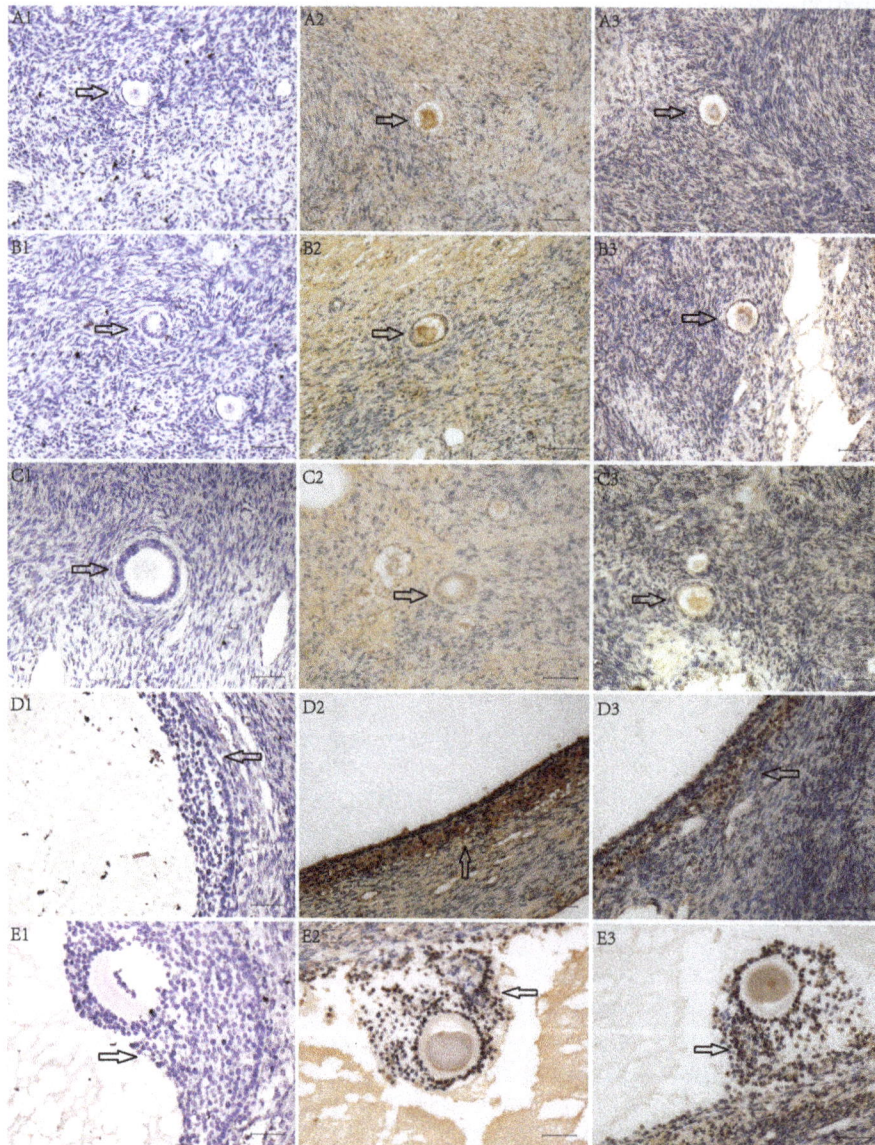

Fig. 1 Immunohistochemistry staining of CLOCK and PER2 in paraffin sections of human ovaries. Staining of CLOCK was detected in the cumulus cells and mural granulosa cells, absent in the theca cells of the dominant antral follicles (D2, E2), and present in the interstitial cells, but absent in primordial follicles (A2), primary follicles (B2), and preantral follicles (C2). Staining of PER2 was present in the cumulus cells, mural granulosa cells, weak in the theca cells of dominant antral follicles (D3, E3), and present in the interstitial cells, but absent in the primordial follicles (A3), primary follicles (B3), and preantral follicles (C3). A1 to E1 are negative controls (no primary antibody) of the primordial, primary, preantral, and antral follicles and the cumulus complex, respectively. Bars = 50 μm. Original magnification, ×200

and corpora lutea of human ovary indicated that expression of circadian gene may also be involved in steroidogenesis in human ovary.

The present study showed that testosterone can induce oscillating expression of *PER2* in human granulosa cells. Although the exact mechanism is unclear, there is some evidence pointing to an association between testosterone and the circadian clock. Testosterone stimulation was shown to promote the association of androgen receptor localized in the plasma membrane with Src kinase, which activated Src kinase [13]. Src-family tyrosine kinases can regulate the expression level of the clock protein Timeless and regulate its function [14]. Moreover, Src activity is involved in the progesterone production of granulosa cells [15]. However, further studies are needed to confirm these relationships.

An experiment on quail in vivo showed that expression of the *Star* gene presented 24-h changes in the largest preovulatory follicle, coinciding with changes in *Per2*. Furthermore, these authors demonstrated that the 5′ flanking region of *Star* contains E-box enhancers that can bind to CLOCK–BMAL1 heterodimers and activate

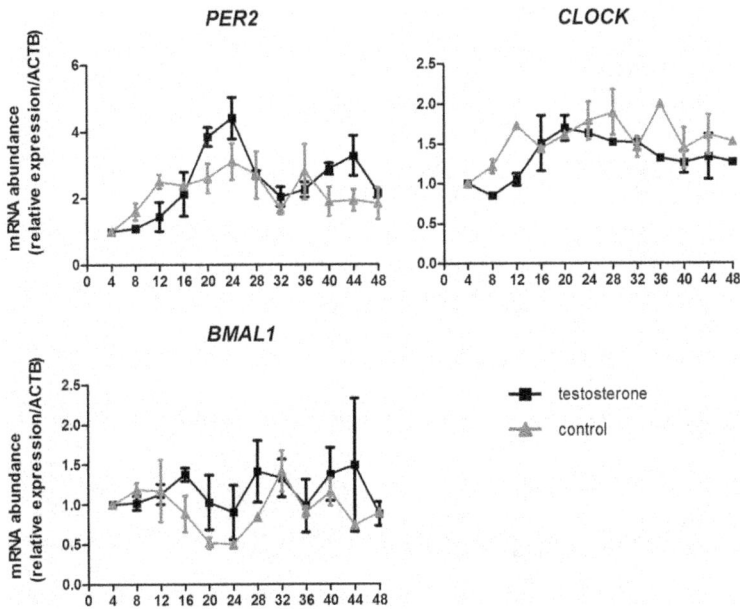

Fig. 2 Expression patterns of circadian genes after testosterone treatment in human luteinized granulosa cells. Human luteinized granulosa cells were exposed to 100 ng/mL testosterone dissolved in serum-free medium for 2 h and cells in the control group were cultured in serum-free medium without treatment. Samples were harvested every 4 h from the beginning of treatment for 48 h. Each value represents the mean ± SEM of three independent experiments. Significant statistical differences are shown as below: the testosterone group *PER2* $P_{4 \text{ vs. } 24} = 0.028$, $P_{24 \text{ vs. } 32} = 0.041$, $P_{24 \text{ vs. } 48} = 0.039$, $P_{4 \text{ vs. } 44} = 0.024$, *CLOCK* $P_{4 \text{ vs. } 24} = 0.04$; the control group *PER2* $P_{4 \text{ vs. } 16} = 0.016$, *CLOCK* $P_{4 \text{ vs. } 12} = 0.022$, $P_{4 \text{ vs. } 16} = 0.031$, $P_{4 \text{ vs. } 20} = 0.006$, $P_{4 \text{ vs. } 36} = 0.011$

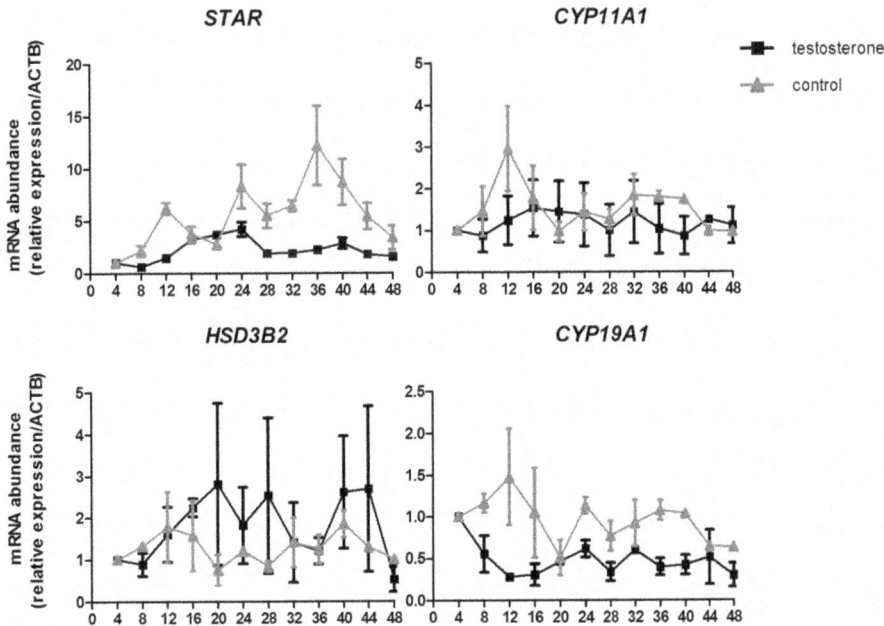

Fig. 3 Expression patterns of steroidogenesis-related genes after testosterone treatment in human luteinized granulosa cells. Human luteinized granulosa cells were exposed to 100 ng/mL testosterone dissolved in serum-free medium for 2 h and cells in the control group were cultured in serum-free medium without treatment. Samples were harvested every 4 h from the beginning of treatment for 48 h. Each value represents the mean ± SEM from three independent experiments. Significant statistical differences are shown as below: the testosterone group *STAR* $P_{4 \text{ vs. } 24} < 0.001$, $P_{24 \text{ vs. } 32} < 0.001$, $P_{4 \text{ vs. } 40} = 0.001$), *CYP19A1* $P_{4 \text{ vs. } 12} = 0.003$; the control group *STAR* $P_{4 \text{ vs. } 24} = 0.028$, $P_{4 \text{ vs. } 36} = 0.001$, $P_{4 \text{ vs. } 40} = 0.021$

gene transcription [16]. Therefore, these findings indicated that *Star* is a clock-driven gene. Similarly, we found that *STAR* expression showed an oscillating pattern in cultured human granulosa cells after testosterone stimulation, but the pattern did not completely coincide with that of *PER2*. The difference between the results of the present study and those of the quail study may be caused by species-specific differences, the in vivo vs. in vitro study design, or the stimulus used. In addition, we found testosterone can decrease *CYP19A1* expression in human granulosa cells. Our results are in accordance with a recent study which showed that exposure to high level of testosterone could decrease both mRNA and protein levels of aromatase in cultured luteinized granulosa cells isolated from non-PCOS women [17]. However, effect of testosterone on aromatase expression in granulosa cells is different in different species. It has been reported that testosterone stimulates *Cyp19* promoter activity and the expression of *Cyp19* in granulosa cells from immature female rats [18].

A recent study pointed to the important role of circadian genes in the development of PCOS and indicated that circadian clock is likely involved in steroidogenesis in granulosa cells [10]. Our results showed that testosterone can affect circadian gene expression in human granulosa cells. Therefore, hyperandrogenemia can affect circadian gene expression, resulting in the disorder of steroidogenesis in granulosa cells leading to the development of PCOS. However, a limitation of the present study is that we used granulosa cells from hormonally stimulated patients, because it is difficult to obtain granulosa cells from hormonally unstimulated patients. Furthermore, this study represents preliminary research on the expression patterns of circadian genes and their relationship with steroidogenesis in the human ovary. Therefore, further studies are needed to elucidate the molecular mechanism.

Conclusions

We found that the circadian genes *CLOCK* and *PER2* are expressed in the dominant antral follicles of the human ovary. Testosterone could induce oscillating expression of the circadian gene *PER2* in cultured human granulosa cells. Moreover, expression of *STAR* in human granulosa cells also displayed an oscillating pattern after testosterone stimulation. Our results indicate a potential relationship between the circadian clock and steroidogenesis in the human ovary, and demonstrate the effect of testosterone on circadian gene expression in granulosa cells.

Acknowledgements
We thank Jin-hu Guo for technical advice for sample harvesting, Chang Liu for technical advice for induction of circadian gene expression, Ping Xiao for technical advice on immunohistochemistry, and Ma Xiang for statistical advice.

Funding
This work was supported by grants from the National Basic Research Program of China (973 program, 2012CB947600), Scientific Project of Health Industry (201002013), and Science and Technology Planning Project of Guangdong Province, China (2008A030201028).

Authors' contributions
MHC, YWX, and CQZ contributed to project design. MHC, BYM, and HZ carried out the cell culture and qRT-PCR. MHC, LL and HJS carried out the immunohistochemistry. MHC, YWX, and HZ wrote the manuscript. All authors discussed the results and commented on the manuscript. All authors read and approved the final manuscript.

Competing interests
The authors declare that they have no competing interests.

Author details
[1]Reproductive Medicine Center, The First Affiliated Hospital of Sun Yat-sen University, 58 2nd Zhongshan Road, Guangzhou GD510080, People's Republic of China. [2]Guangdong Provincial Key Laboratory of Reproductive Medicine, The First Affiliated Hospital of Sun Yat-sen University, 58 2nd Zhongshan Road, Guangzhou GD510080, People's Republic of China. [3]Department of Pathology, The First Affiliated Hospital of Sun Yat-sen University, 58 2nd Zhongshan Road, Guangzhou GD510080, People's Republic of China. [4]Department of Hepatic Surgery, The Third Affiliated Hospital of Sun Yat-sen University, 600 Tianhe Road, Guangzhou GD510630, People's Republic of China.

References
1. Hastings MH. Circadian clocks. Curr Biol. 1997;7:R670–2.
2. Ko CH, Takahashi JS. Molecular components of the mammalian circadian clock. Hum Mol Genet. 2006;15:R271–7.
3. Takahashi JS, Hong HK, Ko CH, McDearmon EL. The genetics of mammalian circadian order and disorder: implications for physiology and disease. Nat Rev Genet. 2008;9:764–75.
4. Gekakis N, Staknis D, Nguyen HB, Davis FC, Wilsbacher LD, King DP, et al. Role of the CLOCK protein in the mammalian circadian mechanism. Science. 1998;280:1564–9.
5. Shearman LP, Sriram S, Weaver DR, Maywood ES, Chaves I, Zheng B, et al. Interacting molecular loops in the mammalian circadian clock. Science. 2000;288:1013–9.
6. Ueda HR, Hayashi S, Chen W, Sano M, Machida M, Shigeyoshi Y, et al. System-level identification of transcriptional circuits underlying mammalian circadian clocks. Nat Genet. 2005;37:187–92.
7. Karman BN, Tischkau SA. Circadian clock gene expression in the ovary: effects of luteinizing hormone. Biol Reprod. 2006;75:624–32.
8. Fahrenkrug J, Georg B, Hannibal J, Hindersson P, Gräs S. Diurnal rhythmicity of the clock genes *Per1* and *Per2* in the rat ovary. Endocrinology. 2006;147:3769–76.
9. Tischkau SA, Howell RE, Hickok JR, Krager SL, Bahr JM. The luteinizing hormone surge regulates circadian clock gene expression in the chicken ovary. Chronobiol Int. 2011;28:10–20.

10. Zhang J, Liu J, Zhu K, Hong Y, Sun Y, Zhao X, Du Y, Chen ZJ. Effects of BMAL1-SIRT1-positive cycle on estrogen synthesis in human ovarian granulosa cells: an implicative role of BMAL1 in PCOS. Endocrine. 2016;53: 574-84.

11. Eisner JR, Barnett MA, Dumesic DA, Abbott DH. Ovarian hyperandrogenism in adult female rhesus monkeys exposed to prenatal androgen excess. Fertil Steril. 2002;1:167–72.

12. Shimizu T, Hirai Y, Murayama C, Miyamoto A, Miyazaki H, Miyazaki K. Circadian Clock genes Per2 and clock regulate steroid production, cell proliferation, and luteinizing hormone receptor transcription in ovarian granulosa cells. Biochem Biophys Res Commun. 2011;412:132–5.

13. Cheng J, Watkins SC, Walker WH. Testosterone activates mitogen-activated protein kinase via Src kinase and the epidermal growth factor receptor in sertoli cells. Endocrinology. 2007;148:2066–74.

14. O'Reilly LP, Zhang X, Smithgall TE. Individual Src-family tyrosine kinases direct the degradation or protection of the clock protein Timeless via differential ubiquitylation. Cell Signal. 2013;25:860–6.

15. Rice VM, Chaudhery AR, Oluola O, Limback SD, Roby KF, Terranova PF. Herbimycin, a tyrosine kinase inhibitor with Src selectivity, reduces progesterone and estradiol secretion by human granulosa cells. Endocrine. 2001;15:271–6.

16. Nakao N, Yasuo S, Nishimura A, Rupp GP, Echternkamp SE. Circadian clock gene regulation of steroidogenic acute regulatory protein gene expression in preovulatory ovarian follicles. Endocrinology. 2007;148:3031–8.

17. Yang F, Ruan YC, Yang YJ, Wang K, Liang SS, Han YB, Teng XM. Yang JZ Follicular hyperandrogenism downregulates aromatase in luteinized granulosa cells in polycystic ovary syndrome women. Reproduction. 2015; 150:289–96.

18. Wu YG, Bennett J, Talla D, Stocco C. Testosterone, not 5α-dihydrotestosterone, stimulates LRH-1 leading to FSH-independent expression of Cyp19 and P450scc in granulosa cells. Mol Endocrinol. 2011; 25:656–68.

18

Ameliorative effects of rutin against metabolic, biochemical and hormonal disturbances in polycystic ovary syndrome in rats

Sarwat Jahan[1], Faryal Munir[1], Suhail Razak[1,2*], Anam Mehboob[1], Qurat Ul Ain[1], Hizb Ullah[1], Tayyaba Afsar[3], Ghazala Shaheen[1] and Ali Almajwal[2]

Abstract

Background: Polycystic ovary syndrome (PCOS) is the most prevalent endocrinopathy in women of reproductive age. The study was commenced to assess the favorable effects of Rutin against metabolic, biochemical, histological, and androgenic aspects of polycystic ovary syndrome in rats.

Methods: Female Sprague-Dawley rats were administered letrozole (1 mg/kg) per orally (p.o) for a period of 21 days for the induction of PCOS, followed by dose of rutin (100 mg/kg and 150 mg/kg, p.o) for 15 days using 0. 5% w/v CMC as vehicle. Metformin was also given as a standard control to one of the rat groups.
Serum estradiol, progesterone, testosterone, serum lipid parameters, CRP and glucose levels were evaluated. Furthermore, antioxidant activity was tested using superoxide dismutase, catalase, glutathione per-oxidase and reactive-oxygen species level.

Results: Rutin flavonoid had a dose-dependent effect on androgenic levels depicting more recovery in the rutin-I treated group, while rutin-II treated groups showed better antioxidant and lipid profiles as compared with PCOS groups. A decrease in the value of C reactive protein (CRP) and a restoration in the proportion of estrous phase smears were observed in the rutin treated groups. Histopathological examination of ovary revealed a significant decrease in the number of cystic follicles in post treated groups. The effects observed with rutin were moderately similar to that with standard metformin, a widely used treatment drug for PCOS.

Conclusion: The study provides evidence for the potential ameliorative effects of rutin against clinical and biochemical features of PCOS.

Keywords: Rutin, Letrozole, Polycystic ovary syndrome, Oxidative stress

Background

Polycystic ovary syndrome (PCOS) is the most prevalent endocrinopathy in women of reproductive age. PCOS are distinguished by hyperandrogenism showing symptoms of hirsutism, acne, androgenic alopecia; irregularities of menstrual cycle such as polymenorrhea, oestrogen-replete amenorrhoea, metrorrhagia and oligomenorrhea, dyslipidemia, insulin resistance, chronic anovulation, hormonal imbalances and reduced fertility [1–4].

Various metabolic and clinical complications are associated with PCOS such as impaired glucose tolerance and diabetes, extensive coronary artery disease, hypertension, chronic oligo-ovulation, anovulation, infertility, endometrial, ovarian and breast cancers [5–11].

PCOS patients usually have a high oxidative profile which causes disturbance in antioxidants balance, leading to harmful effects of reactive oxygen species (ROS)

* Correspondence: ruhail12345@yahoo.com
[1]Reproductive Physiology Laboratory, Department Of Animal Sciences, Quaid-i-Azam University, Islamabad, Pakistan
[2]Department of Community Health Sciences, College of Applied Medical Sciences, King Saud University, Riyadh, Saudi Arabia
Full list of author information is available at the end of the article

including infertility, endometriosis, abortion, birth defects, preeclampsia, injury to ovarian epithelium's DNA, excessive apoptosis and alteration in cell signalling process [12, 13].

Letrozole, known as Femara, inhibits the cytochrome P450 enzyme, aromatase, by the catalytic action of which estrogen is synthesized by the androgens. The absence of aromatase enzyme causes disturbance in the steroidogenesis, thus causing increase in the production of androgens developing PCOS [14].

Metformin is commonly known as Glucophage and it belongs to the biguanide class of drugs. It has the chemical formula of $C_4H_{11}N_5$ and molecular weight of 129.1636 g/mol. Metformin suppresses the process of gluconeogenesis and results in the decrease in blood sugar levels, reduce body weight and may improve the *fibrinolysis* activity, lipid profile, insulin sensitivity and glucose uptake and utilization in peripheral tissues of skeletal muscle and adipocytes [15]. Metformin is also a best drug for PCOS treatment [16].

Flavonoids were chosen as a drug of choice for the cure of antiandrogenic, hyperlipidemic, hyperglycemic and oxidative stress consequences of PCOS. Flavonoids show a variety of biological actions including antimicrobial, antiviral, antiulcerogenic, cytotoxic, antineoplastic, anti-inflammatory, antioxidant, antihypertensive, hepatoprotective, hypolipidemic and antiplatelet activities [17].

The natural rutin (3′,4′,5,7-tetrahydroxyflavone-3-rutinoside) is one of the important phytochemicals. Rutin is a bioflavonoid which is necessary for the absorption of vitamin C and acts as an anti-oxidizer [18]. Rutin has a noteworthy range of scavenging characteristics on oxidizing species such as hydroxy radical, superoxide radical, and peroxyl radical by donating hydrogen atoms to peroxy radicals, superoxide anions, and singlet oxygen and hydroxyl radicals, it also functions as a terminator and chelator of metal ions that are able of oxidizing lipid peroxidation [19–21].

In this study, PCOS was induced by the use of aromatase inhibitor, letrozole, in the rodent model. Rutin was selected to be used as a therapy against polycystic ovary syndrome in the present study. Its comparative effects with metformin were assessed and it is anticipated to recover the complications caused due to PCOS.

The present study was designed to scrutinize whether rutin is effective in treating the endocrine, oxidative and reproductive dysfunctions in letrozole induced PCOS and to assess the prognostic power of this flavonoid in improving the clinical and biochemical features of PCOS.

Methods
Experimental animals
Six weeks old female Sprague-Dawley rats (*Rattus norvegicus*), having weight of about 155 ± 10 g and exhibiting normal estrous cycle of 6 days were taken from Animal house of Quaid-i-Azam University, Islamabad. Animals were supplied with pellets of feed and drinking water *ad libitum* and maintained in controlled experimental conditions in stainless steel cages. They were subjected to a 12:12 h light/dark cycles (relative humidity 60–65%) with room temperature of about 20 ± 5 °C for a period of 36 days. Animal handling, treatments and scarification was approved by the ethical committee of Department of Animal Sciences Quaid-i-Azam University, Islamabad.

PCOS was induced by oral administration of aromatase inhibitor, letrozole (1 mg/kg) dissolved in 0.5% CMC (2 mg/kg) for 21 days. This dose was selected using the previous studies of Kafali et al. [22] and Rezvanfar et al. [23]. During the experiment, the estrous cycle phases were monitored by the analyses of relative proportion of leukocytes, epithelial and cornified cells. All rats were randomly divided into following five groups consisting of five rats in each group: (i) control group (CMC; 2 mg/kg/day, p.o.), (ii) PCOS group (letrozole; 01 mg/kg/day, p.o.), (iii) Metformin group (metformin; 2 mg/100 g/day, p.o.), (iv) Rutin-I group (rutin; 100 mg/kg/day, p.o.), and (v) Rutin-II group (rutin; 150 mg/kg/day, p.o.). Letrozole and CMC were administered for 36 days while metformin and the two rutin doses were administered from day 21 to the day 36 of the experiment.

Rats were sacrificed on 37th day, 24 h later the termination of the experiment. Blood was collected from the aorta of the rats under anesthesia in heparinized syringes and kept at -20 °C. It was then centrifuged at 3000 rpm for 15 min. Blood plasma was separated for biochemical and hormonal analysis and ovaries were taken out for histopathological and antioxidant assessments.

Assessment of experimentally induced PCOS
Anthropometrical parameters
Changes in body weight were recorded every week in control, PCOS, metformin and rutin treated groups throughout the experiment.

Weight gain, body length, body mass index (BMI), the abdominal circumference to thoracic circumference (AC/TC) ratio, Lee index and specific rate of body mass gain were determined during the day of dissection using standard measurement methods.

Ovarian weight, diameter and ovarian organ index were also evaluated using usual measurement procedures. From the first day of study until termination, every morning colypocytological examination was performed to check estrous cyclicity in rats.

Biochemical analysis
The concentration of blood glucose was evaluated on day 1, 21 and 36 of experiment using Accu Chek glucometer.

Antioxidant enzymes and protein levels were estimated in ovarian tissue of control and treated animals.

ROS value was determined using the protocol used by Hayashi et al. [24]. Catalase (CAT), Guaiacol peroxidase (POD) levels were analyzed as described in Chance and Maehly [25] with some modifications. Superoxide dismutase (SOD) was assessed by the protocol adopted by Kakkar et al. [26] and Thiobarbituric reactive acid substances (TBARS) levels were measured using Wright et al. [27] method. Gluthathione reductase (GSR); Carlberg & Mannervik [28], Glutathione-S-transferase (GST); Habig et al. [29], reduced Glutathione (GSH); Tietze et al. [30], Glutathione peroxidase (GSH-px); Mohandas et al. [31] and lipid hydroperoxide (LOOH) levels were measured using standard protocols used by (Jiang et al. [32]) on Smart Spec TM plus spectrophotometer.

Total cholesterol (TC), Triglycerides (TG), High-density lipoprotein (HDL-C), total protein and CRP were analyzed using commercially available kits of AMP diagnostics AMEDA Labordiagnostik GmbH, Austria. All the procedures were carried out using the manufacturer's instructions.

Very low-density lipoprotein cholesterol (VLDL-C) and low density lipoprotein cholesterol (LDL-C) were calculated using Friedewald's formula. Non-HDL cholesterol (non-HDL-C) was calculated as the difference between TC and HDL-C while TC/HDL, TG/HDL and LDL/HDL were also assessed.

Hormonal analysis

Serum total testosterone, progesterone and estradiol were evaluated using commercially available ELISA kits of Microlisa AMGENIX Int, Inc. USA. All the procedures were carried out using manual instructions.

Histopathological analysis

The ovaries were processed for paraffin embedding, sectioned at 7 μm, stained with hematoxylin and eosin, and observed under microscope at 100 × s magnification. All the ovarian follicles were examined depending upon their granulosa and morphology. The presence or absence of corpus luteum and thickness of peripheral theca and granulosa layer were also observed.

Statistical analysis

Data were represented as Mean ± Standard Error of Mean (SEM). Graph Pad PRISM 5 (San Diego, CA, USA) was used to describe the results statistically. Comparison of mean was done by using one-way analysis of variance (ANOVA), followed by Tukey test.

Results

Effect of metformin and rutin on anthropometrical parameters

Administartion of letrozole to female rats for 36 days resulted in a significant increase in final body weights of PCOS group as compared to control ($P < 0.05$), however all the other anthropometrical parameters including weight gain, AC, TC, AC/TC ratio, BMI, Lee index and specific rate of body mass gain remained non-significant among rats in the various groups. Body length showed a significant increase in the PCOS group as compared to control group ($P < 0.05$) (Table 1).

Effect of metformin and rutin on colpocytological examination

Administration of letrozole to rats for 36 days caused disturbance of normal estrous cycle starting from day 17th till the end, in the PCOS group, resulting into a profuse vaginal secretion. Mainly diestrus stage remained dominant in it, exhibiting irregularity of the estrous cycle as compared to control group. In rats treated with metformin, rutin (100 mg/kg) and rutin (150 mg/kg), the normal

Table 1 Effect of Rutin-I (100 mg/kg) and Rutin-II (150 mg/kg) on anthropometrical parameters in Letrozole induced PCOS rats after 36 days of experiment

Parameters	Control	PCOS	Metformin	Rutin-I	Rutin-II
Weight gain (g)	25.20 ± 3.32	62.00 ± 10.61	46.20 ± 8.73	52.40 ± 5.16	36.01 ± 15.72
AC	14.78 ± 0.42	15.82 ± 0.27	15.74 ± 0.29	15.2 ± 0.34	15.02 ± 0.29
TC	13.86 ± 0.27	14.94 ± 0.18	14.78 ± 0.29	14.92 ± 0.18	14.36 ± 0.15
AC/TC ratio	1.06 ± 0.02	1.05 ± 0.01	1.06 ± 0.01	1.01 ± 0.01	1.04 ± 0.02
Body Length (cm)	19.24 ± 0.35	20.62 ± 0.36[a]*	20.42 ± 0.29	20.50 ± 0.27	20.12 ± 0.28
Body mass Index (g/cm^2)	0.491 ± 0.016	0.545 ± 0.023	0.477 ± 0.018	0.522 ± 0.025	0.493 ± 0.029
Lee Index	0.294 ± 0.004	0.292 ± 0.006	0.288 ± 0.003	0.293 ± 0.005	0.287 ± 0.004
Specific Rate of Body mass gain (g/kg)	4.343 ± 0.945	27.760 ± 8.616	16.211 ± 5.041	26.660 ± 5.475	16.170 ± 9.213

AC/TC, abdominal circumference to thoracic circumference; PCOS, polycystic ovary sundrome
Values are expressed as Mean ± SEM
*p< 0.05
[a]Value vs control

Table 2 Effect of Rutin-I (100 mg/kg) and Rutin-II (150 mg/kg) on weights, diameter and ovarian organ index of ovaries in Letrozole induced PCOS rats after 36 days of experiment

Groups (n=5)	Control	PCOS	Metformin	Rutin-I	Rutin-II
Weight of left ovary (mg)	57.03 ± 3.23	66.67 ± 4.53	57.67 ± 5.08	66.33 ± 2.54	61.44 ± 4.23
Weight of right ovary (mg)	56.01 ± 2.44	65.25 ± 5.09	59.20 ± 4.01	64.03 ± 6.78	60.41 ± 3.72
Diameter of right ovary (mm)	4.80 ± 0.37	5.10 ± 0.24	4.60 ± 0.24	5.00 ± 0.31	4.80 ± 0.20
Diameter of left ovary (mm)	5.00 ± 0.44	5.60 ± 0.24	5.20 ± 0.20	5.50 ± 0.22	5.30 ± 0.20
Ovary organ index	0.31 ± 0.01	0.29 ± 0.02	0.28 ± 0.01	0.29 ± 0.01	0.31 ± 0.02

Values are expressed as Mean±SEM

estrous cycle depicted a restoration of regular phases when compared with control and PCOS groups.

Effect of metformin and rutin on weights of ovaries

There was no significant difference noted in weights, diameter and ovarian organ index among the different groups (Table 2).

Effect of metformin and rutin on glucose concentration

On the initial day of experiment blood glucose levels were measured. Mean ± SEM is given in Table 3. There was no major change in the mean values among the groups on the initiation of PCOS induction. On day 21, before the start of post treatment, glucose levels were again measured. PCOS and metformin group depicted significant increase ($P < 0.001$) when compared with control group, whereas, rutin–I and rutin–II groups illustrated significant increase ($P < 0.05$) as compared to control group. On the termination of experiment i.e., on day 36, highly significant increase ($P < 0.001$) in glucose concentration was noticed in PCOS group as compared to control group. On contrary to this, the metformin, rutin-I (100 mg/kg) and rutin-II (150 mg/kg) post treated groups showed highly significant decrease ($P < 0.001$) when compared with PCOS group.

Effect of metformin and rutin on total protein and C reactive protein

In PCOS group, the total protein values increased significantly as compared with the control group ($P < 0.05$) while they were significantly reduced in the rutin-II group ($P < 0.05$) when compared with PCOS group.

The values of C-reactive protein (CRP) increased significantly ($P < 0.05$) in the PCOS group when compared with the control group. None of the other groups i.e., metformin, rutin-I (100 mg/kg) and rutin-II (150 mg/kg) exhibited any significant change in the CRP values when compared with control, PCOS and among themselves (Table 4).

Effect of metformin and rutin on ROS

The value of ROS in PCOS group increased significantly as compared to that of control group ($P < 0.05$) but the change was not significant when taken into comparison with metformin and rutin groups. The values of metformin, rutin-I and rutin-II groups varied significantly as compared with that of the PCOS group ($P < 0.05$). But there was non-significant change in metformin, rutin-I and rutin-II groups as compared with that of the control group and also among each other (Table 5).

Effect of metformin and rutin on antioxidant profile

The results regarding the protective effects of rutin against PCOS in rat ovaries and activities of antioxidant enzymes such as CAT, POD, SOD, TBARS, LOOH, GSH-Px, GSR, GSH and GST are shown in Table 5. Activities of antioxidant enzymes such as CAT, POD, SOD, GSR, GST, GSH and GSH-Px were significantly reduced in PCOS group as compared to control group. This reduction in enzymes activity was reversed non significantly by the treatment of metformin while significant increase was seen in the values of SOD, GSR and GSH ($P < 0.05$). Rutin (100 mg/kg) did not show any significant difference ($P < 0.05$) among various groups except the significant increase in the SOD and GSH value as

Table 3 Effect of Rutin-I (100 mg/kg) and Rutin-II (150 mg/kg) on glucose levels measured on day 1, 21 and 36 of experiment in Letrozole induced PCOS rats

Glucose levels (mg/dL)	Control	PCOS	Metformin	Rutin-I	Rutin-II
Day 1	74.21 ± 1.93	73.23 ± 2.81	73.40 ± 3.29	73.01 ± 2.98	72.61 ± 2.42
Day 21	79.22 ± 3.21	95.61 ± 3.18[a]**	95.83 ± 1.93[a]**	93.21 ± 3.30[a]*	92.80 ± 2.72[a]*
Day 36	79.20 ± 3.11	96.44 ± 2.00[a]***	77.21 ± 1.90[b]***	79.80 ± 1.01[b]***	76.40 ± 1.60[b]***

Values are expressed as Mean ± SEM
*=$p< 0.05$, **=$p< 0.01$, ***=$p< 0.001$
[a]Value vs control, [b]Value vs PCOS

Table 4 Effect of Rutin-I (100 mg/kg) and Rutin-II (150 mg/kg) on total protein and CRP concentration in Letrozole induced PCOS rats after 36 days of experiment

Protein values	Control	PCOS	Metformin	Rutin-I	Rutin-II
Total Protein (mg/g of tissue)	25.371 ± 1.852	40.242 ± 1.771[a*]	25.491 ± 2.423[b*]	26.701 ± 6.264	25.342 ± 2.944[b*]
CRP (mg/dL)	0.051 ± 0.004	0.069 ± 0.001[a*]	0.060 ± 0.006	0.062 ± 0.002	0.059 ± 0.004

Values are expressed as Mean ± SEM
*$p< 0.05$
[a]Value vs control
[b]Value vs PCOs

compared to the PCOS group. Alteration in the ovarian enzyme activities with the treatment of Rutin (150 mg/kg) showed statistically significant increase ($P < 0.05$) as compared to PCOS group.

Letrozole increased the TBARS ($P < 0.01$) and LOOH ($P < 0.05$) levels significantly in PCOS as compared to control. Metformin did not show any significance while rutin (100 mg/kg), rutin (150 mg/kg) treatment exhibited significant decrease ($P < 0.05$) in both antioxidants.

Effect of metformin and rutin on serum testosterone, progesterone and estradiol values
Administration of letrozole to female rats for 36 days resulted in a highly significant increase in the serum testosterone as compared with the control ($P < 0.001$) while the metformin, rutin-I (100 mg/kg) and rutin-II (150 mg/kg) exhibited a moderately significant decrease ($P < 0.01$) in comparison with the PCOS group but remained non-significant when compared with the control group. There was no significant difference in the values of estradiol among rats of all the groups. Letrozole administration resulted in a very significant decrease ($P < 0.01$) in the progesterone value in the PCOS group when compared with the control group (Table 6).

Effect of metformin and rutin on lipid profile
Administration of letrozole (1 mg/kg) to female rats for 36 days resulted in a significant increase in serum TG, VLDL-C, LDL-C and non-HDL-C, whereas HDL-C was significantly decreased when compared with vehicle control ($P < 0.05$). Metformin significantly reduced TC ($P < 0.05$), LDL-C and non-HDL-C ($P < 0.01$). Rutin-I (100 mg/kg) treatment caused significant reduction in TC and non-HDL ($P < 0.05$). While rutin-II (150 mg/kg) significantly lowered TC, TG, VLDL-C, LDL-C and non-HDL-C but did not affect the level of HDL-C (Table 7).

Effect of metformin and rutin on histopathology of ovary
The histological changes studied were as follows: (Fig. 1).

The diameter of developing follicles
The diameter of developing follicles (D20 μm –D > 600 μm) did not depict any significant difference among the various groups.

Number of cystic and atretic follicles
The number of cystic and atretic follicles were increased significantly ($P < 0.001$) in the PCOS group as compared with the control group. Metformin, rutin (100 mg/kg)

Table 5 Effect of Rutin-I (100 mg/kg) and Rutin-II (150 mg/kg) on ROS, TBARS, LOOH, CAT, POD, SOD, GSR, GST, GSH, GSH-px concentrations in Letrozole induced PCOS rats after 36 days of experiment

Parameters	Control	PCOS	Metformin	Rutin-I	Rutin-II
ROS (U/min)	0.20 ± 0.04	0.39 ± 0.09[a*]	0.17 ± 0.02[b*]	0.19 ± 0.02[b*]	0.16 ± 0.01[b*]
TBARS (nmol/min/mg)	5.69 ± 1.07	16.06 ± 1.25[a**]	10.78 ± 1.07	8.93 ± 2.45[b*]	8.15 ± 0.82[b*]
LOOH (nmol/min/mg)	3.29 ± 0.48	5.39 ± 0.29[a*]	3.44 ± 0.47	3.59 ± 0.63	3.23 ± 0.42[b*]
CAT(U/min)	4.93 ± 0.08	3.49 ± 0.33[a*]	4.15 ± 0.47	4.22 ± 0.28	4.49 ± 0.38
POD(nmole)	12.09 ± 0.72	9.29 ± 0.01[a*]	10.44 ± 0.62	10.11 ± 0.58	11.87 ± 0.59[b*]
SOD (U/min)	5.81 ± 0.24	2.74 ± 0.29[a*]	5.51 ± 0.51[b*]	5.41 ± 1.08[b*]	5.72 ± 0.51[b*]
GSR (U/mol/mg)	3.96 ± 0.38	1.79 ± 0.09[a*]	3.89 ± 0.29[b*]	3.46 ± 0.71	4.67 ± 0.52[b*]
GST (U/mol/mg)	10.85 ± 0.21	8.02 ± 0.83[a**]	9.47 ± 0.28	9.37 ± 0.48	10.91 ± 0.22[b*]
GSH (U/mol/mg)	6.91 ± 0.50	4.97 ± 0.14[a**]	6.55 ± 0.48[b*]	6.39 ± 0.02[b*]	6.77 ± 0.88[b**]
GSH-px (U/mol/mg)	29.87 ± 2.14	20.35 ± 0.64[a**]	25.34 ± 2.11	24.24 ± 1.76	30.10 ± 1.29[b**]

Values are expressed as Mean ± SEM
*$=p< 0.05$, **$=p< 0.01$
[a]Value vs control, [b]Value vs PCOS

Table 6 Effect of Rutin-I (100 mg/kg) and Rutin-II (150 mg/kg) on serum testosterone, estradioland progesterone concentrations in Letrozole induced PCOS rats after 36 days of experiment

Hormonal concentrations	Control	PCOS	Metformin	Rutin-I	Rutin-II
Testosterone (ng/ml)	1.88 ± 0.71	10.19 ± 0.76[a***]	4.51 ± 0.30 [b**]	5.77 ± 0.68[b*]	8.21 ± 1.85[a**]
Estradiol (ng/ml)	19.41 ± 2.21	14.26 ± 2.70	28.57 ± 4.32	34.83 ± 8.26	27.25 ± 0.48
Progesterone (pg/ml)	43.43 ± 8.81	12.76 ± 3.75[a**]	22.98 ± 4.85	19.66 ± 5.34[a*]	24.63 ± 3.46

Values are expressed as Mean ± SEM
*=p< 0.05, **=p< 0.01, ***=p< 0.001
[a]Value vs control, [b]Value vs PCOS

and rutin (150 mg/kg) significantly reduced the number of cystic follicles ($P < 0.001$) and atretic follicles ($P < 0.05$) as compared to PCOS group (Table 8).

Number of corpus luteum
The number of corpus luteum was significantly decreased in the PCOS group as compared to control ($P < 0.001$) whereas significant recovery was shown in the metformin, rutin-I and rutin-II groups ($P < 0.05$) (Table 8).

Thickness of peripheral thecal and granulosa layer in normal and cystic follicles
The thickness of peripheral thecal layer (D200 μm -D > 600 μm) remained non-significant in the normal follicles among the various groups but its thickness increased significantly ($P < 0.001$) in the PCOS group when compared with control group. The thickness was restored significantly ($P < 0.001$) in metformin and rutin post treated groups when compared with PCOS group.

PCOS group showed highly significant ($P < 0.001$) reduction in peripheral granulosa thickness in follicles when compared with control group whereas in cystic follicles width of granulose layer increased non-significantly in metformin, rutin-I and rutin-II group as compare to PCOS group (Table 9).

Discussion
Letrozole, an aromatase inhibitor, was used to induce PCOS in the rats. Subsequently the increased weights of rats and irregular estrous cycle in the positive control substantiated the induction of PCOS and also signified that the rat model is anoestrous, as it imitated anovulatory characteristic [33]. Treatment of PCOS induced rats with flavonoid rutin possibly restored the estrous cyclicity in rats. The rutin treated groups, however, did not depict any significant increase in body weight which suggested that rutin might have reduced the expression levels of adipogenic genes thus reducing the weight of adipose tissues [34].

Surprisingly, the ovarian weights, ovarian diameter and ovarian organ index displayed no significant increase. The non-significant anthropometrical results might be due to the fast metabolic response of the animals, suggesting that other genetic or environmental factors or longer time of exposure to aromatase inhibitor was necessary to achieve the full spectrum of ovarian pathology.

The glucose levels increased significantly when measured in the PCOS group during the day 21 and 36 of the experiment. Letrozole seems to create a disturbance in the hormonal profile of the animals mainly because of increased androgen levels. This increased androgen levels in turn induced insulin resistance hence creating a decreased glucose tolerance [35]. Meanwhile, metformin

Table 7 Effect of Rutin-I (100 mg/kg) and Rutin-II (150 mg/kg) on total cholesterol, triglycerides, HDL- C, LDL-C, VLDL-C, Non-HDL-C, TC/HDL, TG/HDL and LDL/HDL concentrations in Letrozole induced PCOS rats after 36 days of experiment

Parameters	Control	PCOS	Metformin	Rutin-I	Rutin-II
Total Cholesterol(mg/dL)	215.60 ± 3.43	231.10 ± 4.27	211.30 ± 6.81[b*]	212.21 ± 1.53[b*]	207.10 ± 2.24[b**]
Triglycerides (mg/dL)	185.11 ± 4.23	213.10 ± 5.16[a*]	197.40 ± 5.82	199.20 ± 6.93	186.12 ± 4.62[b*]
HDL-C (mg/dL)	160.70 ± 4.17	144.41 ± 3.63[a*]	153.21 ± 1.80	146.43 ± 4.52	159.80 ± 3.14[b*]
LDL-C (mg/dL)	17.83 ± 3.98	42.99 ± 1.99[a***]	18.58 ± 7.22[b**]	25.81 ± 5.11	10.05 ± 2.29[b***]
VLDL-C (mg/dL)	37.03 ± 0.85	42.61 ± 1.03[a*]	39.49 ± 1.16	39.83 ± 1.39	37.20 ± 0.92[b*]
Non-HDL-C(mg/dL)	54.86 ± 4.48	85.61 ± 1.50[a**]	58.07 ± 7.32[b**]	65.65 ± 4.75[b*]	47.24 ± 2.64[b***]
TC/HDL	1.34 ± 0.03	1.59 ± 0.02[a***]	1.38 ± 0.05[b**]	1.45 ± 0.04	1.29 ± 0.02[b***c*]
TG/HDL	1.16 ± 0.04	1.48 ± 0.06[a**]	1.29 ± 0.03	1.37 ± 0.06	1.17 ± 0.04[b**]
LDL/HDL	0.11 ± 0.03	0.29 ± 0.01[a**]	0.12 ± 0.05[b**]	0.18 ± 0.04	0.06 ± 0.02[b***]

Values are expressed as Mean ± SEM
* = p < 0.05, ** = p < 0.01, *** = p < 0.001
[a] Value vs control, [b] Value vs PCOS, [c] Value vs Metformin

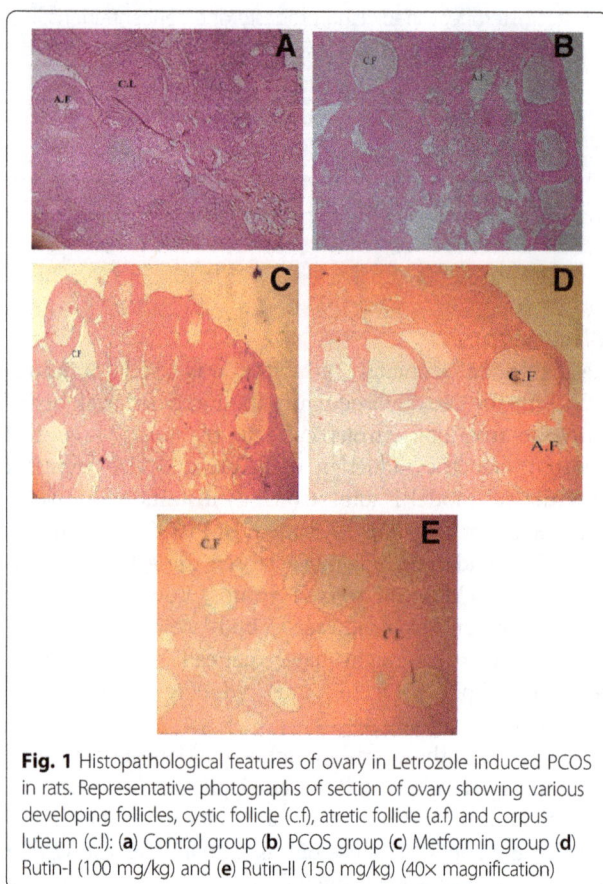

Fig. 1 Histopathological features of ovary in Letrozole induced PCOS in rats. Representative photographs of section of ovary showing various developing follicles, cystic follicle (c.f), atretic follicle (a.f) and corpus luteum (c.l): (**a**) Control group (**b**) PCOS group (**c**) Metformin group (**d**) Rutin-I (100 mg/kg) and (**e**) Rutin-II (150 mg/kg) (40× magnification)

Table 9 Effect of Rutin-I (100 mg/kg) and Rutin-II (150 mg/kg) on thickness of thecal layer and peripheral granulosa layer in Letrozole induced PCOS rats after 36 days of experiment

Thickness (μm) Rutin I	Control Rutin II	PCOS	Metformin
Thecal Layer	–	27.56±2.10	21.25±3.09
18.11±1.28^{a***}	16.78±1.25^{a***}		
Granulosa Layer	–	22.00±2.55	30.00±2.73
26.00±2.91	25.00±3.16		

Values are expressed as Mean ± SEM
***=$p<0.001$
^{a}Value vs PCOS

thus inducing the insulin signalling pathway, and consequently causing increased glucose transporter 4 translocation and increased glucose uptake [38].

The total protein index increased significantly in the PCOS group. This abnormal level of total protein might suggest infectious and chronic inflammation in the PCOS group which might be due to the abnormal androgen secretions. However, metformin significantly lowered the amount of total protein as compared with the positive vehicle group. The improved sensitivity of proteins and protein hormones after the metformin therapy down regulate the increased circulating levels of protein in the blood [39]. Rutin flavonoid significantly decreased the total protein level by inhibiting the eicosanoids and cytokines due to its pharmacologic actions [40]. The C- reactive protein (CRP) is an acute phase protein and a very expedient indicator of inflammation in a tissue. In present study, the CRP levels increased significantly in the PCOS group thus exhibiting severe infection [41].

Elevated testosterone levels in PCOS most probably reflect build-up of androgens because conversion of androgen substrates into estrogens was blocked by aromatase inhibitor. The decrease in testosterone concentration in metformin group reflect diminished androgen biosynthesis by the ovary [42]. The diminution of estrogen production by aromatase inhibition can cause enhanced secretion of LH in hypothalamus and pituitary most likely by negative feedback of estrogens.

Oxidative stress is generally regarded as the phenomena where the generation of reactive oxygen species

reduced the glucose levels significantly as compared to PCOS group. This may be due to the fact that metformin treatment decreased the glucose resistance by maintaining the glucose homeostasis and also by improving the insulin-mediated uptake of glucose [35, 36]. Rutin flavonoid significantly reduces the glucose values in the treated groups as compared with PCOS group because of its antihyperglycemic effect and caused a decrease in the glycaemic levels by conceivably playing its role as potentiating the insulin secretion by the β-cells of Islets of Langerhans thus promoting a balanced uptake of glucose by the cells [37]. It also suggested that rutin might be a potential agent for glycaemic control through enhancement of insulin-dependent receptor kinase activity,

Table 8 Effect of Rutin-I (100 mg/kg) and Rutin-II (150 mg/kg) on number of cystic follicles, atretic follicles and corpus luteum in Letrozole induced PCOS rats after 36 days of experiment

Number of follicles	Control	PCOS	Metformin	Rutin-I	Rutin-II
Cystic follicles	0.0 ± 0.0	10.17 ± 0.70^{a***}	5.16 ± 0.30^{a***b***}	6.16 ± 0.47 ^{a***b***}	7.33 ± 0.42^{a***b**c*}
Atreticfollicles	2.00 ± 0.25	4.50 ± 0.34^{a***}	2.83 ± 0.47^{b*}	2.66 ± 0.33^{b*}	2.83 ± 0.40^{b*}
Corpousluteum	6.80 ± 0.37	2.40 ± 0.24^{a***}	4.20 ± 0.58^{a**b*}	2.40 ± 0.50^{a***c*}	4.40 ± 0.24^{a**b*d*}

Values are expressed as Mean ± SEM
*$p<0.05$, **$p<0.01$, ***$p<0.001$
^{a}Value vs control, ^{b}Value vs PCOS, ^{c}Value vs Metformin, ^{d}Value vsRutin-I

(ROS) cause disruption in the normal functionality of biological system. The aerobic cells have a counter mechanism to deal with oxidative stress by trapping the reactive oxygen intermediates but the inequity in terms of the rate of the production of ROS and their protective systems can cause oxidative stress over time. In present study, the ROS level increased significantly in the PCOS group which depicted an increase in the oxidative stress [43]. The increase in ROS level indicates the molecular damage in the cellular structure and the tissue was mainly due to the over production of free oxidative radicals. ROS value was also decreased significantly in the rutin groups, which is due to the antioxidant activity of rutin. The exact mechanism through which rutin induces antioxidative action is not clear but it reduces the causative agents of oxidative stress [44].

Lipid peroxidation is a free-radical mediated promulgation of oxidative offence inserted to polyunsaturated fatty acids involving numerous types of free radicals. The cessation of lipid peroxidation occurs by antioxidants through their enzymatic action or by free radical scavenging activity [45]. The increase in the lipid per hydroxide levels might be due to the termination of antioxidant effect which caused pathogenesis of the disease.

Histopathological observation of ovaries taken from Letrozole treated animals displayed remarkable resemblance to human PCOS, revealing sub capsular cysts lined with a thin layer of granulosa cells and hyperplasia of theca cells [12]. It has been observed that the increased levels of intra-ovarian androgens lead to abnormal follicular growth and an increase in follicular artesia [46, 47]. Number of corpus luteum and different developing follicles measuring in diameter from 20 μm to more than 600 μm also decreased non-significantly in PCOS group. Cystic follicles were much larger in size as compared to other follicles of ovary with a clear antrum but lacked oocyte. Thickness of peripheral granulosa layer was decreased while that of theca layer was increased significantly in different follicles of PCOS group, as compared to control group. Contrary to this, post treated groups exhibited non-significant increase when compared with PCOS group. These histological findings were pinpointing towards the existence of biologically active levels of FSH, increased LH, and lack of interplay between granulosa and theca cells, which would otherwise lead to ovulation, in the PCOS group.

Conclusions

Concluding our work, present study demonstrates antiandrogenic properties of rutin. It showed estrogenic, antiandrogenic and anti hyperglycemic effects and recovered ovarian cysts and its protective properties was seen to be comparable to that of metformin. The restoration of ovarian function and hormonal profile by rutin treatment could be supportive in managing PCOS. Outcomes of the study also revealed that letrozole induced PCOS had an enhanced level of oxidative stress along with hyperglycemia and hyperlipidemia. Oxidative stress in turn damaged the tissue by reactive oxygen species (ROS) and the rutin flavonoid was able to antidote the oxidative stress. Meanwhile, rutin also played an imperative role in reducing the oxidative stress, boosting the antioxidant status, and possibly reducing the ROS and lipid peroxidation. It displayed a significant role in subsiding the hyperlipidemic state and hyperglycemic state and it can be used as a possible ameliorative medication for curing clinical and biochemical characteristics of polycystic ovary syndrome, its properties were analogous to that of standard metformin. Further research is prerequisite to investigate the pharmacologic and therapeutic potentials of rutin so that it can be used as an adjunct therapy sideways to currently used drugs in PCOS management.

Acknowledgements
We acknowledge Higher Education Commission (HEC) of Pakistan for funding. Furthermore we are grateful to the Deanship of Scientific Research at King Saud University for its funding of this research through Research Group Project number 193.

Funding
The project was partially funded by the Higher Education Commission (HEC) of Pakistan. We are grateful to the Deanship of Scientific Research at King Saud University for its funding of this research through Research Group Project number 193.

Authors' contributions
SJ, FM and HZ made significant contributions to conception, design, experimentation, acquisition and interpretation of data and drafting of the manuscript. SR, TA, AA has made substantial contributions to analyzing, and revising the manuscript for intellectual content. SR, GA, AM and QA made a contribution into revising and editing the manuscript. All authors read and approved the final manuscript.

Competing interests
The authors declare that they have no competing interests.

Author details
[1]Reproductive Physiology Laboratory, Department Of Animal Sciences, Quaid-i-Azam University, Islamabad, Pakistan. [2]Department of Community Health Sciences, College of Applied Medical Sciences, King Saud University, Riyadh, Saudi Arabia. [3]Department of Biochemistry, Quaid-i-Azam University, Islamabad, Pakistan.

References
1. Lobo RA, Carmina E. The importance of diagnosing the polycystic ovary syndrome. Ann Intern Med. 2000;132(12):989–93.

2. Goodarzi MO, Dumesic DA, Chazenbalk G, Azziz R. Polycystic ovary syndrome: etiology, pathogenesis and diagnosis. Nat Rev Endocrinol. 2011;7(4):219–31.

3. Pasquali R, Stener-Victorin E, Yildiz BO, Duleba AJ, Hoeger K, Mason H, Homburg R, Hickey T, Franks S, Tapanainen JS. Polycystic ovary syndrome. Clin Endocrinol. 2011;74(4):424–33.

4. Zawadzki J, Dunaif A. PCOS Forum: research in polycystic ovary syndrome today and tomorrow. PCOS. 1992;4:377–84.

5. Sharma A, Atiomo W. Recent developments in polycystic ovary syndrome. Curr Obstet Gynaecol. 2003;13(5):281–6.

6. Rossing MA, Daling JR, Weiss NS, Moore DE, Self SG. Ovarian tumors in a cohort of infertile women. New Engl J Med. 1994;331(12):771–6.

7. Cheung AP. Ultrasound and menstrual history in predicting endometrial hyperplasia in polycystic ovary syndrome. Obstet Gynecol. 2001;98(2):325–31.

8. Cho LW, Jayagopal V, Kilpatrick ES, Atkin SL. The biological variation of C-reactive protein in polycystic ovarian syndrome. Clin Chem. 2005;51(10):1905a–7.

9. Broekmans F, Knauff E, Valkenburg O, Laven J, Eijkemans M, Fauser B. PCOS according to the Rotterdam consensus criteria: change in prevalence among WHO-II anovulation and association with metabolic factors. BJOG. 2006;113(10):1210–7.

10. Barry JA, Azizia MM, Hardiman PJ. Risk of endometrial, ovarian and breast cancer in women with polycystic ovary syndrome: a systematic review and meta-analysis. Hum Reprod Update. 2014;20(5):748–58.

11. Ladrón DGA, Fux-Otta C, Crisosto N, Szafryk DMP, Echiburu B, Iraci G, Perez-Bravo F, Petermann T. Metabolic profile of the different phenotypes of polycystic ovary syndrome in two Latin American populations. Fertil Steril. 2014;101(6):1732–9. e1731-1732.

12. Riley JC, Behrman HR. Oxygen radicals and reactive oxygen species in reproduction. Exp Biol Med. 1991;198(3):781–91.

13. Agarwal A, Gupta S, Sharma RK. Role of oxidative stress in female reproduction. Reprod Biol Endocrinol. 2005;3(1):1.

14. Corbin C, Trant J, Walters K, Conley AJ. Changes in Testosterone Metabolism Associated with the Evolution of Placental and Gonadal Isozymes of Porcine Aromatase Cytochrome P450 1. Endocrinology. 1999;140(11):5202–10.

15. Del Barco S, Vazquez-Martin A, Cufí S, Oliveras-Ferraros C, Bosch-Barrera J, Joven J, Martin-Castillo B, Menendez JA. Metformin: multi-faceted protection against cancer. Oncotarget. 2011;2(12):896–917.

16. Nawrocka J, Starczewski A. Effects of metformin treatment in women with polycystic ovary syndrome depends on insulin resistance. Gynecol Endocrinol. 2007;23(4):231–7.

17. Formica J, Regelson W. Review of the biology of quercetin and related bioflavonoids. Food Chem Toxicol. 1995;33(12):1061–80.

18. Buszewski B, Kawka S, Suprynowicz Z, Wolski T, Pharm J. Simultaneous isolation of rutin and esculin from plant material and drugs using solid-phase extraction. Biomed Anal. 1993;11(3):211–5.

19. Henry F, Danoux L, Pauly G, Charrouf Z. A plant extract and its pharmaceutical and cosmetic use. Patent Applied WO. 2005; 39610.

20. Middleton E, Kandaswami C, Theoharides TC. The effects of plant flavonoids on mammalian cells: implications for inflammation, heart disease, and cancer. Pharmacol Rev. 2000;52(4):673–751.

21. Wang Q, Ogura T, Wang L. Research and development of new products from bitter-buckwheat. Curr AdvBuckwheat Res. 1995;1:873–9.

22. Kafali H, Iriadam M, Ozardalı I, Demir N. Letrozole-induced polycystic ovaries in the rat: a new model for cystic ovarian disease. Arch Med Res. 2004;35(2):103-108.

23. Rezvanfar MA, Ahmadi A, Shojaei-Saadi HA, Baeeri M, Abdollahi M. Molecular mechanisms of a novel selenium-based complementary medicine which confers protection against hyperandrogenism-induced polycystic ovary. Theriogenology. 2012;78(3):620-631.

24. Hayashi I, Morishita Y, Imai K, Nakamura M, Nakachi K, Hayashi T. High-throughput spectrophotometric assay of reactive oxygen species in serum. Mutation Research/Genetic Toxicology and Environmental Mutagenesis. 2007;631(1):55–61.

25. Chance B, Maehly AC. [136] Assay of catalases and peroxidases. Methods in Enzymol. 1955;2:764–775.

26. Kakkar P, Das B, Viswanathan PN. A modified spectrophotometric assay of superoxide. dismutase. Indian J Biochem Biophys. 1984;21(2):130–2.

27. Wright D, Sutherland L. Antioxidant supplemention in the treatment of skeletal muscle insulin resistance: potential mechanisms and clinical relevance. Appl Physiol Nutr Metab. 2008;33(1):21–31.

28. Carlberg I.N.C.E.R. Mannervik B.E.N.G.T. Purification and characterization of the flavoenzyme glutathione reductase from rat liver. J Biol Chem. 1975;250(14):5475–5480.

29. Habig WH, Pabst MJ, Jakoby WB. Glutathione S-transferases the first enzymatic step in mercapturic acid formation. J Biol Chem. 1974;249(22):7130–7139.

30. Tietze F. Enzymic method for quantitative determination of nanogram amounts of total and oxidized glutathione: applications to mammalian blood and other tissues. Anal Biochem. 1969;27(3):502–522.

31. Mohandas J, Marshall JJ, Duggin GG, Horvath JS, Tiller DJ. Differential distribution of glutathione and glutathione-related enzymes in rabbit kidney: possible implications in analgesic nephropathy. Biochem Pharmacol. 1984;33(11):1801–1807.

32. Jiang Z-Y, Woollard AC, Wolff SP. Lipid hydroperoxide measurement by oxidation of Fe2+ in the presence of xylenol orange. Comparison with the TBA assay and an iodometric method. Lipids. 1991;26(10):853-856.

33. Manneras L, Cajander S, Holmang A, Seleskovic Z, Lystig T, Lönn M, Stener-Victorin E. A new rat model exhibiting both ovarian and metabolic characteristics of polycystic ovary syndrome. Endocrinology. 2007;148(8):3781–91.

34. Kim S, Seo S, Lee M-S, Jang E, Shin Y, Oh S, Kim Y. Rutin Reduces Body Weight with an Increase of Muscle Mitochondria Biogenesis and Activation of AMPK in Diet-induced Obese Rats. FASEB J. 2015;29((1 Supplement):595. 594.

35. Desai NR, Shrank WH, Fischer MA, Avorn J, Liberman JN, Schneeweiss S, Pakes J, Brennan TA, Choudhry NK. Patterns of medication initiation in newly diagnosed diabetes mellitus: quality and cost implications. Am J Med. 2012;125(3):302. e301–7.

36. Pai SA, Majumdar AS. J Pharm Pharmacol. Protective effects of melatonin against metabolic and reproductive disturbances in polycystic ovary syndrome in rats. 2014;66(12):1710–21.

37. Kamalakkannan N, Stanely Mainzen Prince P. Antihyperlipidaemic effect of Aegle marmelos fruit extract in streptozotocin-induced diabetes in rats. J Sci Food Agric. 2005;85(4):569–73.

38. Hsu CY, Shih HY, Chia YC, Lee CH, Ashida H, Lai YK, Weng CF. Rutin potentiates insulin receptor kinase to enhance insulin-dependent glucose transporter 4 translocation. Mol Nutr Food Res. 2014;58(6):1168–76.

39. Oktenli C, Ozgurtas T, Dede M, Sanisoglu YS, Yenen MC, Yesilova Z, Kenar L, Kurt YG, Baser I, Smith J. Metformin decreases circulating acylation-stimulating protein levels in polycystic ovary syndrome. Gynecol Endocrinol. 2007;23(12):710–5.

40. Umar S, Mishra NK, Pal K, Sajad M, Ansari MM, Ahmad S, Katiyar CK, Khan HA. Protective effect of rutin in attenuation of collagen-induced arthritis in Wistar rat by inhibiting inflammation and oxidative stress. Indian J Rheumatol. 2012;7(4):191–8.

41. Boulman N, Levy Y, Leiba R, Shachar S, Linn R, Zinder O, Blumenfeld Z. Increased C-reactive protein levels in the polycystic ovary syndrome: a marker of cardiovascular disease. J Clin Endocrinol Metabol. 2004;89(5):2160–5.

42. Attia GR, Rainey WE, Carr BR. Metformin directly inhibits androgen production in human thecal cells. Fertil Steril. 2001;76(3):517–24.

43. Fenkci V, Fenkci S, Yilmazer M, Serteser M. Decreased total antioxidant status and increased oxidative stress in women with polycystic ovary syndrome may contribute to the risk of cardiovascular disease. Fertil Steril. 2003;80(1):123–7.

44. Yang J, Guo J, Yuan J. In vitro antioxidant properties of rutin. LWT-Food Sci Technol. 2008;41(6):1060–6.

45. Korkina LG, Afanas' Ev IB. Advances in pharmacology. 1996;38:151–63.

46. V Mahesh, T Mills, C Bagnell, B Conway. Animal models for study of polycystic ovaries and ovarian atresia. In: Regulation of Ovarian and Testicular Function. edn.: Springer; 1987: 237-257.

47. Homburg R. Androgen circle of polycystic ovary syndrome. Human Reproduction. 2009. doi: 10.1093/humrep/dep049.

19

Circulatory microRNA 23a and microRNA 23b and polycystic ovary syndrome (PCOS): the effects of body mass index and sex hormones in an Eastern Han Chinese population

Weixi Xiong[1,2,3†], Ying Lin[1,2,4†], Lili Xu[1,2,5†], Amin Tamadon[1†], Shien Zou[6], Fubo Tian[6], Ruijin Shao[7], Xin Li[6*] and Yi Feng[1*] (iD)

Abstract

Background: MicroRNAs (miRNAs) regulate the expression of genes involved in various cellular functions related to metabolism, inflammation, and reproduction. This study evaluated the effects of sex hormones and obesity on the expression of circulating miR-23a and miR-23b in women with polycystic ovary syndrome (PCOS) and healthy women.

Methods: Serum sex hormones concentrations and body mass index (BMI) were measured in 18 women with PCOS and in 30 healthy women from the East China area and these measurements were correlated with serum miR-23a/b levels. The effect of miR-23a and miR-23b risk factors on occurrence of PCOS and predisposing factors of PCOS on these miRNA expressions were evaluated.

Results: The expressions of miR-23a/b were significantly lower in the women with PCOS than the normal women, and the expression levels of miR-23a/b were positively correlated with each other in the normal women ($p = 0.001$) but not in the women with PCOS ($p > 0.05$). In the women with PCOS, miR-23a was positively correlated with BMI ($p = 0.03$). However, no correlations were found between the levels of miR-23a/b and the sex hormones in the normal and PCOS women. On the other hand, without considering the presence or absence of PCOS, increase in BMI had a positive effect on the levels of circulating miR-23b; while testosterone had negative effects on the levels of circulating miR-23a. Furthermore, the likelihood of women with PCOS decreased by 0.01-fold for every 1 fold increase of miR-23a expression.

Conclusions: Both reduced levels and discordance between the expressions of miR-23a/b were observed in the women with PCOS and miR-23a/b were affected from testosterone and BMI, reversely. Therefore, miR-23a alteration in contrast with miR-23b is a better indicator for evaluation of PCOS than the miR-23b.

Keywords: microRNAs, miR-23a/b, Obesity, Sex hormones, Polycystic ovary syndrome

* Correspondence: lxsure@fudan.edu.cn; fengyi17@fudan.edu.cn
†Equal contributors
[6]Department of Gynecology, Obstetrics and Gynecology Hospital, Fudan University, Shanghai 200011, China
[1]Department of Integrative Medicine and Neurobiology, State Key Lab of Medical Neurobiology, School of Basic Medical Sciences, Shanghai Medical College; Institute of Acupuncture Research (WHO collaborating center for traditional medicine) and Institute of Brain Science, Brain Science Collaborative Innovation Center, Fudan University, Shanghai 200032, China
Full list of author information is available at the end of the article

Background

Polycystic ovary syndrome (PCOS) is one of the most common reproductive, endocrine, and metabolic disorders in women. It affects about 5 to 10% of women of reproductive age and is usually a lifelong disease. PCOS is characterized by chronic anovulation, hyperandrogenism, and, consequently, infertility [1]. Metabolic disorders, including obesity, insulin resistance, and diabetes, are cofactors as well as predisposing factors of PCOS [2]. Therefore, understanding the molecular mechanisms of the metabolic diseases underlying the pathophysiology of PCOS will help to identify novel diagnostic and therapeutic strategies.

Previously, it was shown that microRNAs (miRNAs) play an important role in follicular development and fertility [3]. The miRNAs are highly conserved, 19 to 25 nucleotide-long, single-stranded RNA molecules that post-transcriptionally regulate gene expression, and they perform their functions by mediating translational repression or by directing the cleavage of target mRNAs. Recent evidence suggests that miRNAs play fundamental roles in all cellular and tissue activities under both normal and pathological conditions, but the currently available information on the expression and function of miRNAs in the ovary, especially in oocyte development, is still very limited. It was discovered, however, that miRNAs might be involved in the turnover of many maternal transcripts whose degradation might be essential for the successful completion of meiotic maturation by oocytes [3].

The analysis of expression of miR-23a and miR-23b in follicular cells from women undergoing assisted reproductive technology (ART) including the patients with tubal factor and endometriosis showed that significant increase in the levels of miR-23b directly correlated with CYP19A1 (aromatase gene) expression, miR-23a, compared to normal women [4]. Aromatase which convert androgens to estrogen has role in pathogenesis of PCOS [5]. Therefore, in the present study, serum samples and other information were collected from women with PCOS and healthy controls to study the correlation between serum miR-23a/b expression, obesity, and sex hormones in women with PCOS.

Results

Expression of miR-23a/b in controls and PCOS patients

The expression of miR-23a and miR-23b was downregulated in the women with PCOS compared to the healthy controls ($C_v = 73.2$, $p = 0.008$, and $C_v = 93.3$, $p = 0.04$, respectively, Fig. 1a and b). Comparison of the healthy women according to the different phases of the endometrial cycle (proliferative, early secretory,

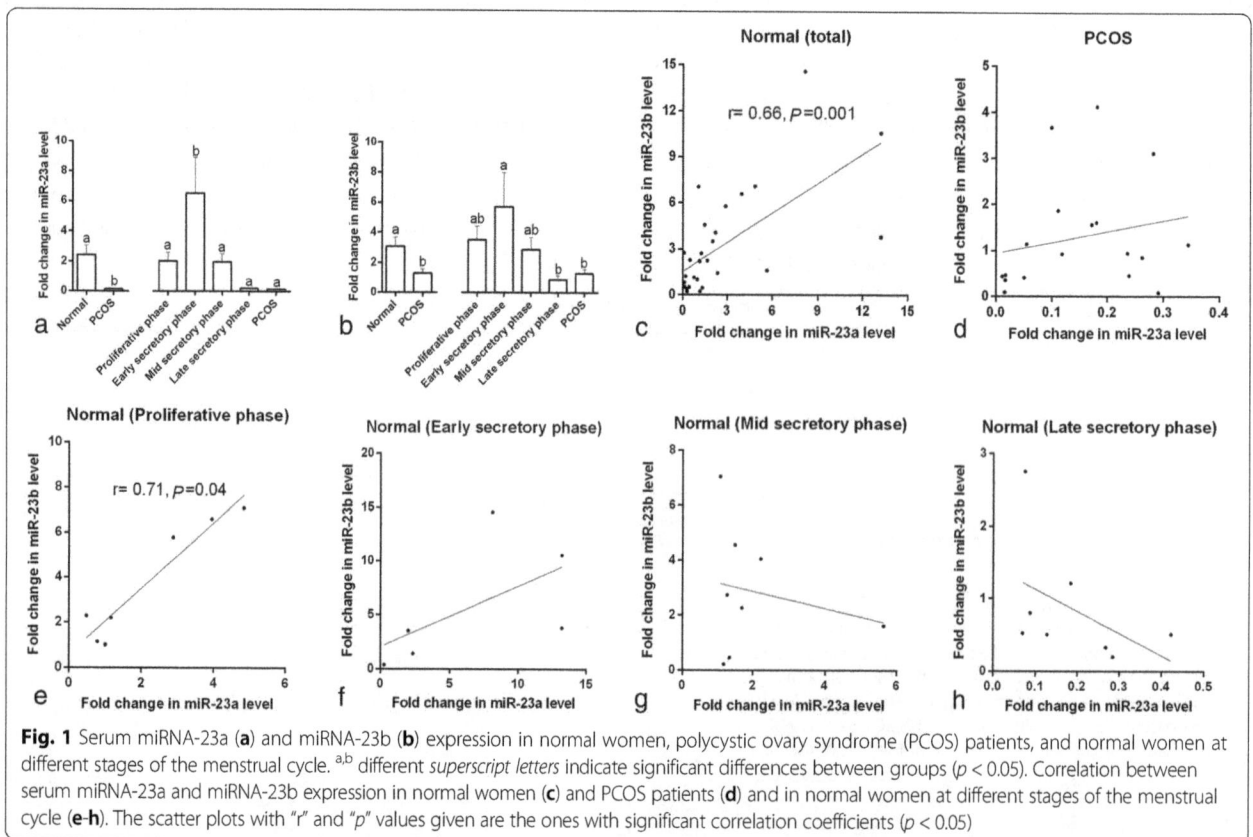

Fig. 1 Serum miRNA-23a (**a**) and miRNA-23b (**b**) expression in normal women, polycystic ovary syndrome (PCOS) patients, and normal women at different stages of the menstrual cycle. [a,b] different *superscript letters* indicate significant differences between groups ($p < 0.05$). Correlation between serum miRNA-23a and miRNA-23b expression in normal women (**c**) and PCOS patients (**d**) and in normal women at different stages of the menstrual cycle (**e-h**). The scatter plots with "r" and "p" values given are the ones with significant correlation coefficients ($p < 0.05$)

mid-secretory, and late secretory) showed that miR-23a and miR-23b reached peak concentrations in the early secretory phase and were at their lowest level in the late secretory phase ($p < 0.05$, Fig. 1a and b). Furthermore, there was a positive correlation between the expression of miR-23a and miR-23b in the serum of the healthy controls and in the subgroup of controls in the proliferative phase ($C_v = 142.4$ and $C_v = 108.9$, respectively, $p < 0.05$, Fig. 1c and e), but there was no significant correlation between the expression of the two miRNAs in the women with PCOS ($r = 0.3$) or in healthy controls in the mid-secretory ($r = -0.1$), early secretory ($r = 0.7$), or late secretory ($r = -0.6$) phases.

Body mass index (BMI) and expression of miR-23a/b in PCOS patients and healthy controls

The BMI in the women with PCOS was higher than in the healthy controls as a group ($C_v = 18.5$ vs. $C_v = 8.4$, respectively; $p = 0.001$) and in the proliferative, early secretory, and late secretory subgroups ($p < 0.05$, Fig. 2a). There was a positive correlation between BMI and the expression of miR-23a in the serum of PCOS patients ($p < 0.05$, Fig. 2l), but no such correlation was seen in any of the healthy controls ($p > 0.05$). On the other hand, BMI and serum miR-23b expression showed significant negative and positive correlations in the

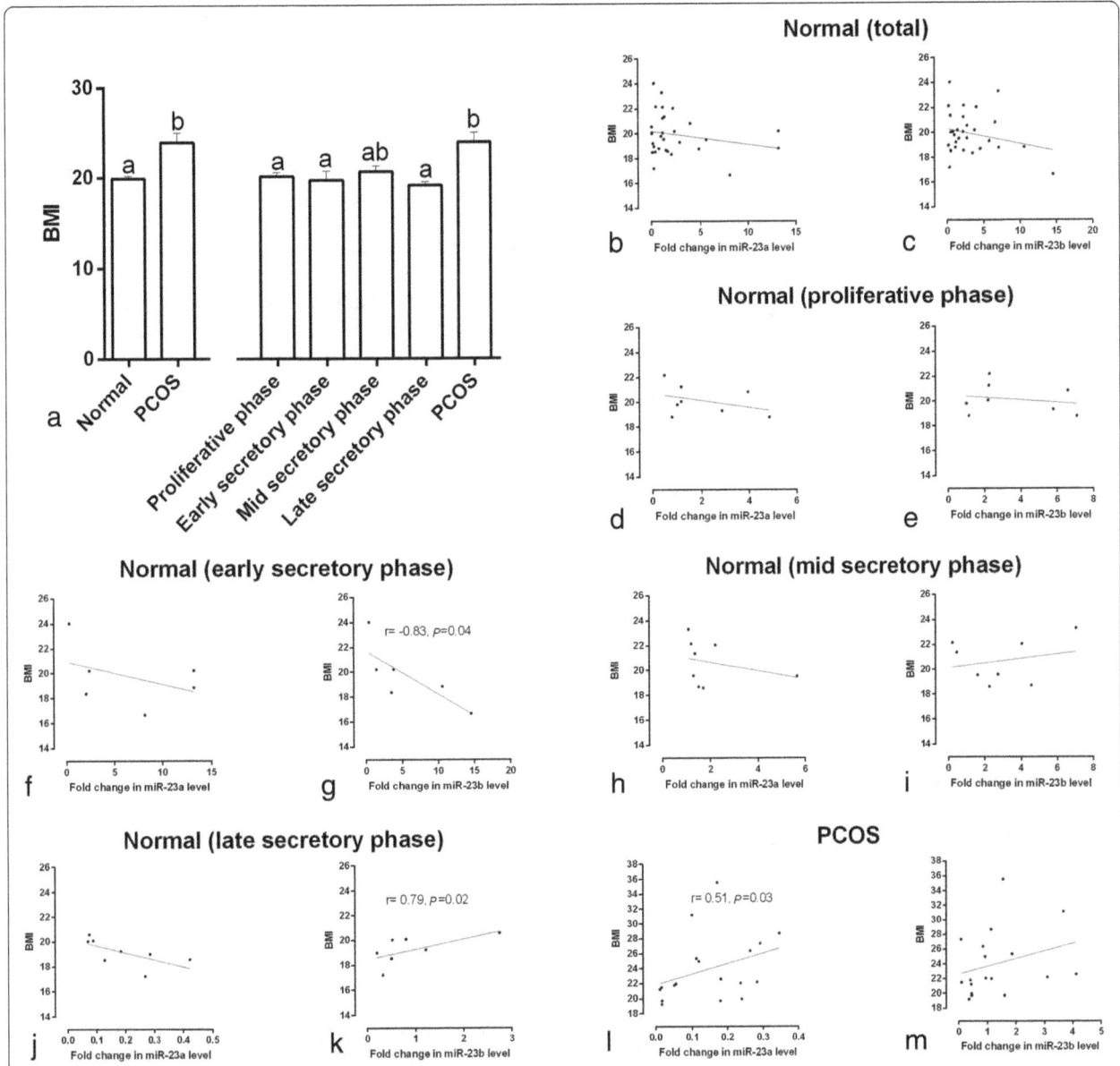

Fig. 2 Body mass index (BMI, kg/m^2) (**a**) in normal women, polycystic ovary syndrome (PCOS) patients, and normal women at different stages of the menstrual cycle. [a,b] different *superscript letters* indicate significant differences between groups ($p < 0.05$). Correlation of serum miRNA-23a and miRNA-23b expression with BMI in normal women (**a** and **b**), normal women at different stages of the menstrual cycle (**c–k**), and PCOS patients (**l** and **m**). The scatter plots with "r" and "p" values given are the ones that had significant correlation coefficients ($p < 0.05$)

early and late secretory phases in normal women, respectively, ($p < 0.05$, Fig. 2g and k), but not in the proliferative or mid-secretory subgroups or in the PCOS patients ($r = 0.4$, $p = 0.09$, Fig. 2m).

Testosterone and expression of miR-23a/b in PCOS patients and healthy controls

The serum testosterone concentrations in the PCOS patients were about four times higher than in the healthy controls ($C_v = 31.6$ vs. $C_v = 46.2$, respectively) and in the four subgroups of healthy controls ($p < 0.001$, Fig. 3a). However, there was no correlation between miR-23a or

miR-23b expression and testosterone concentrations in the serum of the PCOS patients or the healthy controls in any phase of the endometrial cycle ($p > 0.05$, Fig. 3b to m).

P_4 and E_2 and expression of miR-23a/b in healthy controls

Similarly to what has been demonstrated in previous studies, the serum P_4 and E_2 concentrations reached their peak levels in the mid-secretory phase and proliferative phase, respectively ($p < 0.05$, Figs. 4a and 5a), and were at their the lowest concentrations in the proliferative phase and mid-secretory phase, respectively ($p < 0.05$).

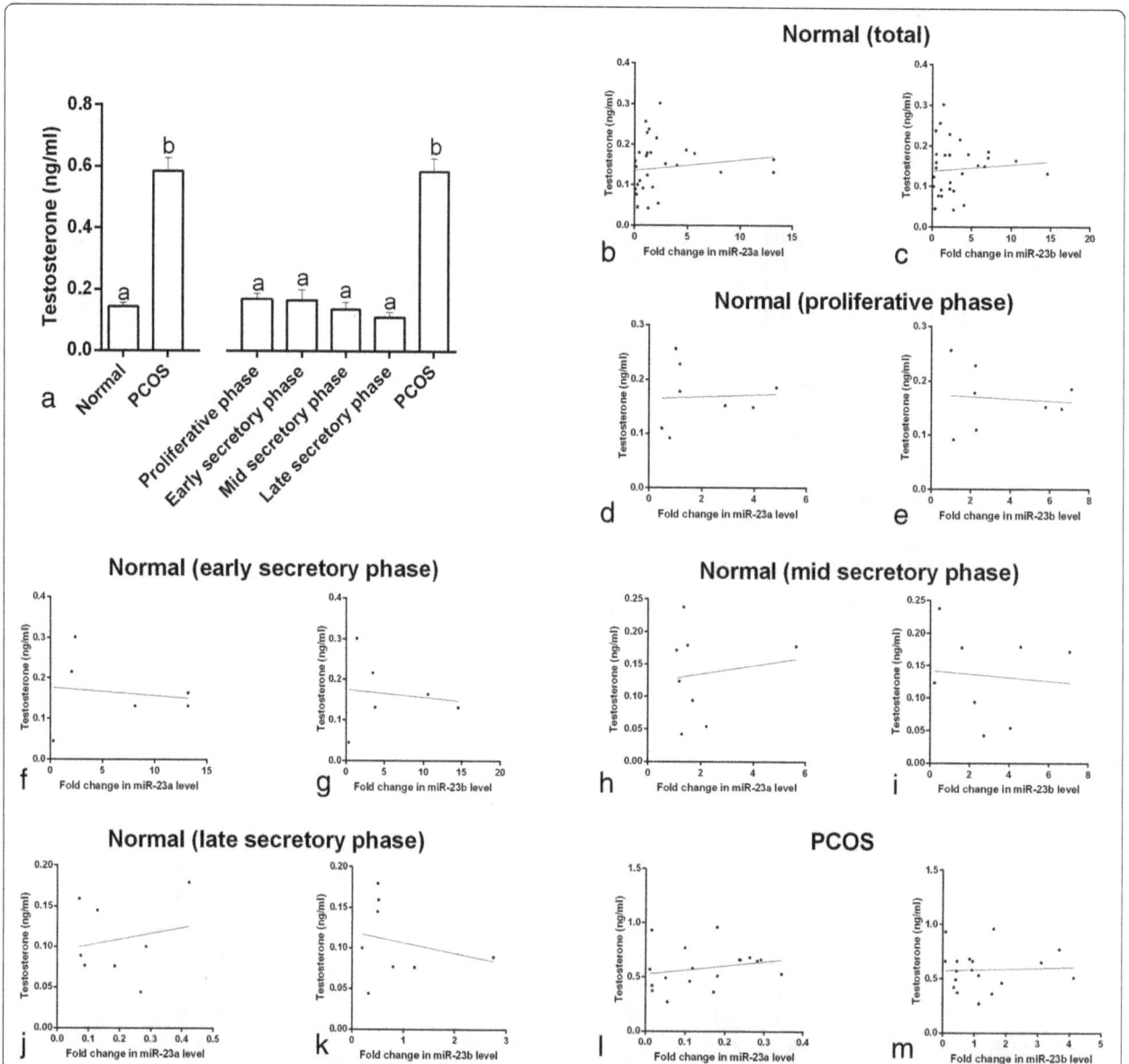

Fig. 3 Serum testosterone concentrations (a) in normal women, polycystic ovary syndrome (PCOS) patients, and normal women at different stages of the menstrual cycle. [a,b] different *superscript letters* indicate significant differences between groups ($p < 0.05$). Correlation of serum miRNA-23a and miRNA-23b expression with testosterone concentrations in normal women (a and b), in normal women at different stages of the menstrual cycle (c–k), and in PCOS patients (l and m). None of the scatter plots showed significant correlation coefficients ($p > 0.05$)

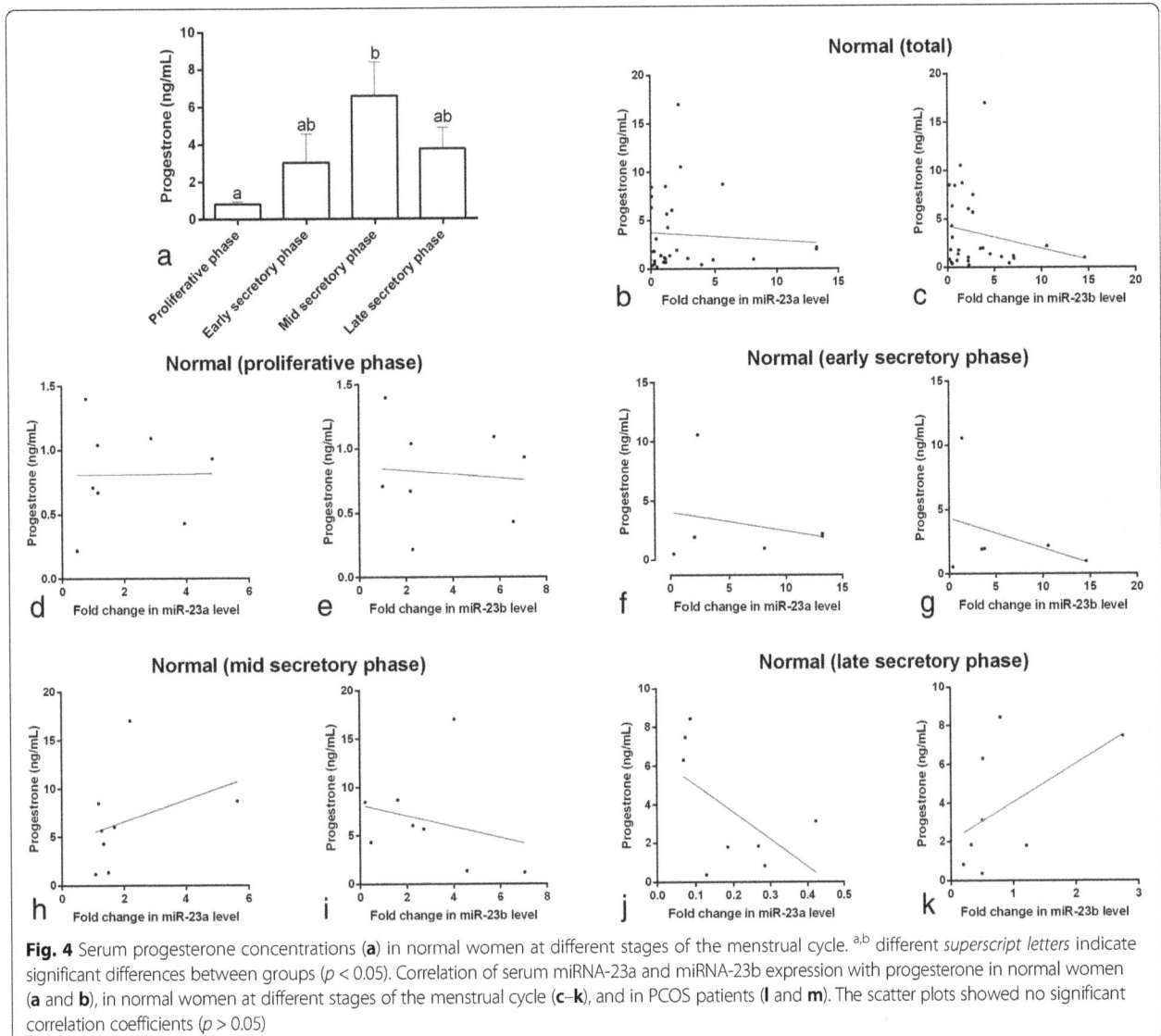

Fig. 4 Serum progesterone concentrations (**a**) in normal women at different stages of the menstrual cycle. [a,b] different *superscript letters* indicate significant differences between groups ($p < 0.05$). Correlation of serum miRNA-23a and miRNA-23b expression with progesterone in normal women (**a** and **b**), in normal women at different stages of the menstrual cycle (**c–k**), and in PCOS patients (**l** and **m**). The scatter plots showed no significant correlation coefficients ($p > 0.05$)

In the healthy controls in the proliferative phase, the E_2 concentrations were negatively correlated with the expression of miR-23a ($p = 0.04$, Fig. 5d), but not with the expression of miR-23b ($p > 0.05$, Fig. 5e). There was no correlation between P_4 concentration and miR-23a or miR-23b expression ($p > 0.05$) in the proliferative phase nor were there any correlations between E_2 and P_4 and miR-23a or miR-23b expression in any of the other phases.

Luteinizing hormone (LH) and follicle stimulating hormone (FSH) and expression of miR-23a/b in PCOS patients

The mean and SE values of LH and FSH concentrations in PCOS patients were 10.8 ± 1.6 ng/mL and 5.9 ± 0.5 ng/mL, respectively, and did not significantly correlate with miR-23a or miR-23b expression (Fig. 6).

Hormones and BMI in healthy controls and PCOS patients

Concentrations of testosterone ($r = 0.04$), LH ($r = -0.06$), and FSH ($r = -0.3$) did not correlate with BMI in the PCOS patients ($p > 0.05$). The correlation coefficients between testosterone concentrations and BMI were negative in all four subgroups of healthy women, but none of the correlations were statistically significant ($p > 0.05$). Among the healthy controls, the correlation coefficients between E_2 and P_4 concentrations and BMI were not significant, except for the correlation between P_4 concentrations and BMI in the late secretory phase ($r = 0.71$, $p = 0.04$).

Power of study and odds ratio of effective factors on PCOS and expression of miR-23a/b

The observed powers of analysis in the risk factors (miR-23a/b expression, BMI and testosterone concentrations) of PCOS were more than 80% (Table 1).

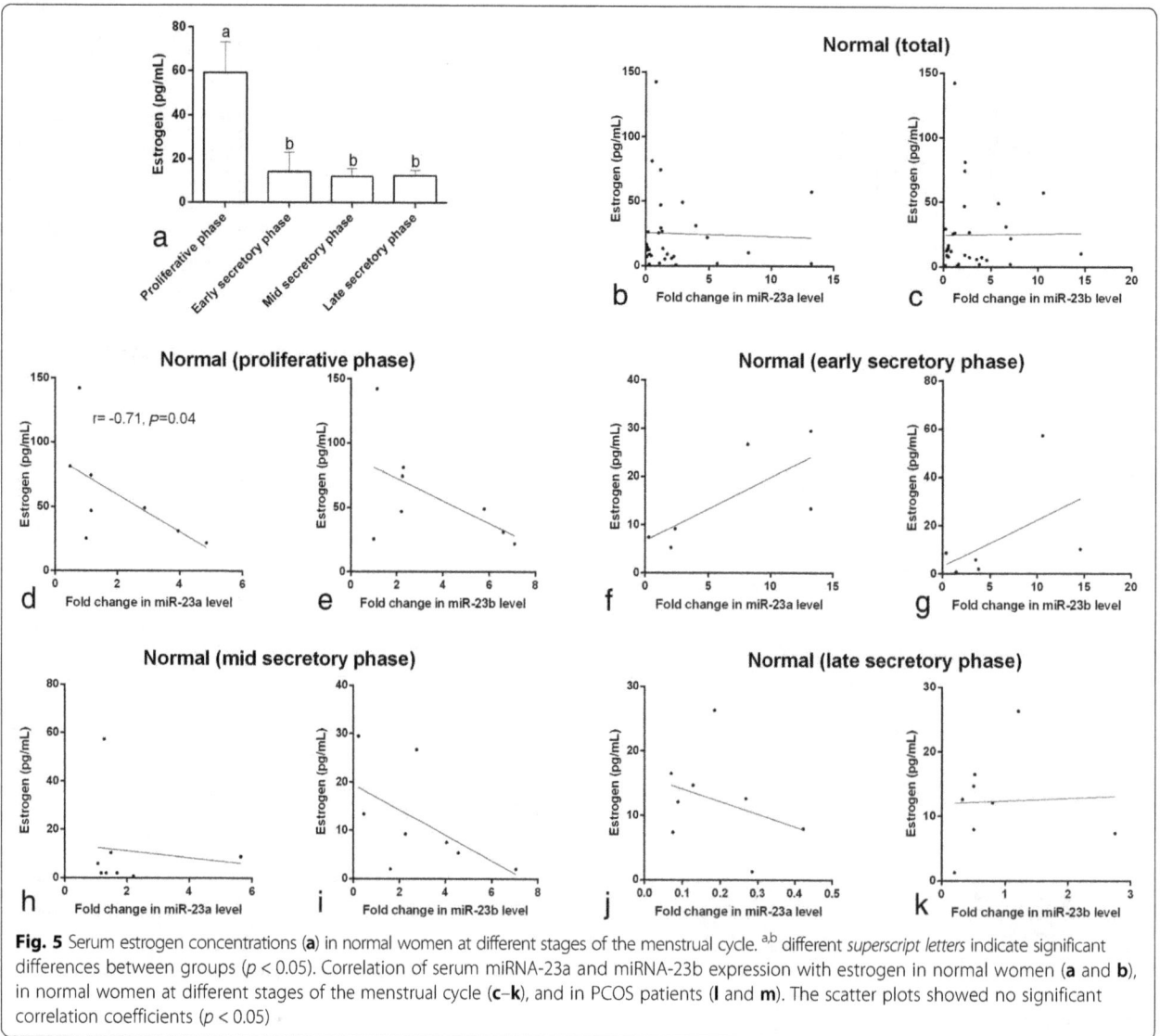

Fig. 5 Serum estrogen concentrations (**a**) in normal women at different stages of the menstrual cycle. [a,b] different *superscript letters* indicate significant differences between groups (*p* < 0.05). Correlation of serum miRNA-23a and miRNA-23b expression with estrogen in normal women (**a** and **b**), in normal women at different stages of the menstrual cycle (**c–k**), and in PCOS patients (**l** and **m**). The scatter plots showed no significant correlation coefficients (*p* < 0.05)

Furthermore, the adjusted odds ratios of the variables finally included in the logistic model are shown in Tables 2 and 3. Logistic regression analysis indicated significant effects of the fold changes of miR-23a/b on the likelihood of women with PCOS. The likelihood of women with PCOS decreased by 0.01-fold for every 1 fold increase of miR-23a expression (*P* = 0.02; Table 2). On the other hand, the miR-23b expression on the PCOS was not significant in the equation (*P* > 0.05; Table 2).

Without considering the presence or absence of PCOS, logistic regression analysis indicated significant negative effects of the testosterone concentrations on the likelihood of fold changes of miR-23a (Table 3). The likelihood of more than 1 in fold changes of miR-23a would be 0.003-fold for each 1 fold decrease in testosterone concentration (*P* = 0.01). While, BMI significant positive effect was observed only on the likelihood of fold changes of miR-23b. The likelihood of more than 1

in fold changes of miR-23b would be 1.056-fold for each 1 fold increase in BMI (*P* = 0.03).

Biological functions of the predicted targets of miR-23a/b

The predicted target genes for miR-23a and miR-23b were screened in *Homo sapiens* using the MicroCosm Targets software. The list of predicted target genes included 1078 genes for miR-23a and 1049 genes for miRNA-23b, from which 377 and 356 target genes, respectively, were mapped to biological functions and processes, including hormone synthesis, metabolic functions, and sexual reproduction. Of these target genes, the analysis revealed 309 common target genes for both miR-23a and miR-23b, 68 genes related exclusively to miR-23a, and 47 genes related exclusively to miR-23b, and these genes are involved in eight biological processes (Fig. 7).

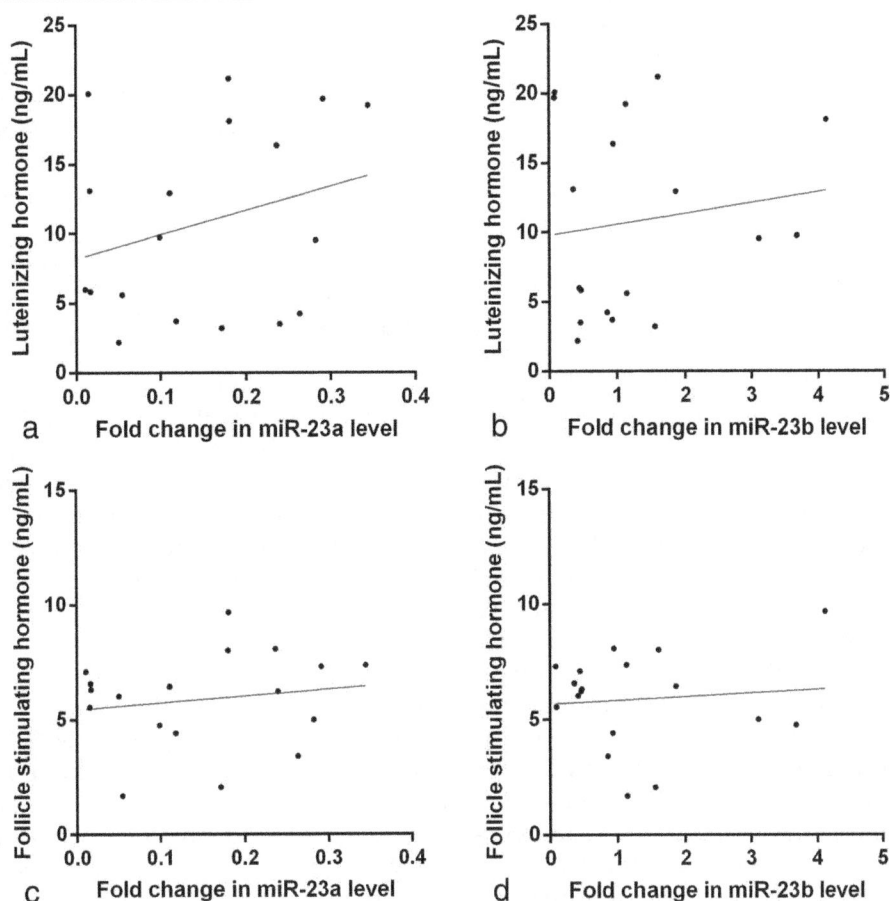

Fig. 6 Correlation of serum miRNA-23a and miRNA-23b expression with luteinizing hormone (LH, **a** and **b**) and follicle stimulating hormone (FSH, **c** and **d**) concentrations in PCOS patients. The scatter plots showed no significant correlation coefficients ($p > 0.05$)

Discussion

We found a negative influence of decrease of miR-23a on occurrence of PCOS and increase of testosterone. On the other hand, although a positive effect of BMI on the expression levels of miR-23b (without considering presence or absence of PCOS) was observed in logistic regression analysis, but decrease in miR-23b fold-changes as well as miR-23a decrease was observed in PCOS women. Considering this fact that miR-23a alterations was not affected by BMI in contrast with miR-23b, suggests it as a better indicator for evaluation of PCOS than the miR-23b.

Furthermore, the BMI among the women with PCOS was higher on average compared with the healthy controls. The mean BMI of healthy women of the same ethnicity and in the same age range (20.99 ± 3.31 kg/m^2) [6] is similar to the BMI among healthy controls in the current study. Therefore, all of the PCOS patients in this study could be considered to be obese (the mean BMI of the PCOS patients was 23.96 ± 4.44 kg/m^2). Obesity in the PCOS patients increased the expression of both miR-23a and miR23b, but BMI was correlated with decreased expression of these miRNAs in the healthy controls. The pattern of correlations between obesity

Table 1 Observed powers of analysis regarding to different dependent variables in five groups of normal and polycystic ovary syndrome women

Variables	Observed power (%)
miRNA-23a	100
miRNA-23b	93
Body mass index	95
Testosterone	100

Table 2 Odds ratios of the variables included in the final logistic regression model for the polycystic ovary syndrome and serum miRNA-23a and miRNA-23b expression

Variables	Odds ratio	95% Confidence interval	P-value
miRNA-23a	0.012	0.0–0.46	0.017
miRNA-23b	1.803	0.99–3.54	0.053

Backward likelihood ratio test = 28.57, 2 df, $P = 0.0001$; Hosmer and Lemeshow goodness-of-fit test = 2.81, 8 df, $P = 0.95$; the model fits

Table 3 Odds ratios of the variables included in the final logistic regression model for the serum miRNA-23a or miRNA-23b expression and body mass index and testosterone concentration

Variables	Odds ratio	95% Confidence interval	P-value
miRNA-23a			
Body mass index	1.051	0.99–1.11	0.08
Testosterone	0.003	0.00–0.24	0.01
miRNA-23b			
Body mass index	1.056	1.01–1.11	0.03
Testosterone	0.100	0.01–1.47	0.09

miRNA-23a: Backward likelihood ratio test = 14.08, 2 df, $P = 0.001$; Hosmer and Lemeshow goodness-of-fit test = 18.67, 8 df, $P = 0.02$; the model fits
miRNA-23b: Backward likelihood ratio test = 5.17, 2 df, $P = 0.08$; Hosmer and Lemeshow goodness-of-fit test = 8.47, 8 df, $P = 0.39$; the model fits

and the expression of miR-23a and miR23b that was observed in the present study resembles the pattern of correlations of serum testosterone, LH, and FSH concentrations with the expression of the miR-23a and miR23b, but the effects of obesity on the relationship with miR-23a/b expression in the women with PCOS was greater than the association of hormone changes with miR-23a/b expression. In the healthy controls and the endometrial-phase subgroups, obesity and testosterone concentrations had negative correlation coefficients, whereas in the women with PCOS a positive but non-significant correlation in increased BMI and testosterone concentrations was observed. Consistent with our findings, Murri et al. [7] reported opposite patterns of association between obesity and testosterone concentrations in PCOS patients and healthy controls. According to the normal range of testosterone levels among healthy women of the same ethnicity and in the same age range of the current study (0.32 ± 0.16 ng/mL) [6], all of the PCOS patients who were selected in this study based on the Rotterdam consensus criteria were defined as having hyperandrogenemia (0.59 ± 0.19 ng/mL).

The patterns of changes in the expression of miR-23a and miR-23b were the same in the PCOS patients and in the healthy controls and in the endometrial-phase subgroups, and in the present study the expressions of both miR-23a and miR-23b in serum were significantly lower in the women with PCOS compared to the healthy controls. The one exception was that the mean expression of miR-23b in the women with PCOS was higher than that in the healthy controls in the late secretory phase, and it can be speculated that this difference might be due to the involvement of miR-23b in ovulation. In support of this, it has been shown that miR-23b targets the X-linked inhibitor of apoptosis and can induce apoptosis in human granulosa cells in vitro [8]. In addition, a comparison of seasonally ovulatory and anovulatory follicles in horses revealed increased expression of miR-23b in the anovulatory follicles [9]. Furthermore, in our current

work we found that the pattern of expression of miR-23a and miR-23b changed from a positive correlation in the proliferative phase to a negative correlation in the late secretory phase; whereas the women with PCOS showed a positive correlation in the expressions of miR-23a and miR-23b.

In the present study, the increase in serum E_2 concentrations in the proliferative phase was negatively correlated with the expression of miR-23a and miR-23b in the healthy controls. Furthermore, in the evaluated population, a negative influence of increase of testosterone concentrations on miR-23a expression was observed. In addition, the same non-significant effect of testosterone was observed on miR-23 expression in whole blood. A previous study on the expression of miR-23a and miR-23b in follicular fluid showed that expression of these miRNAs along with the expression of their target gene could regulate the expression of aromatase, CYP19A1, in ovarian cells and, therefore, might have a role in E_2 biosynthesis [4]. Therefore, it can be speculated that alterations in the expression of these miRNAs in serum might affect follicular growth and ovulation via other target genes than those that play a role in E_2 hormone synthesis, including target genes that are functionally related to cell growth and apoptosis. In the present study, a decrease in miR-23a expression in women with PCOS was observed, and overexpression of pre-miR-23 has previously been shown to play a role in apoptosis in cultured human luteinized granulosa cells [8]. Therefore, altered miR-23a expression in PCOS patients might induce down-regulation of apoptotic processes in ovarian cells.

With the help of bioinformatics tools, we have shown that miR-23a and miR-23b target large numbers of genes and that many of these genes are targeted by several other miRNAs. Target genes of miR-23a and miR-23b are involved in many biological functions, including metabolic, cellular, and reproductive processes that are important in PCOS pathogenesis [2, 10]. One of the metabolic disorders that has a definite role in PCOS is obesity [11], and several studies have shown that cellular communication can be altered in PCOS and obesity, including communication between inflammatory cells and metabolic cells [12–14]. Additionally, inflammatory and immune gene targets that regulate cellular processes such as apoptosis can influence follicular function and steroid production [10, 15].

The major limitation of the present study was possibly the evaluation of serum miRNA expression, which represents miRNAs from several unknown origin cell types. However, several studies have highlighted the potential of serum samples to act as developmental markers of diseases, including PCOS [7, 16–18]. Therefore, sampling of serum might represent the overall

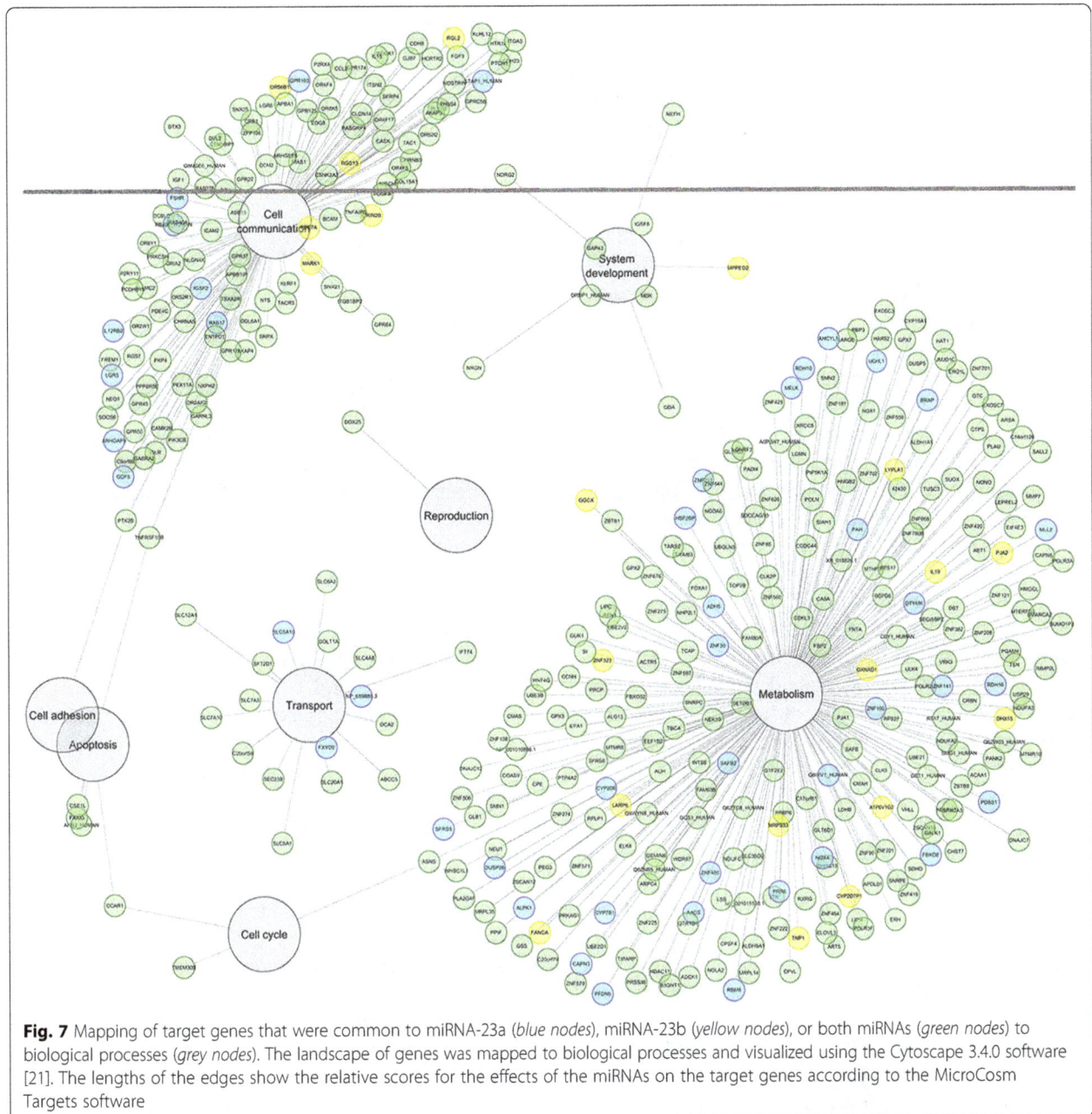

Fig. 7 Mapping of target genes that were common to miRNA-23a (*blue nodes*), miRNA-23b (*yellow nodes*), or both miRNAs (*green nodes*) to biological processes (*grey nodes*). The landscape of genes was mapped to biological processes and visualized using the Cytoscape 3.4.0 software [21]. The lengths of the edges show the relative scores for the effects of the miRNAs on the target genes according to the MicroCosm Targets software

state of the entire body instead of specific cells at the time of collection.

Conclusions

The present research showed lower concentrations of miR-23a and miR-23b in the serum of PCOS patients compared to healthy controls. Furthermore, we demonstrated the positive influence of obesity on the serum expression of miR-23b related to metabolic and cell function disorders. In addition, testosterone had negative effects on the levels of circulating miR-23a. Exploring the target genes and pathways of miR-23a/b and other differentially expressed miRNAs will contribute to a

better understanding of the roles of miRNAs in the pathogenesis of PCOS. In terms of new biomarkers for the detection of PCOS in patients, miR-23a might be a better choice, but the correlation between the levels of these miRNAs in the serum and in the follicular cells needs further investigation.

Methods

Subjects and selection criteria

In the current study, 18 Han Chinese women (with a mean ± SD age of 25.8 ± 4.5 years) were recruited from the Affiliated Obstetrical and Gynecological Hospital of Fudan University between September 2011 and

January 2012. The women were all diagnosed with PCOS based on the revised diagnostic criteria announced in the Rotterdam consensus [1], and patients with Cushing syndrome, late-onset congenital adrenal hyperplasia, thyroid dysfunction, hyperprolactinemia, or androgen-secreting tumors were excluded. Other exclusion criteria included diabetes, hypertension, chronic renal disease, smoking, and the use of alcohol or medications. Thirty healthy age-matched Han Chinese women (25.5 ± 2.3 years old) with no previous history of reproductive system diseases or appendicitis served as controls. The control women had normal and regularly cycling menstrual periods, and their ovaries appeared normal on ultrasound. The exclusion criteria of the healthy women in the study were taking drugs, including oral contraceptives or other hormone drugs, intrauterine device placement, smoking, and/or pregnancy in the past 3 months. Control subjects were divided into four groups according to their endometrial cycle phase – proliferative phase (days 4–14, $n = 8$), early secretory phase (days 15–18, $n = 6$), mid-secretory phase (days 19–24, $n = 8$), and late secretory phase (days 25–30, $n = 8$).

Assessment of BMI and sex hormones

The BMI in both normal women and PCOS patients was calculated as weight (kg) divided by the square of the height (m^2). Measurements and blood samples were conducted within the first 10 days from the onset of menstruation in PCOS cases with mild oligomenorrhea, and they were conducted at random times for PCOS cases with severe oligomenorrhea or amenorrhea. Measurements and blood samples were conducted at different phases of the endometrial cycle in controls as described above. Total testosterone, LH, and FSH were measured by radioimmunoassay (RigorBio Scientific and Technology Co., Beijing) according to the manufacturer's instructions.

Quantification of miR 23a/b in peripheral blood

Venous blood samples (5 ml) were drawn from every subject. Serum was separated by centrifuging at $3000 \times g$ for 10 min at 4 °C and was stored at –20 °C. Whole RNA was extracted from 200 μL of serum with the miRcute miRNA Isolation kit (DP501, Tiangen Biotech, Beijing) according to the manufacturer's instructions. The RNA was then reverse transcribed using the miRcute miRNA first-strand cDNA synthesis kit (KR201, Tiangen Biotech, Beijing), and quantitative real-time polymerase chain reaction (qPCR) was performed using the miRcute miRNA qPCR detection kit (Tiangen Biotech, Beijing). The qPCR was performed under the following conditions: initial PCR denaturation at 94 °C for 120 s followed by 42 combined cycles of denaturation of 20 s at 94 °C and annealing and extension of 34 s at 60 °C. Fluorescence was measured at 55 °C in

81 cycles of 10 s. Results were calculated using the $2^{-\Delta\Delta Ct}$ method, and U6 was used as the controls for miR-23a and miR-23b. The sequences of primers were as follows (Invitrogen, Shanghai):

Primer sequence of miR-23a: 5′-ATCACATTGCCA GGGATTTCCA-3′

Primer sequence of miR-23b: 5′-GCACATTGCCA GGGATTACCA-3′

U6 as the internal control: 5′-CTCGCTTGGGCAGC ACA-3

Statistical analysis

Data are described as the mean $\pm$ SD. An independent sample t-test or one-way ANOVA with correction of p-values with the Bonferroni *post-hoc* test was used to test for differences in demographic variables and laboratory measurements between PCOS patients and healthy controls. Spearman correlation coefficients were calculated to evaluate the relationship between miRNA levels and other measurements in both the PCOS and control groups. All data were analyzed using SPSS version 22.0 (SPSS, Inc., Chicago, IL), and $p < 0.05$ was considered statistically significant.

To evaluate the power of study regarding to the selected sample size and the five groups of normal and PCOS women, the observed power of the dependent variables (miR-23a/b expression, BMI and testosterone concentrations) were estimated using univariate analysis of variance in general linear model of SPSS [19].

Possible effects of the miR-23a and miR-23b on occurrence of PCOS were explored using logistic regression analysis. The data of the normal women was used as reference. The data were compared by logistic regression analysis using the presence of PCOS as the dependent variable (0 denotes normal and 1 denotes PCOS) and the expression of miR-23a and the expression of miR-23b as the independent factors were entered into equation. Furthermore, possible effects of the BMI and serum testosterone concentration on the fold change of miR-23a and miR-23b were explored using logistic regression analysis. The data of the fold change of miR-23a/b less than 1 was used as reference. The data were compared by logistic regression analysis using the fold change of miR-23a or miR-23b as the dependent variable (0 denotes less than 1 fold change and 1 denotes more than or equal 1 fold change) and the BMI and serum testosterone, concentration as the independent factors were entered into equation.

Regression analyses were conducted according to the method of Hosmer and Lemeshow [20]. The p-values for data inclusion and exclusion were set at 0.05 and 0.10, respectively. The variable that had been selected or retained entered the final likelihood ratio (LR), in which the final odds ratio estimates with 95% confidence intervals were derived. The constants were not included in the model.

Abbreviations

BMI: Body mass index; FSH: Follicle stimulating hormone; LH: Luteinizing hormone; miRNA: microRNA; PCOS: Polycystic ovary syndrome; qPCR: Quantitative real-time polymerase chain reaction

Acknowledgements

Not applicable.

Funding

This study was supported by grants from the Zhengyi Fund of Shanghai Medical School, Fudan University, and the National Natural Science Foundation of China for Talents (No. J1210041 to WX, YL, and LX); the Swedish Medical Research Council, Fredrik and Ingrid Thurings Foundation, Göteborgs Läkaresällskap, the Tore Nilson Foundation, and The Swedish federal government under the LUA/ALF agreement (Project no. 5859 and ALFGBG-147791 2014 to RS); the Chinese Special Fund for Postdocs (No. 2014T70392 to YF), the National Natural Science Foundation of China (No. 81673766 to YF, No. 81572555 to XL), the New Teacher Priming Fund, the Zuoxue Foundation of Fudan University (to YF), and the Development Project of Shanghai Peak Disciplines-Integrated Chinese and Western Medicine (to YF).

Authors' contributions

Conceived and designed the experiments: WX, YL, LX, RS, XL, and YF. Performed the experiments: WX, YL, LX, SZ, FT, and RS. Analyzed the data: WX, YL, LX, AT, and YF. Wrote the paper: AT, XL, and YF. All authors read and approved the final manuscript.

Competing interests

The authors declare that they have no competing interests.

Author details

[1]Department of Integrative Medicine and Neurobiology, State Key Lab of Medical Neurobiology, School of Basic Medical Sciences, Shanghai Medical College; Institute of Acupuncture Research (WHO collaborating center for traditional medicine) and Institute of Brain Science, Brain Science Collaborative Innovation Center, Fudan University, Shanghai 200032, China. [2]Grade 2008 Clinical Medicine, Shanghai Medicine School, Fudan University, Shanghai 200032, China. [3]Department of Neurology, West China Hospital of Sichuan University, Chengdu, Sichuan 610041, China. [4]Department of Medical Oncology, Fudan University Shanghai Cancer Center, Shanghai 200032, China. [5]Department of Cardiology, Zhongshan Hospital, Fudan University, Shanghai 200032, China. [6]Department of Gynecology, Obstetrics and Gynecology Hospital, Fudan University, Shanghai 200011, China. [7]Institute of Neuroscience and Physiology, Department of Physiology, Sahlgrenska Academy, University of Gothenburg, Gothenburg 40530, Sweden.

References

1. The Rotterdam ESHRE/ASRM-sponsored PCOS consensus workshop group. Revised 2003 consensus on diagnostic criteria and long-term health risks related to polycystic ovary syndrome (PCOS). Hum Reprod. 2004;19:41–7.
2. Escobar-Morreale HF, San Millán JL. Abdominal adiposity and the polycystic ovary syndrome. Trends Endocrinol Metab. 2007;18:266–72.
3. Toloubeydokhti T, Bukulmez O, Chegini N. Potential regulatory functions of microRNAs in the ovary. Semin Reprod Med. 2008;26:469–78.
4. Alford C, Toloubeydokhti T, Al-Katanani Y, Drury KC, Williams R, Chenini N. The expression of microRNA (miRNA) mir-23a and 23b and their target gene, CYP19A1 (aromatase) in follicular cells obtained from women undergoing ART. Fertil Steril. 2007;88:S166–7.
5. Hemimi N, Shaafie I, Alshawa H. The study of the impact of genetic polymorphism of aromatase (CYP19) enzyme and the susceptibility to polycystic ovary syndrome (575.5). FASEB J. 2014;28:575-5.
6. Du X, Ding T, Zhang H, Zhang C, Ma W, Zhong Y, Qu W, Zheng J, Liu Y, Li Z, et al. Age-specific normal reference range for serum anti-müllerian hormone in healthy Chinese Han women: a nationwide population-based study. Reprod Sci. 2016;23:1019–27.
7. Murri M, Insenser M, Fernández-Durán E, San-Millán JL, Escobar-Morreale HF. Effects of polycystic ovary syndrome (PCOS), sex hormones, and obesity on circulating miRNA-21, miRNA-27b, miRNA-103, and miRNA-155 expression. J Clin Endocrinol Metab. 2013;98:E1835–44.
8. Yang X, Zhou Y, Peng S, Wu L, Lin H-Y, Wang S, Wang H. Differentially expressed plasma microRNAs in premature ovarian failure patients and the potential regulatory function of mir-23a in granulosa cell apoptosis. Reproduction. 2012;144:235–44.
9. Donadeu FX, Schauer SN. Differential miRNA expression between equine ovulatory and anovulatory follicles. Domest Anim Endocrinol. 2013;45:122–5.
10. Escobar-Morreale H, Luque-Ramírez M, González F. Circulating inflammatory markers in polycystic ovary syndrome: a systematic review and metaanalysis. Fertil Steril. 2011;95:1048–58. e1-2.
11. Escobar-Morreale HF, Samino S, Insenser M, Vinaixa M, Luque-Ramarez M, Lasunción MA, Correig X. Metabolic heterogeneity in polycystic ovary syndrome is determined by obesity: plasma metabolomic approach using GC-MS. Clin Chem. 2012;58:999–1009.
12. Tarantino G, Valentino R, Somma CD, D'Esposito V, Passaretti F, Pizza G, Brancato V, Orio F, Formisano P, Colao A, et al. Bisphenol A in polycystic ovary syndrome and its association with liver–spleen axis. Clin Endocrinol (Oxf). 2013;78:447–53.
13. Lumeng CN, DelProposto JB, Westcott DJ, Saltiel AR. Phenotypic switching of adipose tissue macrophages with obesity is generated by spatiotemporal differences in macrophage subtypes. Diabetes. 2008;57:3239–46.
14. Feuerer M, Herrero L, Cipolletta D, Naaz A, Wong J, Nayer A, Lee J, Goldfine A, Benoist C, Shoelson S, et al. Fat T(reg) cells: a liaison between the immune and metabolic systems. Nat Med. 2009;15:930–9.
15. Wu R, Van der Hoek KH, Ryan NK, Norman RJ, Robker RL. Macrophage contributions to ovarian function. Hum Reprod Update. 2004;10:119–33.
16. Creemers EE, Tijsen AJ, Pinto YM. Circulating microRNAs: novel biomarkers and extracellular communicators in cardiovascular disease? Circ Res. 2012; 110:483–95.
17. Tan KS, Armugam A, Sepramaniam S, Lim KY, Setyowati KD, Wang CW, Jeyaseelan K. Expression profile of MicroRNAs in young stroke patients. PLoS One. 2009;4:e7689.
18. Wang H, Peng W, Shen X, Huang Y, Ouyang X, Dai Y. Circulating levels of inflammation-associated miR-155 and endothelial-enriched miR-126 in patients with end-stage renal disease. Braz J Med Biol Res. 2012;45:1308–14.
19. D'Amico EJ, Neilands TB, Zambarano R. Power analysis for multivariate and repeated measures designs: a flexible approach using the SPSS MANOVA procedure. Behav Res Methods Instrum Comput. 2001;33:479–84.
20. Hosmer DW, Lemeshow S. Applied logistic regression. New York: Wiley; 1989.
21. Shannon P, Markiel A, Ozier O, Baliga NS, Wang JT, Ramage D, Amin N, Schwikowski B, Ideker T. Cytoscape: a software environment for integrated models of biomolecular interaction networks. Genome Res. 2003;13:2498–504.

Androstenedione response to recombinant human FSH is the most valid predictor of the number of selected follicles in polycystic ovarian syndrome: (a case-control study)

Eser Sefik Ozyurek[1*], Tevfik Yoldemir[2] and Gokhan Artar[1]

Abstract

Background: We aimed to test the hypothesis that the correlation of the changes in the blood Androstenedione (A_4) levels to the number of selected follicles during ovulation induction with low-dose recombinant human follicle stimulating hormone (rhFSH) is as strong as the correlation to changes in the blood Estradiol (E_2) levels in polycystic ovary syndrome (PCOS).

Methods: Prospective Case-control study conducted from October 2014 to January 2016. 61 non-PCOS control (Group I) and 46 PCOS (Group II) patients treated with the chronic low-dose step up protocosl with rhFSH. A_4, E_2, progesterone blood levels and follicular growth were monitored.. Univariate and hierarchical multivariable analysis were performed for age, BMI, HOMA-IR, A_4 and E_2 (with the number of selected follicles as the dependent variable in both groups). ROC analysis was performed to define threshold values for the significant determinants of the number of selected follicles to predict cyle cancellations due to excessive ovarian response.

Results: The control group (Group I) was comprised of 61 cycles from a group of primary infertile non-PCOS patients, and the study group (Group II) of 46 cycles of PCOS patients. The analysis revealed that the strongest independent predictor of the total number of selected follicles in Group I was the E_2(AUC) (B = 0.0006[0.0003-0.001]; $P < 0.001$); whereas for Group II, it was the A_4 (AUC) (B = 0.114[0.04-0.25]; $P = 0.01$). Optimum thresholds for the A_4 related parameters were defined to predict excessive response within Group II were 88.7%, 3.1 ng/mL and 5.4 ng*days for the percentage increase in A_4, the maximum A_4 value and area under the curve values for A_4, respectively.

Conclusion: A_4 response to low-dose rhFSH in PCOS has a stronger association with the number of follicles selected than the E_2 reponse. A_4 response preceding the E_2 response is essential for progressive follicle development. Monitoring A_4 rather than E_2 may be more preemptive to define the initial ovarian response and accurate titration of the rhFSH doses.

Trial registration: The study was registered as a prospective case-control study in the ClinicalTrials.gov registry with the identifier NCT02329483.

Keywords: Androgens, Androstenedione, Polycystic ovary syndrome, Ovulation induction, Folliculogenesis, Human FSH, Gonadotropins

* Correspondence: eozyurek@yahoo.com
[1]Bagcilar Research and Training Hospital Obgyn Department, Merkez Mh., Mimar Sinan Caddesi, 6. Sokak, 34100 Bagcilar, Istanbul, Turkey
Full list of author information is available at the end of the article

Background

Oligoovulation related to polycystic ovarian syndrome is treated with ovulation induction medications [1]. These patients have an increased risk of excessive ovarian response which is closely associated with the number of selected follicles [2]. Therefore, milder protocols have been developed [3]. In PCOS cases, the estradiol response to gonadotropin treatment is delayed and discordant with the visualized follicular responses [3]. Androstenedione (A_4), mostly synthesized in the ovaries is a precursor of E_2 [4, 5].

In this study, we aimed to test the hypothesis that the cumulative changes in A_4 during ovulation induction with low dose rhFSH in PCOS cases are correlated to the number of selected follicles (follicles sized ≥ 12 mm) comparable to the the cumulative changes in E_2.

Methods

This is a prospective case-control study conducted between October 2014 and January 2016. Ethical permission was obtained from the Bagcilar Research and Training Hospital Research Ethics Committee. It was recorded as a prospective case-control study in the ClinicalTrials.gov registry with the identifier NCT02329483. The study was conducted in accordance with the Declaration of Helsinki. Informed consent for participation was obtained from all patients.

Study setting

The study was conducted at the Bagcilar Research and Training Hospital Gynecology and Obstetrics Department, Infertility Section. Cycle monitoring was done with folliculometry with transvaginal sonography, E_2, P_4 and A_4 measurements.

Study population

A total of 107 cycles of 61 Control-nonPCOS infertile (Group I) and 46 Study-PCOS infertile (Group II) women were included in the study. The study group was comprised of patients with anti-Müllerian hormone (AMH) levels ≥ 5 ng/mL (which is equivalent to PCOM (polycystic ovary morphology sonographically confirmed) [6–8]. PCOS was defined as the copresence of at least one of two of the following criteria combined with the PCOM; *(1): oligoamenorrhea-OA*: cycle length > 35 days, *(2): hyperandrogenism (HA)*: presence of clinical findings including hirsutism defined as the presence of coarse [long/pigmented] terminal hair over the most commonly encountered three or more regions within the Modified Ferriman-Gallwey Score System (the buttocks/perineum, sideburn, and neck areas which contributed greatly to the score in the geographic locale where this study was conducted) with or without elevated blood testosterone levels (>0.5 ng/mL) [7–12]. The control group was comprised of unexplained primary/secondary infertile women with

AMH levels <5 ng/mL, not displaying any clinical findings associated with hyperandrogenism (HA) and with regular menstrual cycles. The inclusion criteria for both groups included ages within 20-35, with normal spermiograms or with mild male factor infertility (i.e.: male partners with only one the following abnormalities: sperm counts being lower than 20 million/ml *or* showing a normal morphology quotient of less than 4% *or* having a sperm motility lower than 40%; *AND* with post-wash total motile sperm counts equal to or higher than 5 million/ml), normal anatomic findings with the hysterosalpingography (no bilateral tubal obstruction or Müllerian anomalies), hormonally eugonadotropic, normal blood prolactin/thyroid-stimulating hormone (TSH) levels and being planned for controlled ovarian hyperstimulation and intrauterine insemination treatment. Exclusion criteria included: diabetes mellitus, BMI < 20 or >30, hypo or hypergonadotropism, other causes for hyperandrogenism, ≥ 2 abortions or ectopic pregnancy, additional medical disorders, ovarian cysts or previous pelvic surgery.

Controlled ovarian hyperstimulation and intrauterine insemination

Ovulation induction was conducted with follitropin alpha (Gonal-f Multidose 450 IU; Merck-Serono-Turkey) starting with a dose of 37.5 U/day or 50 U/day as described by Homburg et al. [2]. Ovulation induction was started on the 3rd or the 4th day of a menstrual cycle having early cycle blood E_2 levels <50 pg/mL and blood Progesterone levels <0.5 ng/mL and in the absence of any ovarian residual follicles larger than 15 mm to rule out the presence of a corpus luteum or any other cystic ovarian structure which could require further clarification. If a primary follicle response characterised by the appearance of a selected growing follicle of ≥ 10 mm and a rise $\geq 25\%$ in blood E_2 levels was not observed despite 14 days of rhFSH stimulation, the initial dose was increased initially to 75 U/day and +37.5 U/day, weekly at each additional incremental step (i.e. 112.5, 150 U/day). Blood E_2, P_4, and A_4 levels were measured and follicle growth was monitored with transvaginal sonography at every visit (every 2-3 days) starting on day 2 or 3 of the cycles. Once 1 or 2 mature follicles ≥ 18 mm were observed, rhCG (Ovitrelle 150 μg; Merck-Serono-Turkey) s.c. was administered. Sperm washing and intrauterine insemination were carried within [36th–40th] hours. On the 15th day postinsemination, blood beta-hCG levels were measured and conception confirmed if the beta-hCG blood level was higher than 20mIU/mL.

Cycle cancellation policy

Cycle cancellations were due to excessive ovarian responses (more than 2 selected follicles ≥ 16 mm or blood E_2 level > 1500 pg/mL on the rhCG trigger day), no ovarian response despite dose step-up and stimulation for 28-30 days, or premature luteinisation (P$_4$ blood level ≥ 1.3 ng/mL).

Laboratory analysis of blood samples

Blood samples for hormone measurement were collected from the antecubital vein with a single puncture at every visit during ovulation induction. Samples were collected in a sterile tube and transferred to the lab on the same day. All except the A$_4$ blood level measurement results were reported to the physicians on the afternoon of the same day. A$_4$ blood levels were available 7-10 days later, and did not provide any guidance to management. A colorimetric ELISA assay (Abcam-USA; Kimera Istanbul-Turkey) was used to measure A$_4$ levels. Measurements of AMH were made by using the AMH/MIS enzyme-linked immunosorbent assay. Testosterone values were assayed with the competitive immunoenzymatic colorimetric method. The serum FSH, luteinising hormone (LH), TSH, E$_2$, and prolactin levels were measured using a chemiluminescent microparticle immunoassay.

Data analysis

Univariate parametric tests were used for group comparisons. Significance was defined as a P-value <0.05. A$_4$ (AUC) was calculated as the sum of the areas of trapezoids. Primary A$_4$ response during ovulation induction was considered when a rise of ≥25% was observed in the basal A$_4$ level. HOMA-IR (Homeostatic Model Assessment of Insulin Resistance) Index was calculated for each patient by using an online calculator.

Hierarchial multivariable regression analysis was conducted in both groups to study in a three level linear regression model the contribution of *three sets of independent variables* including the (Model 1) age, BMI and HOMA-IR variables; (Model 2) the E$_2$(AUC) values and (Model 3) (the androstenedione related variables: the primary blood androstenedione level and the A$_4$ (AUC) values); stepwise, defining *changes in R²values* (ΔR^2) representing the additional effect of each of these newly added independent variable sets, on *the total number of selected follicles*. The SPSS 20.0 and Microsoft Excel 2010 were used.

ROC analysis was performed to define threshold values of the significant determinants of the number of selected follicles to predict cyle cancellations due to excessive ovarian response.

Results

A total of 107 cycles of infertile women Group I: 61 non-PCOS and Group II: 46 PCOS were followed in 16-months. The PCOS phenotypes were: PCOM (polycystic ovarian morphology:AMH ≥ 5 ng/mL)/OA (oligo/amenorrhea): 4 patients; PCOM/HA (Hyperandrogenism): 27

patients; PCOM/HA/OA: 15 patients. Mild male factor infertility was present in (22/61) 36% of Group I and (15/46) 32.6% in Group II (P = 0.5). The HOMA-IR score was ≥4.5 in 6/61 (9,8%) and 9/46 (19,6%) of patients in Groups I and II, respectively. The patient characteristics are summarised in (Table 1). There were 6/61 (9.8%) and 9/46 (19.5%) conceptions in Groups I and II, respectively. The comparison of hormonal characteristics among the conceived and the nonconceived subjects within Groups I and II are summarized in (Table 2). No conception was achieved in the absence of a primary androstenedione response earlier than the primary estradiol response. Cancelled cycles were not included in this comparison.

Table 1 Cycles analysed in this study

	Group I (Control Group)	Group II (PCOS Group)
Age	29.8 ± 0.6	28.7 ± 0.6
Duration of infertility (years)	3.5 ± 0.3	3.4 ± 0.4
BMI (kg/m²)^a	25 ± 0.7	27.7 ± 0.6
AMH(ng/mL)^a	2.4 ± 0.2	9 ± 0.9
HOMA^a	2.8 ± 0.4	3.8 ± 0.4
FSH (mIU/ml)^a	7.2 ± 0.3	6.3 ± 0.2
LH (mIU/ml)^a	6.5 ± 0.5	9.8 ± 0.6
TSH (μIU/mL)	2.7 ± 0.2	3.3 ± 0.7
PRL (ng/ml)	20.9 ± 1.2	22 ± 1.9
Initial Dose (IU/day)	70 ± 4.1	65 ± 3.7
Cycle Length (days)	12.2 ± 4.1	17 ± 0.6
Primary follicular/E$_2$ response day^a	6.7 ± 0.4	9.4 ± 0.4
EM at trigger day (mm)	9.9 ± 0.3	9.4 ± 0.3
Maximum E$_2$ (pg/dl)	453 ± 42.1	556.9 ± 89.3
Follicles >16 mm (n)	1.1 ± 0.1	1.4 ± 0.2
Follicles 12-16 mm (n)	1.2 ± 0.2	1.6 ± 0.3
Total number of follicles	1.9 ± 0.2	2.2 ± 0.3
P$_4$ at trigger day (ng/mL)	0.7 ± 0.1	0.8 ± 0.1
Day 3 Total Testosterone (ng/mL)^a	0.34 ± 0.28	0.87 ± 0.3
Primary androstenedione level (ng/mL)^a	0.9 ± 0.1	1.4 ± 0.1
Primary androstenedione respond day^a	6.2 ± 0.3	7.4 ± 0.4
Time Lag (A$_4$ → E$_2$) initial responses (days)^a	0.5 ± 0.4	2 ± 0.5
Maximum A$_4$(ng/mL)^a	1.8 ± 0.1	2.6 ± 0.3
Rise in A$_4$ (%)^a	66.5 ± 6.9	84.1 ± 7.4
A$_4$ (AUC) (ng*days)^a	3.6 ± 0.3	5.5 ± 1.3
A$_4$ on the trigger day (ng/mL)^a	1.3 ± 0.1	2.5 ± 0.4

PCOS polycystic ovarian syndrome, *AMH* Anti-Müllerian hormone, *HOMA* homeostasis model for assesment of insulin resistance, *FSH* follicle-stimulating hormone, *LH* luteinising hormone, *TSH* thyroid-stimulating hormone, *E$_2$* estradiol, *PRL* prolactin, *EM* endometrial thickness, *P$_4$* progesterone, *AUC* area under the curve, *A$_4$* androstenedione
^{a}P < 0.05

Table 2 Comparison of the hormonal characteristics among the conceived and nonconceived subjects

	Group I (Control Group)		Group II (PCOS Group)	
	Did not conceive	Conceived	Did not conceive	Conceived
Primary A_4^a	0,88 ± 0.45	0,96 ± 0.2	1,39 ± 0.08	1.4 ± 0.33
A_4 (AUC)[b]	3,06 ± 2.8	2.8 ± 1.3	4,2 ± 0.7	10.7 ± 7.1
E_2(AUC)[c]	1916,6 ± 206.3	2942.7 ± 1058.4	2654,2 ± 677.3	4212.7 ± 767.2
AMH[d]	2,53 ± 1.2	3.0 ± 0.41	9.23 ± 1	8.6 ± 1.5
HOMA-IR[e]	3,08 ± 0.3	2.4 ± 0.6	3,2 ± 0.34	2.22 ± 0.33
Time Lag A_4-E_2Response	−0,92 ± 0.46	−0,67 ± 0.4	−0,23 ± 0.11[af]	−3.79 ± 0.86[af]

[a]The initial blood androstenedione level (ng/mL)
[b]Area under the curve value for Androstenedione (ng*days)
[c]Area under the curve value for estradiol (pg*days)
[d]Antimüllerian hormone (ng/mL)
[e]Homeostasis Model for Assessment of Insulin Resistance
[f]$P<0.05$

Nineteen cycles were cancelled due to excessive response ($n = 8$), no response ($n = 6$), or premature luteinisation ($n = 5$). In those cycles cancelled due to no response, there was no primary A_4 response.

Univariate analysis revealed that the primary, maximum, and AUC values for A_4 and the primary blood testosterone levels were all higher in Group II than those in Group I (Table 1).

Plateauing or decreasing A_4 levels before the trigger day were observed in 33/61 (54,1%) of completed cycles in Group I and 14/46 (30,4%) of cycles in Group II. None of these made any significant difference in the basic characteristics or outcome parameters.

The correlation of A_4 parameters with the selected follicle numbers and E_2 (AUC) values are summarised in Figs. (1 and 2; and Tables (3 and 4): The A_4(AUC) was

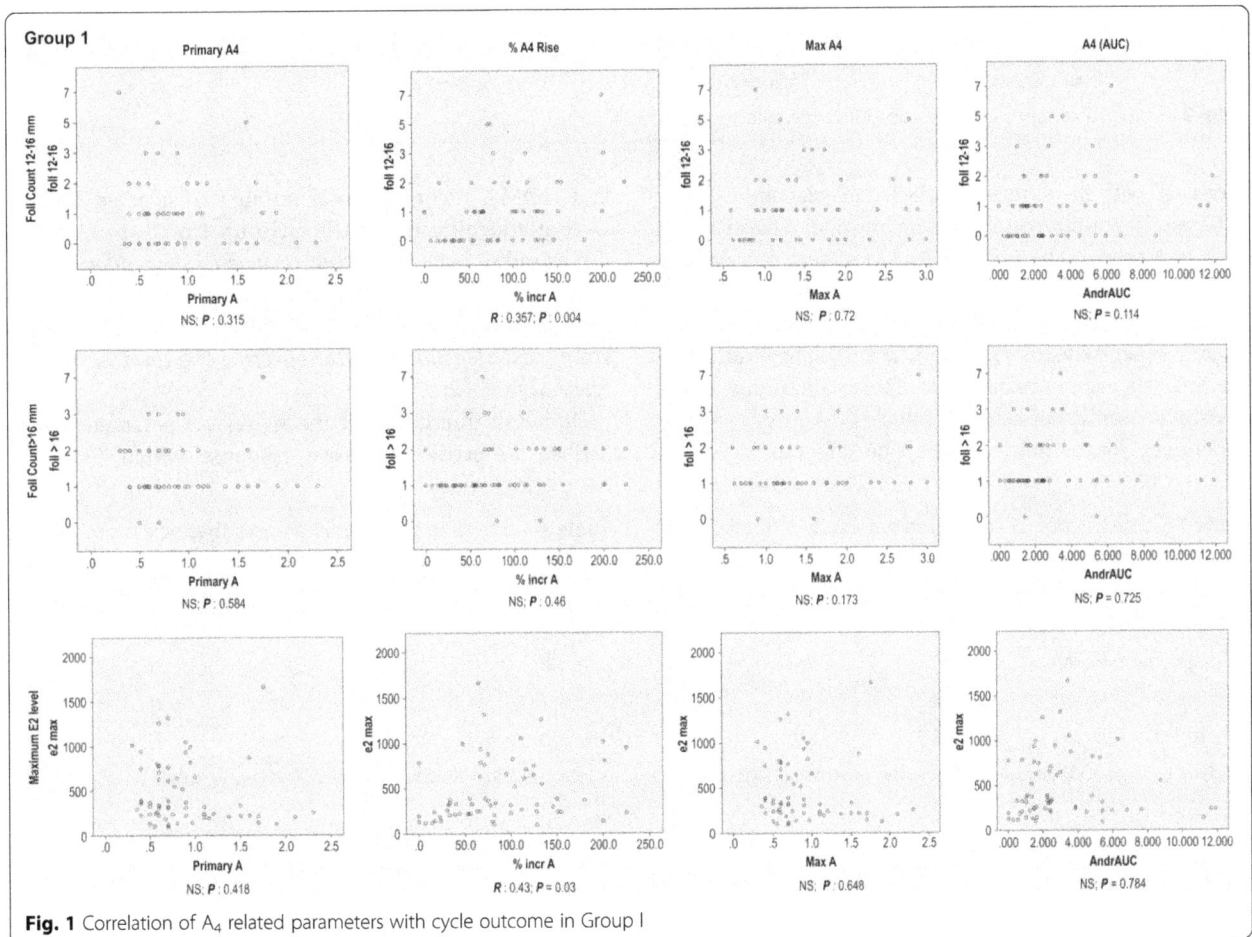

Fig. 1 Correlation of A_4 related parameters with cycle outcome in Group I

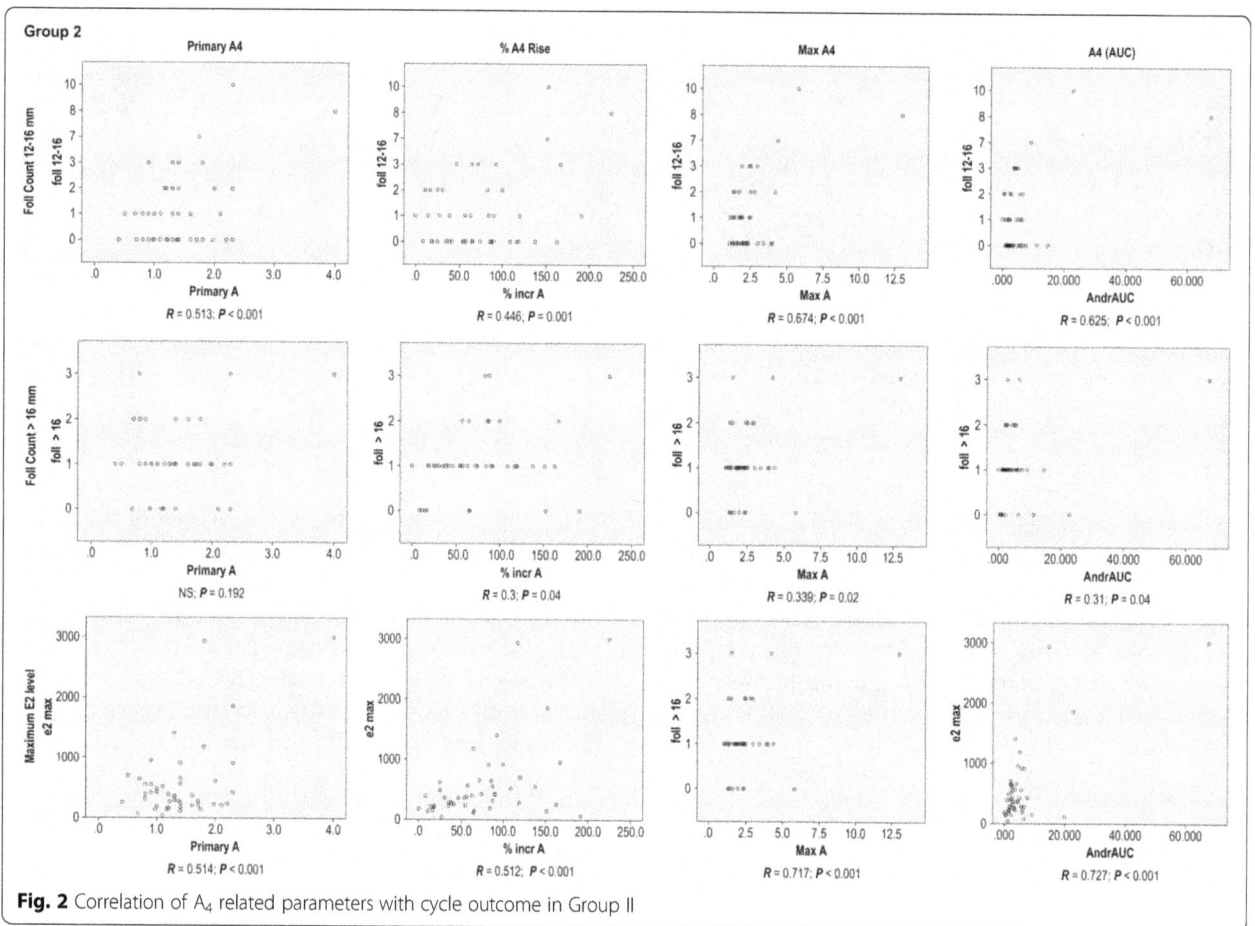

Fig. 2 Correlation of A_4 related parameters with cycle outcome in Group II

correlated with the number of selected follicles and E_2(AUC) in Group II, but not correlated with any one of these parameters in Group I The primary A_4 levels were correlated to the primary testosterone levels in both Groups I and II.

Hierarchical multivariable regression analysis was conducted seperately for *Groups I and II*. The findings of the analysis are summarized in Tables 5(a,b) and 6(a,b). The total number of selected follicles ($\geq$12 mm) was the dependent (outcome) variable. The effect of age, BMI and HOMA-IR on the total number of selected follicles were not significant in either Group I or II. In Group I: the estradiol (AUC) was *the strongest independent factor* (B = 0.0006[0.0003-0.001]; *P* < 0.001), *whereas* in Group II: the A_4(AUC) (B = 0.114 [0.04-0.25]; *P* = 0.01) was *the strongest independent factor effecting the total number of selected follicles.*

Optimum thresholds for the A_4 related parameters were defined to predict excessive response within Group II

Table 3 Correlation of A_4 parameters with cycle outcome parameters in Group I (Control Group)

R^a	Primary A_4	increase A_4%[b]	Max A_4	A_4 AUC
Foll 12-16[d]	NS	0.36[y]	NS	NS
Foll >16[c]	NS	NS	NS	NS
Maximum E_2	NS	0.43[y]	NS	NS
Total Foll[e] Selected	*NS*	*0.32[y]*	*NS*	*NS*

E_2 = Estradiol; A_4 = Androstenedione; AUC = Area under the curve;
Foll = Number of follicles
[y]*P* < 0.005
[a]Pearson Correlation constant
[b]Percentage rise in the A_4 level
[c]number of follicles >16 mm
[d]number of follicles 12-16 mm
[e]number of follicles >12 mm

Table 4 Correlation of A_4 parameters to the cycle outcome parameters in Group II (PCOS Group)

R^a	Primary A_4	increase A_4%[b]	Max A_4	A_4 AUC
Foll 12-16[d]	0.513[y]	0.446[y]	0.674[y]	0.625[y]
Foll >16[c]	NS	0.3	0.339[y]	0.31[y]
Maximum E_2	0.514[y]	0.512[y]	0.717[y]	0.727[y]
Total Foll Selected[e]	*0.542[y]*	*0.5[y]*	*0.73[y]*	*0.673[y]*

E_2 = Estradiol, A_4 = Androstenedione, AUC = Area under the curve,
Foll = Number of follicles
[a]Pearson Correlation constant
[b]Percentage rise in the A_4 level
[c]number of follicles >16 mm
[d]number of follicles 12-16 mm
[e]number of follicles >12 mm
[y]A significant correlation; *P*<0.05

Table 5 Hierarchical multivariable regression analysis of independent variables in Group I (Control Group)

Model Summary for Group I

(A): Model Summary

Models		Change Statistics		
	R Square	R Square Change	F Change	Sig. F Change
1[a]	0,07	0,07	1,1	NS
2[b]	*0,42*	*0,35*	*25,4*	*<0.001*
3[c]	0,44	0,01	0,5	NS

(B): Coefficients

Models		Coefficients		
		B	Std. Error	P
1[a]	(Constant)	3,49	1,78	0,06
	Age	0,0004	0,05	0,99
	BMI	−0,02	0,04	0,59
	HOMA-IR	−0,19	0,13	0,15
2[b]	(Constant)	−0,46	1,63	0,78
	Age	0,06	0,04	0,17
	BMI	−0,01	0,03	0,75
	HOMA-IR	0,03	0,11	0,76
	$E_2(AUC)$	*0,0006*	*0,0001*	*<0.001*
3[c]	(Constant)	−0,50	1,65	0,77
	Age	0,06	0,04	0,20
	BMI	−0,02	0,03	0,66
	HOMA-IR	−0,03	0,13	0,83
	E_2 (AUC)	*0,0006*	*0,0001*	*<0.001*
	Primary A	0,48	0,49	0.68
	$A_4(AUC)$	0,01	0,07	0,85

[a]Model 1: including the independent variables Age, BMI, HOMA-IR
[b]Model 2: adding the independent variable E2 (AUC) to the previous Model 1
[c]Model: adding the independent variables Primary A and A4(AUC) to the previous Model 2

Table 6 Hierarchical multivariable regression analysis of independent variables in Group II (PCOS Group)

Model Summary for Group 2

(A): Model Summary

Models		Change Statistics		
	R Square	R Square Change	F Change	Sig. F Change
1[a]	0,05	0,05	0,3	0.8
2[b]	*0,49*	*0,44*	*16,6*	*<0.001*
3[c]	*0,63*	*0,14*	*15,1*	*0.001*

(B): Coefficients

Models		Coefficients		
		B	Std. Error	P
1[a]	(Constant)	5,68	3,37	0,10
	Age	−0,05	0,08	0,57
	BMI	−0,07	0,10	0,50
	HOMA-IR	−0,10	0,21	0,64
2[b]	(Constant)	6,14	2,52	0,02
	Age	−0,06	0,06	0,36
	BMI	−0,12	0,08	0,13
	HOMA-IR	−0,08	0,15	0,62
	$E_2(AUC)$	*0,002*	*0,001*	*<0,01*
3[c]	(Constant)	4,62	2,43	0,07
	Age	−0,01	0,06	0,89
	BMI	−0,14	0,07	0,05
	HOMA-IR	−0,06	0,14	0,67
	E_2 (AUC)	0,0005	0,0003	0,34
	Primary A	0,57	0,60	0,35
	$A_4(AUC)$	*0,114*	*0,03*	*0.01*

[a]Model 1: including the independent variables Age, BMI, HOMA-IR
[b]Model 2: adding the independent variable E2 (AUC) to the previous Model 1
[c]Model: adding the independent variables Primary A and A4(AUC) to the previous Model 2

combined were as in Table 7: 88.7%, 3.1 ng/mL and 5.4 ng*days for the percentage increase in A_4, the maximum A_4 value and area under the curve values for A_4, respectively.

Discussion

In this study, we observed that in PCOS, the cumulative A_4 response to low-dose rhFSH is a more valid measure of the number of selected follicles than the cumulative Estradiol (E_2) response [13]. The early and midfollicular A_4 variations are more critical determinants than the late follicular variations (following follicle selection), because drops or plateauing observed in A_4 in the late stages did not influence cycle outcome. The A_4 respond to rhFSH was earlier than that of E_2 in cycles with progressive follicular growth and conception.

In six cycles cancelled due to lack of response to rhFSH, there was no A_4 response. In contrast, in four of

the eight cycles cancelled due to excessive response, a dosage step-up had been made due to lack of E_2 response, while there had already been an initial A_4 response. If this corrective information could have been taken into account, an unnecessary step-up could have been avoided.

PCOS is the most common cause of anovulatory infertility, and is reported to comprise 15.3% of the women living in the geographic region where this study was conducted [14]. PCOS is characterised by three main elements: follicular growth arrest, hyperandrogenism and excessive folliculogenesis [15].

The chronic low-dose step up protocol used for ovulation induction in PCOS patients requires up to 14 days of rhFSH treatment to overcome a temporary ovarian refractoriness ending with follicle selection [16]. The follicular growth response initiated by rhFSH in the granulosa cell component when treated with

Table 7 ROC analysis of Androstenedione related parameters (maximum A4, percentage increase in A4 and A4 area under the curve) to define optimum threshold parameters to predict cycle cancellations in Group II

	Area Under Curve ± SEM [5-95p]	Optimum Threshold	Sensitivity (%)	Specificity (%)
A_4 percentage increase	0.73 ± 0.07 [0.6-0.87]	88.7%	75	72
Maximum A_4	0.78 ± 0.19 [0.66-0.9]	3.1 ng/mL	75	74
A_4 (AUC)	0.78 ± 0.06 [0.67-0.9]	5.4 ng*day	70	72

rhFSH is propagated to the theca cell component. During this initial response, in PCOS patients, the reversal of the FSH/LH effect in favour of FSH and aromatisation may not be as hormonally evident with rising E_2 blood levels as the thecal androgen response, especially at earlier stages. Granulosa cells of the antral follicle at this stage normally respond to this early rise in A_4 by increasing their aromatase activities, which is strongly counteracted by high AMH levels in the follicular microenvironment of the PCOS follicles, analogous to the AMH-FSH counteraction at later stages of follicular growth [17]. Thus, the transient follicular growth arrest is observed at this early stage due to the AMH-androgen counteraction [18, 19]. High androgen and AMH concentrations also contribute to the microenvironment that fosters excessive folliculogenesis and follicular growth arrest [11, 20–23].

Basal androgen blood levels measured at the beginning or during induction cycles have been reported in various studies in low responders, patients with diminished ovarian reserves, or normal responders, but not in PCOS cases. Ferrario et al. showed in a group of older women with low response that A_4 levels measured at the beginning of IVF cycles were predictors of positive outcome [24]. Similarly, Sun et al. have shown in a study of 1413 infertile women going through their first cycle of IVF that the testosterone blood levels measured at the beginning of the treatment cycles were predictors of the number of follicles larger than 14 mm on the day of hCG trigger, but were not predictors of conception [25]. It would be interesting and supplementary to monitor the testosterone response to rhFSH during ovulation induction cycles in prospective observational studies.

Our study had some *potential causes of bias and limitations* which need to be addressed. From the perspective of the Rotterdam 2003 definition of PCOS, cases with the nonPCOM/HA/OA (defined as phenotype B) may be being underrepresented in the infertile PCOS patients group (Group II) [26]. Another limitation was that the BMI's in *Group II* were slightly, but significantly higher than *Group I*. However, in the hierarchical multivariable regression conducted, BMI as well as age and HOMA-IR were included in a separate model and their effects on the total number of selected follicles were found to be insignificant in both *Groups I and II*.

Conclusion

The findings in this clinical study suggest that the reactive rise in androstenedione in the early follicular phase is a better predictor of the number of follicles selected than the conventionally used reactive rise in estradiol in PCOS cases. The longer/higher is the increase in its blood levels, the more are the follicles joining the growing cohort with an increasing risk of excessive ovarian response. On the other hand, androstenedione is an earlier and more reliable marker of the initial ovarian response to gonadotropins and this earlier response may be essential for progressive follicle growth and possibly a conception in an ovulation induction and intrauterine insemination cycle (using rhFSH) in PCOS. It still needs to be further studied in prospective studies encompassing induction cycles managed mainly with A_4 monitoring, to provide stronger evidence if androstenedione monitoring provides a more valid and useful information to indicate ovarian response and if an earlier androstenedione response is associated with conception.

Abbreviations

A4: Androstenedione; AMH: Antimüllerian hormone; AUC: Area under the curve; beta-hCG: beta human chorionic gonadotroopin; BMI: Body mass index; E2: Estradiol.; FSH: Follicle stimulating hormone; HA: Hyperandrogenism; HOMA-IR: Homeostatic model assessment of insulin resistance; IVF: In vitro fertilization; OA: Oligo/amenorrhea; P4: Progesterone; PCOM: polycystic ovarian morphology; PCOS: Polycystic ovary syndrome; rhFSH: Recombinant human follicle stimulating hormone; ROC: Receiver operating curve; TSH: Thryoid stimulating hormone

Acknowledgements

Not applicable.

Funding

The Funding of the study was provided by the Bagcilar Research and Training Hospital Education Planning Committee.

Authors' contributions

SEO conceptualized and suggested a plan for the study. TY then joined the study group and helped improve the plan and theoretically better defined the study plan and its connotations of possible results. With contribution of GA the study was started. The data collection and input was carried out by SEO and GA. The data analysis and manuscript writing was done by SEO and the manuscript read and approved by the three authors.

Competing interests

The authors declare that they have no competing interests.

Author details

[1]Bagcilar Research and Training Hospital Obgyn Department, Merkez Mh., Mimar Sinan Caddesi, 6. Sokak, 34100 Bagcilar, Istanbul, Turkey. [2]Marmara University Teaching and Research Hospital Obgyn Department, Fevzicakmak District Muhsin Yazicioglu Street 10 Ustkaynarca Pendik, Istanbul, Turkey.

References

1. Homburg R, Howles CM. Low-dose FSH therapy for anovulatory infertility associated with polycystic ovary syndrome: rationale, results, reflections and refinements. Hum Reprod Update. 1999;5:493–9.
2. Nastri CO, Teixeira DM, Moroni RM, Leitão VM, Martins WP. Ovarian hyperstimulation syndrome: pathophysiology, staging, prediction and prevention. Ultrasound Obstet Gynecol. 2015;45(4):377–93.
3. White DM, Polson DW, Kiddy D, Sagle P, Watson H, Gilling-Smith C, et al. Induction of ovulation with low-dose gonadotropins in polycystic ovary syndrome: an analysis of 109 pregnancies in 225 women. J Clin Endocrinol Metab. 1996;81:3821–4.
4. Tsang BK, Taheri A, Ainsworth L, Downey BR. Secretion of 17 alpha-hydroxyprogesterone, androstenedione, and estrogens by porcine granulosa and theca interna cells in culture. Can J Physiol Pharmacol. 1987;65:1951–6.
5. Arai S, Ito K. Androstenedione. Nihon Rinsho. 2010;68(Suppl 7):374–6.
6. Dewailly D, Lujan ME, Carmina E, Cedars MI, Laven J, Norman RJ, et al. Definition and significance of polycystic ovarian morphology: a task force report from the androgen excess and polycystic ovary syndrome society. Hum Reprod Update. 2014;20:334–52.
7. Catteau-Jonard S, Dewailly D. Anti-Mullerian hormone and polycystic ovary syndrome. Gynecol Obstet Fertil. 2011;39:514–7.
8. Dewailly D, Pigny P, Soudan B, Catteau-Jonard S, Decanter C, Poncelet E, Duhamel A. Reconciling the definitions of polycystic ovary syndrome: the ovarian follicle number and serum anti-Müllerian hormone concentrations aggregate with the markers of hyperandrogenism. J Clin Endocrinol Metab. 2010;95:4399–405.
9. Hassa H, Tanir HM, Yildirim A, Senses T, Eskalen M, Mutlu FS. The hirsutism scoring system should be population specific. Fertil Steril. 2005;84:778–80.
10. Yildiz BO, Bolour S, Woods K, Moore A, Azziz R. Visually scoring hirsutism. Hum Reprod Update. 2010;16:51–64.
11. Pasquali R, Zanotti L, Fanelli F, Mezzullo M, Fazzini A, et al. Defining Hyperandrogenism in women with polycystic ovary syndrome: a challenging perspective. J Clin Endocrinol Metab. 2016;101:2013–22.
12. Romualdi D, Di Florio C, Tagliaferri V, De Cicco S, Gagliano D, Immediata V, et al. The role of anti-Müllerian hormone in the characterization of the different polycystic ovary syndrome phenotypes. Reprod Sci. 2016;23:655–1.
13. Azziz R, Carmina E, Dewailly D, Diamanti-Kandarakis E, EscobarMorreale HF, Futterweit W, et al. Positions statement: criteria for defining polycystic ovary syndrome as a predominantly hyperandrogenic syndrome: an androgen excess society guideline. J Clin Endocrinol Metab. 2006;91:4237–45.
14. Yildiz BO, Bozdag G, Yapici Z, Esinler I, Yarali H. Prevalence, phenotype and cardiometabolic risk of polycystic ovary syndrome under different diagnostic criteria. Hum Reprod. 2012;27(10):3067–73.
15. Jonard S, Dewailly D. The follicular excess in polycystic ovaries, due to intra-ovarian hyperandrogenism, may be the main culprit for the follicular arrest. Hum Reprod Update. 2004;10:107–17.
16. Brown JB. Pituitary control of ovarian function–concepts derived from gonadotrophin therapy. Aust N Z J Obstet Gynaecol. 1978;18:46–54.
17. Almahbobi G, Anderiesz C, Hutchinson P, McFarlane JR, Wood C, Trounson AO. Functional integrity of granulosa cells from polycystic ovaries. Clin Endocrinol. 1996;44:571–80.
18. Lenie S, Smitz J. Functional AR signaling is evident in an in vitro mouse follicle culture bioassay that encompasses most stages of folliculogenesis. Biol Reprod. 2009;80:685–95.
19. Li M, Schatten H, Sun QY. Androgen receptor's destiny in mammalian oocytes: a new hypothesis. Mol Hum Reprod. 2009;15:149–54.
20. Weil SJ, Vendola K, Zhou J, Adesanya OO, Wang J, Okafor J, et al. Androgen receptor gene expression in the primate ovary: cellular localization, regulation, and functional correlations. J Clin Endocrinol Metab. 1998;83:2479–85.
21. Pache TD, Fauser BC. Polycystic ovaries in female-to-male transsexuals. Clin Endocrinol. 1993;39:702–3.
22. Murray AA, Gosden RG, Allison V, Spears N. Effect of androgens on the development of mouse follicles growing in vitro. J Reprod Fertil. 1998;113:27–33.
23. Magarelli PC, Zachow RJ, Magoffin DA. Developmental and hormonal regulation of rat theca-cell differentiation factor secretion in ovarian follicles. Biol Reprod. 1996;55:416–20.
24. Ferrario M, Secomandi R, Cappato M, Galbignani E, Frigerio L, Arnoldi M, et al. Ovarian and adrenal androgens may be useful markers to predict oocyte competence and embryo development in older women. Gynecol Endocrinol. 2015;31:125–30.
25. Sun B, Wang F, Sun J, Yu W, Sun Y. Basal serum testosterone levels correlate with ovarian response but do not predict pregnancy outcome in non-PCOS women undergoing IVF. J Assist Reprod Genet. 2014;31(7):829–35.
26. Rotterdam ESHRE/ASRM-Sponsored PCOS Consensus Workshop Group. Revised 2003 consensus on diagnostic criteria and long-term health risks related to polycystic ovary syndrome. Fertil Steril. 2004;1:19–25.

21

Small leucine-rich proteoglycans (SLRPs) in the endometrium of polycystic ovary syndrome women

Ricardo Santos Simões[1], José Maria Soares-Jr[1,4*], Manuel J. Simões[1], Helena B. Nader[2], Maria Cândida P. Baracat[1], Gustavo Arantes R. Maciel[1], Paulo C. Serafini[1], Ricardo Azziz[3] and Edmund C. Baracat[1]

Abstract

Background: Small leucine-rich proteoglycans (SLRPs) play an important role in tissue homeostasis and cell proliferation since these proteoglycans sequester multiple growth factors. However, the content of SLRPs in the endometrium of polycystic ovary syndrome (PCOS) women is unknown. Our purpose was to test the hypothesis that excessive endometrial proliferation in PCOS may be partly related to abnormalities in SLRPs.

Methods: In a cross section study a total of 20 endometrial samples were collected from 10 patients with PCOS and 10 ovulatory women during their proliferative (pre-ovulatory) phase. The study subjects were matched for age, body mass index and race. The age range was 20 to 35 years. All volunteers were evaluated in reproductive endocrinology clinic, Gynecology Division, Clinics Hospital, University of São Paulo Medical School Profile and concentration of small leucine-rich proteoglycans (decorin, lumican, fibromodulin and biglycan) were determined by immunohistochemical testing and Western blotting.

Results: Decorin and lumican demonstrated higher immunoreactivity and relative expression in the endometrium of women with PCOS compared to that of women with regular menstrual cycles.

Conclusion: Our data suggests that the endometrium of PCOS women demonstrate a greater content of SLRP than controls; decorin and lumican, in particular, were found in higher concentrations in the endometrium of PCOS women during the proliferative phase. These differences may, in part, explain the excess of endometrial proliferation frequently observed in PCOS. Further studies are warranted.

Keywords: Polycystic ovary syndrome, Endometrium, Small leucine-rich proteoglycans, Proliferative phase

Background

Polycystic ovary syndrome (PCOS) is an endocrine disorder which affects approximately 5 to 18% of women in childbearing age depending on the study population and the diagnostic criteria [1]. The syndrome is associated with ovulatory dysfunction, which can lead to menstrual cycle disruption including amenorrhea and oligomenorrhea increasing the incidence of infertility [2–4].

Additionally, in most cases PCOS show evidence of insulin resistance and hyperinsulinemia [1].

The incidence of endometrial hyperplasia in PCOS women is significantly higher than in controls and may, in part, be the result of hyperestrogenic anovulation and persistent hyperinsulinemia [5]. However, endometrial function in women with PCOS appears to differ significantly from that of normal endometrium, a difference that may predispose these patients to endometrial hyperplasia and carcinoma [6, 7].

Investigators have reported that in PCOS endometrial metabolism is altered, with local insulin resistance and increased growth factor content [8]. Growth factors mediating inflammation, including cytokines not only affect endometrial epithelial proliferation, but may alter

* Correspondence: jsoares415@hotmail.com
[1]Disciplina de Ginecologia, Departamento de Obstetrícia e Ginecologia, Hospital das Clínicas, Faculdade de Medicina da Universidade de São Paulo, São Paulo, Brazil
[4]Av. Dr. Enéas de Carvalho Aguiar, 255 - 10o.andar - Sala 10.167 - 05403-900, São Paulo, SP, Brazil
Full list of author information is available at the end of the article

factors in the extracellular matrix (ECM), including the production and action of small leucine-rich proteoglycans (SLRPs) [9, 10]. These proteoglycans play an important role in tissue homeostasis and cell proliferation, and protect the endometrium against agents that induce excessive endometrial proliferation [11–14]. Decorin, a specific SLRP, induces cell cycle arrest by activating cyclin-dependent protein kinase inhibitor, decreasing the activity and abundance of multiple cyclins, activating pro-apoptotic pathways and upregulating p21 synthesis in human endometrial stromal cells [14, 15].

The increased risk of endometrial hyperplasia and malignancy in PCOS is believed to be due not only to the reduction in the cyclic effect of progesterone, leading to chronic estrogen exposure, but also to the abnormal production of a large number of growth factors, cytokines, and other elements mediating inflammation [9, 10]. These factors may alter factors in the ECM, including SRLPs. However, the content of SLRPs in the endometrium of PCOS is unknown. Therefore, we designed a pilot study to test the hypothesis that the content of SLRPs, including decorin, lumican, fibromodulin, and biglycan, in the endometrium of PCOS subjects is detectable, and abnormal, which may predispose these patients to the development of endometrial hyperplasia and malignancy.

Methods
Study subjects
PCOS and control women were recruited from an outpatient reproductive endocrinology clinic at an academic tertiary medical care center (Gynecology Division, Clinics Hospital) from 2013 to 2015. We prospectively recruited all PCOS subjects first and then a match among controls was sought (i.e. ±4 kg/m^2 in BMI, ±4 years in age, and similar race to the PCOS subject), either from a previously recruited pool of controls or, if no control with the needed parameters was so identified, then a new control was sought. This recruitment strategy yielded cohorts of PCOS and controls similar in number, mean BMI, mean age and race distribution.

PCOS patients
The diagnosis of PCOS was made in accordance with the Rotterdam 2003 criteria, and subjects were categorized by phenotype (phenotype A-D) [16, 17]. Clinical hyperandrogenism was established by the presence of hirsutism, determined by a modified Ferriman and Gallwey (mFG) score equal to or higher than 8.

Control
Controls were healthy women with confirmed fertility (having had at least one child previously), who had undergone tubal ligation and had a long-term history of menstrual cycles with regular intervals (25–35 days).

These women were not using hormonal contraceptive methods.

All subjects (PCOS patients and control) were 20–35 years of age. Women who had causes of hyperandrogenism other than PCOS, anovulation which had been treated with hormones or other drugs in the 6 months prior to the study, systemic diseases, sexually transmitted diseases, uterine tumors, ovarian cysts or tumors, additional endocrine disorders, or using any hormones, including hormonally active herbal substances, statins, corticoids, or infertility drugs in the previous 6 months were excluded.

All participants of the study were subjected to a detailed history and physical examination, where height, weight, waist circumference (WC), hip circumference (HC), hirsutism by the mFG score, and a transvaginal ultrasound scan of the ovaries was obtained. Waist circumference was measured at the narrowest area between the last rib and the iliac crest, and HC at the most prominent point of the gluteal area.

This study was approved by the Research Ethics Committee of the Clinics Hospital, University of São Paulo School of Medicine (CEP 0164/09) and informed written consent was obtained from all subjects. The study was carried out from April 1, 2012 to August 31, 2015.

Endometrial sampling
Endometrial samples (amount was 1.3 ± 0.45 g) were obtained using the Pipelle de Cornier catheter (Laboratoire CCD, Paris, France). Participants in the PCOS group were generally anovulatory and their endometrial biopsies were performed randomly after a negative pregnancy (β-hCG) result. Biopsies in the control group were scheduled during cycle days eight to twelve of the menstrual cycle. The rationale for this schedule was to avoid the menstruation period and the periovulatory phase [18].

Histological processing of the endometrial samples
Endometrial samples were fixed for 24 h in 10% formaldehyde, dehydrated in increasing concentrations of ethyl alcohol, cleared in xylene, and then imbedded in paraffin. Paraffin-embedded samples were then cut into ten 3-μm sections per subject. Eight of these sections were stained for SLRPs by immunohistochemistry (see below), and the two remaining sections were stained with hematoxylin and eosin (H&E), to confirm the menstrual cycle phase (proliferative) using the criteria suggested by Noyes et al. [19] (Fig. 1).

Sections of endometrium were incubated with the primary antibody for detection of decorin (Abcam 175,404), lumican (Abcam 168,348), fibromodulin (Bioss 12,362), and biglycan (Bioss 7552R), incubated with a second antibody, namely chicken antirabbit immunoglobulin G (DakoCytomation, Glostrup, Denmark), and then incubated in 0.05%

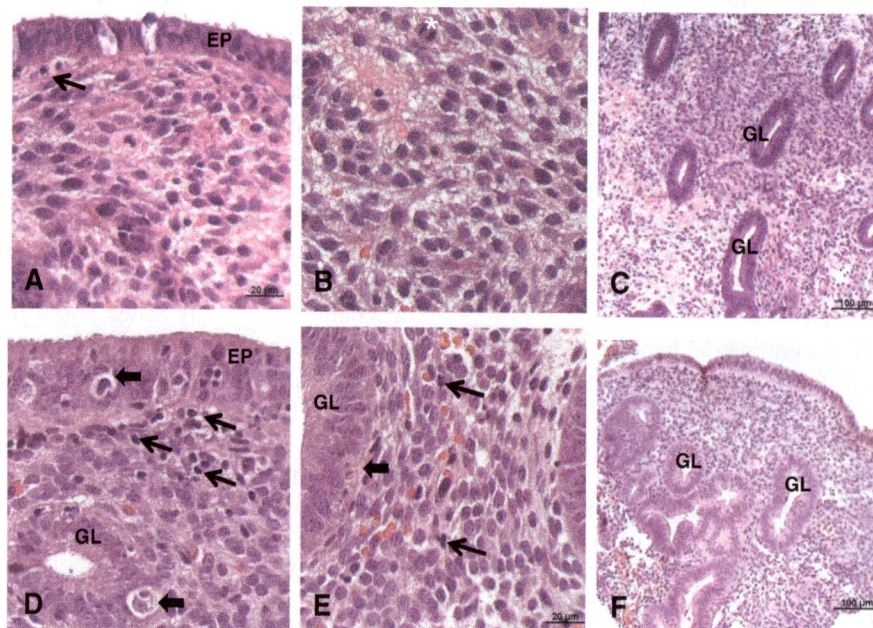

Fig. 1 Photomicrographs of the endometrium in the proliferative phase (**a, b,** and **c**) of the CONTROL and PCOS women (**d, e,** and **f**). Note thicker surface epithelium (EP) and gland (GL) as well as a higher concentration of leukocytes within the lamina propria of the endometrium of PCOS patients in **d** and **e** compared to **a** and **b** (*thin arrows*). Also note typical apoptosis in **d** and **e** (*thick arrows*) (* mitotic figure). Staining with H.E. **d** = 200X, **b** and **e** = 400X, and **c** and **f** = 100X

DAB (3,3′-diaminobenzidine) (Sigma Chemical Co). Negative controls were prepared by incubating the sections with rabbit nonspecific immunoglobulin fraction (DAKOCytomation) instead of the primary antibody and by staining the sections with hematoxylin for nucleous identification.

The images obtained were examined with optical microscope and digitally analyzed with the Carl Zeiss® AxioVision microscopy software (Rel. 4.6. Oberkochen, Baden-Württemberg).

Tissue homogenate preparation and Western blot analysis
Endometrial samples were homogenized, prepared, and sonicated in a buffer of 50 mM Tris-HCl, 150 mM NaCl, and 1% Triton-X pH 7.4 containing a complete protease inhibitor cocktail and PhosSTOP tablets (Roche Applied Science). Protein levels were determined by the Bradford assay and equalized prior to boiling in Laemmli buffer (Bio-Rad Laboratories, Hercules, CA, USA). To detect Gal-1 and MAPKs, protein extracts (40 μg per lane) were loaded onto a 15% SDS-PAGE together with appropriate molecular weight markers (Bio-Rad Laboratories) and transferred to ECL Hybond nitrocellulose membranes. Reversible protein staining of the membranes with 0.1% Ponceau-S in 5% acetic acid (Santa Cruz Biotechnology, Santa Cruz, CA, USA) was performed to verify protein transfer.

Membranes were incubated for 15 min in 5% BSA in Tris-buffered saline (TBS) before the addition of the rabbit polyclonal antibodies anti-decorin (Abcam175404), anti-lumican (Abcam168348), anti-fibromodulin (Bioss-12362R), anti-biglycan (Bioss-7552R), and anti-β-actin (Bs-12362R), all of which were diluted 1:500 in TBS with 0.1% Tween 20 (antibodies were purchased from Santa Cruz Biotechnology). Incubation was followed by 15 min of washing with TBS and 60 min of incubation at room temperature with peroxidase-conjugated goat anti-rabbit IgG (1:1000; Thermo Fisher Scientific, Inc., Rockford, MI, USA). Membranes were again washed for 15 min with TBS. Immunoreactive proteins were detected using an enhanced Supersignal West Pico chemiluminescent substrate kit (Thermo Fisher Scientific).

After exposure of the blots in dark room the resulting x-ray film was developed, imaged and quantified using ImageJ software1.440 (http://imagej.nih.gov/ij/ National Institutes of Health, Bethesda, MD, USA) to determine the relative expression (arbitrary units, AU) of SRPL/β-actin.

Hormonal assays
The serum levels of thyroid-stimulating hormone (TSH), free thyroxine, follicle-stimulating hormone (FSH), lutein hormone (LH), total testosterone (TT), free testosterone (Tfree), androstenedione (A), cortisol, prolactin (PRL), dehydroepiandrosterone sulfate (DHEAS), 17α-hydroxyprogesterone (17-OHP), fasting insulin, fasting glucose, 2-h oral glucose tolerance test, β-human chorionic gonadotropin (β-hCG), and

sex hormone-binding globulin (SHBG) were measured in both groups. Total testosterone levels were determined in triplicate using an electrochemiluminescence immunoassay (Testosterone II Cobas™ kit, Roche Diagnostics GmbH, Mannheim, Germany). The minimum detectable level of TT with this assay is 0.025 ng/ml and the main cross-reaction is with androstenedione (< 2.5%). The intra assay coefficient of variation (CV) was 12.5% and the inter assay CV was 13.8%.

Statistical analysis

All measurements were assessed for normality using the Kolmogorov-Smirnov test. The unpaired Student t-test was used to compare the PCOS and CONTROL groups. Statistical analysis was performed using the GraphPad Prism software version 3.0 for Windows (GraphPad Software, San Diego, CA, USA). The data are presented as mean ± standard deviation (SD), and the significance level was set at $p < 0.05$.

Results

A total of 20 women, aged 20 to 35 years, agreed to participate in this pilot study: a) 10 women with PCOS (PCOS), all phenotype A (hyperandrogenism either clinical and/or biochemical + ovulatory dysfunction + polycystic ovarian morphology), and b) 10 matched controls (CONTROL). The characteristics of these groups are depicted in Table 1.

Morphological analysis of endometrial samples

Morphological analysis confirmed that in CONTROL endometrial tissue obtained was in the proliferative

Table 1 Characteristics of participants

	CONTROL ($n = 10$)	PCOS ($n = 10$)	p-value
Age, years	28.6 ± 2.0	29.6 ± 1.2	NS
Caucasian, n	5	6	NS
BMI, Kg/m²	27.49 ± 2.45	28.01 ± 3.19	NS
TT (ng/dL)	35.9 ± 11.7	83.09 ± 24.8	< 0.05*
DHEAS (mg/mL)	421.5 ± 52.1	520.4 ± 82.1	NS
TSH (µUI/mL)	2.8 ± 1.7	2.9 ± 1.6	NS
Insulin (µUI/mL)	8.8 ± 2.9	15.5 ± 3.5	< 0.05*
Glucose (mg/dL)	81.8 ± 8.6	89.2 ± 11.9	NS
17-OHP (mg/mL)	17.3 ± 8.4	18.3 ± 7.4	NS
FSH (mUI/ml)	5.0 ± 1.2	5.1 ± 1.1	NS
LH (mUI/ml)	5.9 ± 2.9	9.5 ± 3.8	< 0.05*
PRL (ng/dl)	10.8 (4.3–34.5)	11.4 (4.2–33.5)	NS
A (ng/mL)	2.2 ± 0.8	4.2 ± 1.3	< 0.05*
Tfree (pg/dl)	1.7 ± 0.40	2.1 ± 1.0	NS

Data are expressed as median and standard deviation; *BMI* Body mass index, *TT* total testosterone, *TSH* thyroid stimulating hormone, *Tfree* free testosterone, *A* androstenedione, *LH* lutein hormone, *FSH* follicle-stimulating hormone, *PRL* prolactin, *17-OHP* 17α-hydroxyprogesterone, *DHEAS* dehydroepiandrosterone sulfate, *NS* nonsignificant difference ($p > 0.05$). *Significance of P-value <0.05

phase on days 8–12 of the menstrual cycle. Samples demonstrated a simple columnar epithelium lining and well-developed glands with cells in mitosis and endometrial stroma with several fibroblasts with an obvious elliptical nucleus, indicating intense cellular activity and synthesis of extracellular matrix components (Fig. 1), which are normal findings in the proliferative phase of the menstrual cycle in ovulatory patients.

The endometrial tissue of PCOS subjects had the epithelial lining and the glands were thicker, and the endometrial stroma contained many leukocytes, consistent with excessive estrogenic action compared to CONTROL subjects [20]. In some PCOS subjects epithelial cells with signs of apoptosis and well-developed endometrial stroma were observed (Fig. 1).

Immunohistochemical detection and comparison of SLRPs in the endometrium

Immunohistochemical analysis demonstrated SLRPs throughout the ECM of endometrial samples of both CONTROL and PCOS subjects. In both groups, SLRPs were also present throughout the endometrial stroma and could be observed clearly in the basement membrane of blood vessels, the epithelial lining, and the glands.

In CONTROL the intensity of immunoreactivity of biglycan and lumican was increased compared to that of decorin and fibromodulin. Alternatively, in PCOS biglycan, decorin, and lumican immunoreactivity were heightened compared with that of fibromodulin. Overall, the immunoreactivity pattern of SRPLs was higher in PCOS compared to CONTROL subjects (Fig. 2).

Quantification of SLRP expression by Western blotting

The expression of each SRPL studied (i.e. decorin, lumican, fibromodulin, and biglycan) relative to that of β-actin is summarized in Table 2 and Fig. 3. Overall, decorin and lumican had higher relative expressions in the PCOS than in CONTROL subjects ($p < 0.05$).

Discussion

Endometrial growth and differentiation is under the influence of sex hormones such as estrogen, progesterone, and androgens. In women with PCOS there is a deficiency in cyclic progesterone production due to chronic anovulation and a relative increase in other substances, such as insulin, cytokines, and growth factors, which results in an imbalance in endometrial hemostasis in these patients, possibly leading to abnormal uterine bleeding, infertility, and an increased risk of developing endometrial hyperplasia [3, 21–25]. The specific receptors for insulin and Insulin Growth Factors (IGFs) as well as high-affinity IGF-binding proteins (IGFBPs) have been detected in endometrial tissues [26]. IGFs have proliferative effects

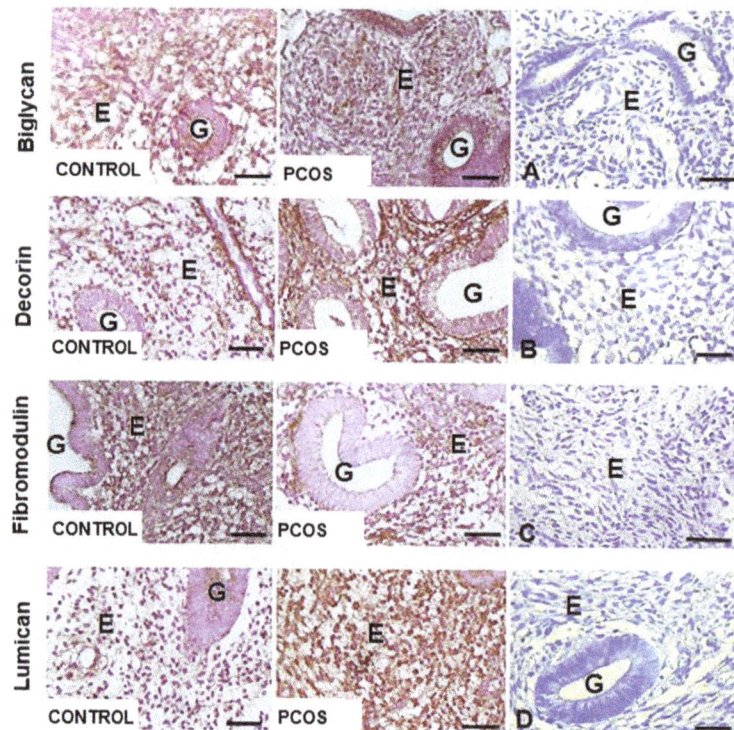

Fig. 2 Photomicrographs of the endometrium in the proliferative phase of CONTROL and PCOS women. Endometrial fragments subjected to immunohistochemical methods for identification of decorin, biglycan, lumican, and fibromodulin. Bar = 20 μm

and the secretion of these IGFBPs, which can modulate the bioavailability of IGFs by competing with the IGF receptor, is stimulated by progesterone and inhibited by insulin. Consequently the action of IGFs may be more intense in endometrial cells [6]. Moreover, both insulin and IGF-I inhibit the hepatic synthesis of sex-hormone binding globulin (SHBG) [27], and insulin stimulates aromatase activity in both endometrial glands and stroma, thus enhancing endogenous endometrial estrogen production [27, 28]. The final result is an excess of estrogen and IGFs action on the endometrium of PCOS.

Furthermore, data on stromal (non-epithelial) structures in the endometrium of women with PCOS are lacking [3, 10, 24, 25]. Therefore, our pilot study has contributed to the scientific literature with the following two findings: a) demonstrating the presence of SLRPs in the endometrium of women with PCOS; and b) demonstrating that the SLRP content in these women appears to be abnormal, specifically appearing to be enhanced relative to normals.

Previous studies have reported that SRLPs in the endometrium are important for embryonic implantation and placentation [24, 29, 30]. However, such studies have not included women with PCOS. In fact, the expression and distribution of endometrial decorin, biglycan, lumican, and fibromodulin are hormone dose dependent [30]. The hyperandrogenism may explain the upregulated production of decorin and lumican. Under the influence of the ovarian hormones estrogen and progesterone, the endometrial SLRPs undergo profound changes during the menstrual cycle in normal women. However, we have not assayed the level of estrogen and progesterone at time of endometrial sampling. It is one limitation of our study.

Increased decorin and lumican in endometrial ECM may have a local antiproliferative activity due to bind cytokines and growth factors [31, 32]. Furthermore, some investigators suggest that decorin and lumican inhibit tumor growth, particularly in prostate and lung cancer [33, 34]. Thus, these SLRPs may partially protect the

Table 2 SLRP content in endometrial stromal cells in PCOS and CONTROL subjects[a]

	Anti-decorin	Anti-biglycan	Anti-lumican	Anti-fibromodulin
CONTROL	3.4 ± 0.3**	17.5 ± 5.7	12.1 ± 0.5**	11.9 ± 2.7
PCOS	7.6 ± 0.5	21.1 ± 4.6	40.7 ± 0.4	15.1 ± 3.2

[a]Western blotting yield relative to beta-actin values of the SLRPs studied (mean ± SD) in endometrial stromal cells. Data are expressed as median and standard deviation. ** Significance of P-value <0.05

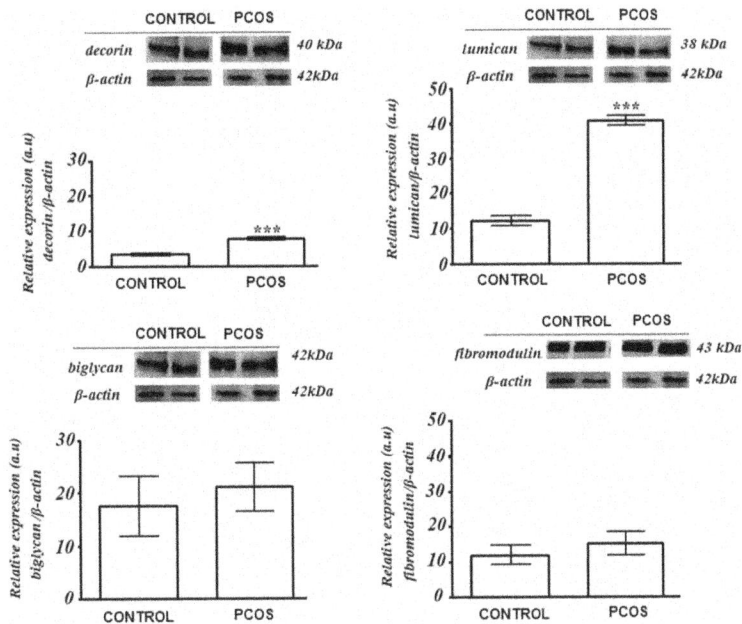

Fig. 3 Western blotting results for decorin, lumican, biglycan, and fibromodulin expression in the endometrium of CONTROL and PCOS women

endometrium of women with PCOS from malignant transformation.

The mechanism of action of decorin and lumican includes blocking tyrosine kinase receptors (TKR) and reducing the influence of EGFR, IGF-IR, HGFR, and VEGFR-2 on the endometrium. Moreover, decorin restrains angiogenesis by binding to thrombospondin-1, TGFβ, VEGFR-2, and possibly IGF-IR, and then halting tumor growth by antagonizing oncogenic TKRs and angiogenesis [35, 36]. These effects may negatively act on the implantation process by inhibiting trophoblast migration and invasion [36].

The collagen fiber is the most abundant component in the extracellular matrix. It is present in the ECM as a fibrillar protein providing structural support to cells and participating in cell-cell and cell-matrix interactions; thus, it has a fundamental role in tissue architecture [37–39]. Collagen fibers interact with extracellular matrix components, such as heparin sulfate. A research carried out by Giordano et al. [40] demonstrate alterations in the endometrial glycosaminoglycan levels – chiefly those of heparan sulfate – in women with PCOS.

Conclusion

Notwithstanding the sex steroid disorder, the exact pathophysiological mechanisms of endometrial PCOS believed to account for excessive endometrial proliferation are not known [41, 42]. Our data suggests that the endometrium of patients with PCOS exhibits higher expressions of decorin and lumican than that of healthy control women in the proliferative phase of the menstrual cycle. It is then possible that this proteoglycan excess may interfere with normal endometrial hemostasis in PCOS. Further studies are warranted.

Abbreviations

17-OHP: 17α-hydroxyprogesterone; A: Androstenedione; CV: Coefficient of variation; DHEAS: Dehydroepiandrosterone sulfate; ECM: Extracellular matrix; EGFR: Epidermal growth factor receptor; FSH: Follicle-stimulating hormone; H&E: Hematoxylin and eosin; HC: Hip circumference; IGFIR: Insulin-like growth factor receptor I; LH: Lutein hormone; MET: Hepatocyte growth factor receptor; mFG: Modified Ferriman and Gallwey; PCOS: Polycystic ovarian syndrome; PRL: Prolactin; SHBG: Sex hormone-binding globulin; SLRPs: Small leucine-rich proteoglycans; TBS: Tris-buffered saline; Tfree: Free testosterone; TGF: Transforming growth factor; TKR: Tyrosine kinase receptors; TSH: Thyroid-stimulating hormone; TT: Total testosterone; WC: Waist circumference; β-hCG: β-human chorionic gonadotropin

Acknowledgements

Not applicable.

Funding

This study was supported by FAPESP (#Fapesp 2009/54019–9) and CAPES (Brasilia – Brazil).

Authors' contributions

RSS, HBN, PCS and ECB contributed to conception, design, text writing and final approval of the version to be published. MJS and MCPB contributed for acquisition of data and text writing. JMS and GRAM analyzed and interpreted data. RA revised the article critically. All authors read and approved the final manuscript.

Authors' information

Not applicable.

Competing interests
The authors declare that they have no competing interests.

Author details
[1]Disciplina de Ginecologia, Departamento de Obstetrícia e Ginecologia, Hospital das Clínicas, Faculdade de Medicina da Universidade de São Paulo, São Paulo, Brazil. [2]Department of Molecular Biology, Federal University of São Paulo, São Paulo, Brazil. [3]Departments of Obstetrics and Gynecology and of Medicine, Medical College of Georgia, Augusta University, Augusta, GA, USA. [4]Av. Dr. Enéas de Carvalho Aguiar, 255 - 10o.andar - Sala 10.167 - 05403-900, São Paulo, SP, Brazil.

References
1. Azziz R. Introduction: Determinants of polycystic ovary syndrome. Fertil Steril. 2016;106:4–5.
2. Hull MG. Epidemiology of infertility and polycystic ovarian disease: endocrinological and demographic studies. Gynecol Endocrinol. 1987;1:235–45.
3. Lopes IM, Maganhin CC, Oliveira-Filho RM, Simões RS, Simões MJ, Iwata MC, et al. Histomorphometric Analysis and Markers of Endometrial Receptivity Embryonic Implantation in Women With Polycystic Ovary Syndrome During the Treatment With Progesterone. Reprod Sci. 2014;21:930–8.
4. Balen AH, Conway GS, Kaltsas G, Techatrasak K, Manning PJ, West C, Jacobs HS. Polycystic ovary syndrome: the spectrum of the disorder in 1741 patients. Hum Reprod. 1995;10:2107–11.
5. Barry JA, Azizia MM, Hardiman PJ. Risk of endometrial, ovarian and breast cancer in women with polycystic ovary syndrome: a systematic review and meta-analysis. Hum Reprod Update. 2014;20:748–58.
6. Gadducci A, Gargini A, Palla E, Fanucchi A, Genazzani AR. Polycystic ovary syndrome and gynecological cancers: is there a link? Gynecol Endocrinol. 2005;20:200–8.
7. Pillay OC, Te Fong LF, Crow JC, Benjamin E, Mould T, Atiomo W, Menon PA, Leonard AJ, Hardiman P. The association between polycystic ovaries and endometrial cancer. Hum Reprod. 2006;21:924–9.
8. Roemer KL, Young SL, Savaris RF. Characterization of GAB1 expression over the menstrual cycle in women with and without polycystic ovarian syndrome provides a new insight into its pathophysiology. J Clin Endocrinol Metab. 2014;99:E2162–8.
9. Lopes IM, Baracat MC, Simões Mde J, Simões RS, Baracat EC, Soares JM Jr. Endometrium in women with polycystic ovary syndrome during the window of implantation. Rev Assoc Med Bras. 2011;57:702–9.
10. Baracat MC, Serafini PC, Simões Rdos S, Maciel GA, Soares JM Jr, Baracat EC. Systematic review of cell adhesion molecules and estrogen receptor expression in the endometrium of patients with polycystic ovary syndrome. Int J Gynaecol Obstet. 2015;129(1):1–4.
11. Mauviel A, Santra M, Chen YQ, Uitto J, Iozzo RV. Transcriptional regulation of decorin gene expression. Induction by quiescence and repression by tumor necrosis factor-alpha. J Biol Chem. 1995;270:11692–700.
12. Seidler DG, Dreier R. Decorin and its galactosaminoglycan chain: extracellular regulator of cellular function? IUBMB Life. 2008;60:729–33.
13. Iozzo RV. The family of the small leucine-rich proteoglycans: key regulators of matrix assembly and cellular growth. Crit Rev Biochem Mol Biol. 1997;32:141–74.
14. Iozzo RV, Sanderson RD. Proteoglycans in cancer biology, tumour microenvironment and angiogenesis. J Cell Mol Med. 2011;15:1013–31.
15. Ono YJ, Terai Y, Tanabe A, Hayashi A, Hayashi M, Yamashita Y, Kyo S, Ohmichi M. Decorin induced by progesterone plays a crucial role in suppressing endometriosis. J Endocrinol. 2014;223:203–16.
16. Rotterdam ESHRE/ASRM-Sponsored PCOS Consensus Workshop Group. Revised 2003 consensus on diagnostic criteria and long-term health risks related to polycystic ovary syndrome (PCOS). Hum Reprod. 2004;19:41–7.
17. Lizneva D, Suturina L, Walker W, Brakta S, Gavrilova-Jordan L, Azziz R. Criteria, prevalence, and phenotypes of polycystic ovary syndrome. Fertil Steril. 2016;106:6–15.
18. Fraser IS, Critchley HO, Broder M, Munro MG. The FIGO recommendations
19. Noyes RW, Hertig AT, Rock J. Dating the endometrial biopsy. Am J Obstet Gynecol. 1975;122:262–3.
20. Andrade PM, Baracat EC, Simões MJ, Rodrigues de Lima G. Histomorphometric aspects of adult castrated rat endometrium after the use of estrogen, progesterone and tamoxifen. Clin Exp Obstet Gynecol. 2000;27:138–41.
21. Cheung AP. Ultrasound and menstrual history in predicting endometrial hyperplasia in polycystic ovary syndrome. Obstet Gynecol. 2001;98:325–31.
22. Apparao KBC, Lovely LP, Gui Y, Lininger RA, Lessey BA. Elevated endometrial androgen receptor expression in women with polycystic ovarian syndrome. Biol Reprod. 2002;66:297–304.
23. San Martin S, Soto-Suazo M, Ferreira de Oliveira S, Aplin JD, Abrahamsohn P, TMT Z. Small leucine-rich proteoglycans (SLRPs) in uterine tissues during pregnancy in mice. Reproduction. 2003;125:585–95.
24. Giudice LC. Endometrium in PCOS: Implantation and predisposition to endocrine CA. Best Pract Res Clin Endocrinol Metab. 2006;20:235–44.
25. Iatrakis G, Tsionis C, Adonakis G, Stoikidou M, Anthouli-Anagnostopoulou F, Parava M, et al. Polycystic ovarian syndrome, insulin resistance and thickness of the endometrium. Eur J Obstet Gynecol Reprod Biol. 2006;127:218–21.
26. Rutanen EM. Insulin-like growth factors in endometrial function. Gynecol Endocrinol. 1998;12(6):399–406.
27. Kaaks R. Plasma insulin, IGF-I and breast cancer. Gynecol Obstet Fertil. 2001; 29(3):185–91.
28. Randolph JF Jr, Kipersztok S, Ayers JW, Ansbacher R, Peegel H, Menon KM. The effect of insulin on aromatase activity in isolated human endometrial glands and stroma. Am J Obstet Gynecol. 1987;157(6):1534–9.
29. Kitaya K, Yasuo T. Dermatan sulfate proteoglycan biglycan as a potential selectin L/CD44 ligand involved in selective recruitment of peripheral blood CD16(−) natural killer cells into human endometrium. J Leukoc Biol. 2009;85:391–400.
30. Salgado RM, Favaro RR, Zorn TM. Modulation of small leucine-rich proteoglycans (SLRPs) expression in the mouse uterus by estradiol and progesterone. Reprod Biol Endocrinol. 2011;9:22.
31. Yamaguchi Y, Ruoslahti E. Expression of human proteoglycan in Chinese hamster ovary cells inhibits cell proliferation. Nature. 1988;336:244–6.
32. Vij N, Roberts L, Joyce S, Chakravarti S. Lumican suppresses cell proliferation and aids Fas - Fas ligand mediated apoptosis: implications in the cornea. Exp Eye Res. 2004;78:957–71.
33. Niu C, Liang C, Guo J, Cheng L, Zhang H, Qin X, Zhang Q, Ding L, Yuan B, Xu X, et al. Downregulation and growth inhibitory role of FHL1 in lung cancer. Int J Cancer. 2012;130:2549–56.
34. Coulson-Thomas VJ, Coulson-Thomas YM, Gesteira TF, Andrade de Paula CA, Carneiro CR, Ortiz V, et al. Lumican expression, localization and antitumor activity in prostate cancer. Exp Cell Res. 2013;319:967–81.
35. Hildebrand A, Romarís M, Rasmussen LM, Heinegård D, Twardzik DR, Border WA, Ruoslahti E. Interaction of the small interstitial proteoglycans biglycan, decorin and fibromodulin with transforming growth factor beta. Biochem J. 1994;302:527–34.
36. Lala PK, Nandi P. Mechanisms of trophoblast migration, endometrial angiogenesis in preeclampsia: The role of decorin. Cell Adhes Migr. 2016;10:111–25.
37. Vogel KG, Paulsson M, Heinegard D. Specific inhibition of type I and type II collagen fibrilogenesis by the small proteoglycan of tendon. Biochem J. 1984;222:587–97.
38. Vogel KG, Trotter JA. The effect of proteoglycan on the morphology of collagen fibrils formed in vitro. Coll Relat Res. 1987;7:105–14.
39. Rada JA, Cornuet PK, Hassell JR. Regulation of corneal collagen fibrillogenesis in vitro by corneal proteoglycan (lumican and decorin) core proteins. Exp Eye Res. 1993;56:635–48.
40. Giordano MV, Giordano LA, Gomes RC, Simões RS, Nader HB, Giordano MG, et al. The evaluation of endometrial sulfate glycosaminoglycans in women with polycystic ovary syndrome. Gynecol Endocrinol. 2015;31(4):278–81.
41. Azziz R, Carmina E, Dewailly D, Diamanti-Kandarakis E, Escobar-Morreale HF, Futterweit W, et al. Positions statement: criteria for defining polycystic ovary syndrome as a predominantly hyperandrogenic syndrome: an Androgen Excess Society guideline. J Clin Endocrinol Metab. 2006;91:4237–45.

on terminologies and definitions for normal and abnormal uterine bleeding. Semin Reprod Med. 2011;29(5):383–90.

22

Protective effects of GABA against metabolic and reproductive disturbances in letrozole induced polycystic ovarian syndrome in rats

Asad Ullah[1], Sarwat Jahan[1], Suhail Razak[1,2], Madeeha Pirzada[1], Hizb Ullah[1], Ali Almajwal[2], Naveed Rauf[1] and Tayyaba Afsar[3*]

Abstract

Background: PCOs is a heterogeneous disorder with anovulation/oligo ovulation usually taken as oligo menorrhoea or amenorrhoea, hyperandrogenemia, hirsutism, acne, androgen alopecia and polycystic ovaries as the key diagnostic feathers. The study was undertaken to investigate the possible protective and ameliorating effects of GABA in Letrozole induced PCOS model in rats by targeting insulin resistance.

Methods: PCOs in Adult female rat was induced by the daily gastric administration of letrozole (1 mg/kg/day) in CMC (0.5%) for 36 days. Rats were given metformin (2 mg/kg), GABA (100 mg/kg/day) and GABA (500 mg/kg/day) along with letrozole. One group severed as vehicle control. On the 37 day, the animals were euthanized, and anthropometrical, biochemical (glucose, insulin, lipids, testosterone, Estradiol, Progesterone, oral glucose tolerance test, total protein content in ovary, cholesterol level, triglyceride, HDL, LDL), Antioxidants (CAT, POD, GSR, ROS, GSH, TBARS), and histopathological evaluation of ovaries were carried out. Daily colpocytological examination was also carried out until the termination.

Results: Both the doses of GABA significantly reduced body weight, body mass index and testosterone. While the levels of CAT, SOD, POD and Estradiol (E_2) were significantly increased in the both doses of GABA. A favourable lipid profile, normal glucose tolerance, and decreased in the percentage of estrus smears were observed. Histopathological examination of ovary revealed a decreased in the number of cystic follicles, and decreased in the adipocytes respectively. The effects observed with GABA were comparable to that with metformin.

Conclusion: The results suggest that GABA treatment has shown protective effect in PCOs and provide beneficial effect either by reducing insulin resistance or by inducing antioxidant defence mechanisms.

Keywords: Gamma amino butyric acid, Follicles, Cysts, Oxidative stress, ELISA

Background

The polycystic ovary syndrome (PCOs) is one of the most common endocrine disorder present in women worldwide. PCOs is a heterogeneous disorder with anovulation/oligo ovulation usually taken as oligo menorrhoea or amenorrhoea, hyperandrogenemia, hirsutism, acne, androgen alopecia and polycystic ovaries as the key diagnostic feathers [1, 2]. There is also a great deal of chance for the development of metabolic and cardiovascular abnormalities because of the presence of insulin resistance (IR) as the central pathogenic feature [3].

Obesity and PCOs seems to be in close relation as many family studies have shown that weight gain promotes the chances of PCOs [4]. Lower levels of sex hormone binding globin (SHBG) are also observed [5]. Insulin resistance (IR) is main defining characteristic of PCOs, occurs in 50–70% of the population. Many of the scientists have also suggested that there is a big link between insulin levels and androgens [5]. Insulin stimulates thecal cells to produce androgens, and the higher levels of androgens are related to many problems as the

* Correspondence: Tayyaba_sona@yahoo.com
[3]Department of biochemistry, Quaid-i-Azam University, Islamabad, Pakistan
Full list of author information is available at the end of the article

symptoms seen in PCOs. The hyperinsulinemia which is observed in PCOs is mostly a result of increased secretion of basal insulin along with decreased hepatic insulin clearance [6]. The relationship has been supported by research which stated that reduced androgens were also seen with improvements in insulin sensitivity [7].

Inappropriate gonadotropins secretion is associated with the very classical forms of PCOs. Women with PCOs exhibit a high LH secretion with very low level of FSH secretion [8]. Premature androgen production may also explain the arrested antral follicle development in PCOs [9].

Hyperinsulinemia is a key element in the pathogenesis of PCOS. Insulin sensitizing drugs including metformin and thiazolidinediones (TZDs) have been used as a treatment for this syndrome [10]. It prevents hepatic glucose making and improves peripheral tissue sensitivity to insulin, reducing the androgen synthesis by ovarian theca cells [11]. Metformin also suppresses ovarian steroidogenesis [12, 13].

GABA exerts protective and regenerative effects on islets beta cell and reverses diabetes. Outside of the brain, GAD and GABA receptors have been reported in the pancreatic islets, the gastrointestinal tract, ovaries and adrenal medulla. Treatment with GABA improves glucose tolerance and insulin sensitivity by inhibiting inflammation in fat fed mice [14]. GABA has been reported as a positive regulator of antioxidant enzymes, reduces ROS and reducing cholesterol and triglycerides in the human [15, 16]. The present study was design to investigate the possible protective and ameliorating effects of GABA in Letrozole induced PCOS model in rats by targeting insulin resistance that can effects Glucose levels in PCOS, antioxidants status of the ovaries, production Reactive oxygen species (ROS) in the ovaries, synthesis and secretion of steroid hormones, follicle development and folliculogensis and cholesterol and plasma creatinine levels.

Methods

The study was conducted in the department of animal Sciences, Quaid-i-Azam University, Islamabad, Pakistan and the study was approved by the ethical committee of department of animal sciences and the work was performed in the months of March–May. Adult female rats, weighing 200 ± 15 g were obtained from the department animal facility of Quaid-i-Azam University, and were kept under 12/14 h light/dark cycle in 22–25 °C temperature. Animals were provided with standard laboratory food and tap water. Vaginal smear was examined daily for estrous cyclicity and the animals having two regular cycles were selected and included in the study. Letrozole (Femara) was purchased from novartis. Metformin (Glucophage) was purchased from merck Serrano.

Gamma-Aminobutyric acid (GABA) was purchased from International Labortory, USA and stored at room temperature. Enzyme linked immunosorbent assay (ELISA) kits for estradiol (E_2), testosterone (T) and progesterone (P_4) were purchased from Microlisa (Amgenix USA). Animals ($n = 25$) were divided into five groups according to the treatment. Group 1 animals were control group and were treated with 0.5% corboxymethylcellulose (CMC) through gastric intubation daily throughout the experiment. Animals in group 2 were allocated as PCOs group and received daily gavage of 1 mg/kg/day Letrozole dissolved in 0.5% CMC throughout the experiment. Animals in group 3 received letrozole (1 mg/kg.day) and cotreatment with metformin (2 mg/kg) from day 21 of treatment till the end of experiment. This group was allocated as metformin group. Group 4 animals were treated with daily dose of Letrozole (1 mg/kg/day) and GABA (100 mg/kg/day) from day 21 till the end of experiment. Animals in group 5 received daily dose of Letrozole (1 mg/kg/day) and were treated with GABA (500 mg/kg/day) from day 21 till the end of the experiment.

All the animals were anesthetized with chloroform on day 37, 24 h after the treatment. Blood samples were obtained by cardiac puncture in heparinized syringes and centrifuged at 3000 rpm for 10 min. Plasma was separated and placed at −20 °C until analyzed. Ovaries were removed, weighed and ovarian volume was measured. Left ovaries was placed at −80 °C for analysis of antioxidant enzymes while right ovaries were washed in cold physiological saline and placed in 10% formalin for histological processing. In tissue histology ovaries were placed in 10% formalin for 48 h for fixation. After fixation, tissues were subjected to ascending grades of alcohol for dehydration followed by two washes in xylene for clearing. Tissues were checked for clearance and then embedded in paraffin wax after words the fixed tissues were embedded for microtomy. In the process of microtomy and section cutting 7 micrometer thick sections were obtained from tissue. Every tenth section of the tissue was cut out of the ribbon and placed in warm water at low levels for stretching. Sections were carefully placed on albumenized slides, air dried for 30 min and transferred into paraffin oven for 1 h at 37–40 °C. For tissue staining sections were de-parafinized by placing the slides in xylene for 10 min and xylene washes were changed twice (10 min each). After complete deparaffinization, slices were subjected to descending grades of alcohol for rehydration. Destaining was done when needed with 95% Ethanol and cover slips were placed on the slides. For antioxidant enzymes the ovarian tissues were homogenized in 2 ml of phosphate buffer saline (PBS), centrifuged at 4 °C for 30 min at 3000 rpm. Supernatant was separated and was used for estimation of antioxidant enzymes, protein content and lipid profile.

In antioxidant enzymes Catalase (CAT) activity was determined by the decrease in absorbance due to H_2O_2 consumption by method of Aebi. [17]. Peroxidase (POD) activity in homogenate was determined by spectrophotometric method of [18]. Glutathione reductase (GSR) activity was determined by the method of [19]. Reactive oxygen species (ROS) activity was determined by following method of [20]. Reduced glutathione (GSH) activity was determined by following method of [21] with some modifications by utilizing Ellman's reagent (DTNB).

Estimation of Lipid per oxidation by TBARS was determined by the malondialdehyde in homogenate by reaction with thiobarbituric acid (TBA) by the method of [22].

Total protein content in ovarian tissue was quantitatively determined by using specific protein kit. The kit was purchased from AMEDA Labordiagonstik GmbH Krenngasse, Graz/Austria. Plasma cholesterol level was determined by using AMP diagnostic kit (AMEDA labordiagnostik Gmbh, Austria) and was analyzed on picco 5 chemistry analyzer. Plasma triglyceride levels were determined by using AMP diagnostic kit (AMEDA labordiagnostik Gmbh) and were analyzed on picco 5 chemistry analyser. Plasma HDL Cholesterol level was determined by using AMP diagnostic kit (AMEDA labordiagnostik Gmbh) and were analyzed on picco 5 chemistry analyser. Plasma LDL Cholesterol level was determined by using AMP diagnostic kit (AMEDA labordiagnostik Gmbh) and were analyzed on picco 5 chemistry analyser.

For the hormonal analysis three different kits were purchased form (Amgenix Inc., USA) for the determination of testosterone, Estradiol and progesterone from serum. Testosterone concentrations were quantitatively determined by using EIA tests kits (Amgenix Inc., USA). Estradiol EIA tests kits (Amgenix Inc., USA) were used to determine E_2 concentrations (pg/ml) in the serum. Progesterone (P4) EIA tests kits (Amgenix Inc., USA) were used to determine P4 concentrations (ng/ml) in the serum.

All the data were expressed as Mean ± SEM. One way Analysis of Variance (ANOVA) followed by tukey's test was used for comparing different groups using graph pad prism 5 software. Probability value less than 0.05 was considered statistically significant.

Results
Protective effect of different doses of GABA against Letrozole induced Polycystic Ovarian syndrome was determined by using different parameter.

Determination of estrous cyclicity
Estrous cycle was studied by regular monitoring and collection of vaginal smear from all the experimental groups throughout the experiment. Estrous cycle in the PCOS group was irregular and long as compared to the control animals while the metformin and GABA treated groups showed normal estrous cycle. Changes in the Estrous cycle are represented in Fig. 1.

Body weight and blood glucose
Animals included in the study were of approximately equal initial body weights (Table 1). However, final body weights showed significant difference in PCOS when comparison was made with control and other treated groups. Significant increase in body weight was observed in PCOS group ($P < 0.001$) as compared to control group. Significant difference was also being observed in metformin treated group ($p < 0.05$), GABA 1 treated group ($P < 0.01$) and GABA 2 treated group ($P < 0.01$) as compared to the PCOS group (Table 1).

Blood glucose level as determined at day 1 of the experiment were same in all the groups, but Final blood glucose levels showed significant difference in PCOS when comparison was done with control and other treated groups (Table 1). There was Significant increase ($P < 0.001$) observed in blood glucose of PCOS group as compared to control group. In PCOS group blood glucose was significantly different as compared to metformin treated group ($p < 0.01$), GABA 1 and GABA 2 treated group ($P < 0.05$) and presented in Table 1.

Body length and body mass index (BMI)
There was significant increase ($p < 0.05$) in body length of PCOS group when compared with control group but there was no significant difference observed in the body length of metformin, GABA 1 and GABA 2 treated groups as compared to PCOS group. BMI was not significantly different in all treatment groups and presented in Table 1.

Ovarian diameter, abdominal circumference (AC) and thoracic circumference (TC)
There were no significant differences noticed in ovarian length, abdominal circumference and thoracic circumference in all the treated groups as compared to control group (Table 1).

Total protein, CAT, SOD and POD
Total protein content showed no significant difference in all treated groups. CAT and SOD content of the ovarian tissues in PCOS groups were significantly low ($P < 0.01$) as compared to the control group. It was also observed that the Metformin treated group showed a good recovery of CAT ($P < 0.05$) and SOD ($P < 0.001$) as compared to PCOS group. CAT and SOD levels were significantly high ($P < 0.05, 0.001$) in GABA 2 treated groups as compared to PCOS, but there was no significant difference observed in GABA 1 treated group (Table 2). POD activity in PCOS group was significantly

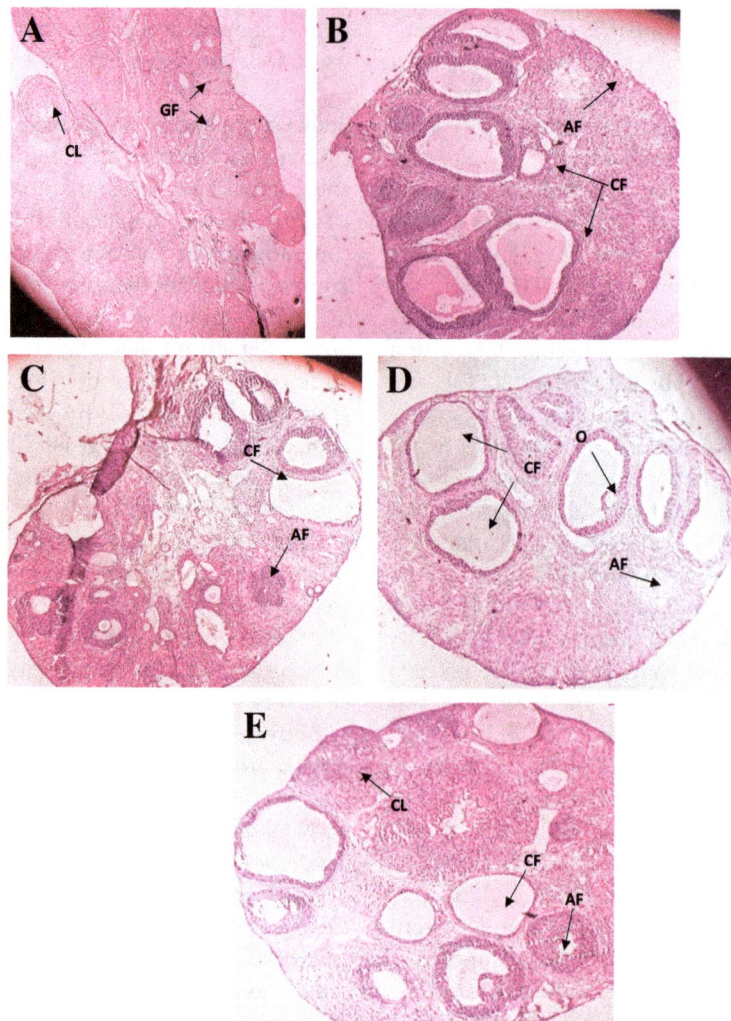

Fig. 1 Histopathological features of ovary in Letrozole induced PCOS in rats and (**a**) Control group (**b**) PCOS group (**c**) Metformin group (**d**) GABA 1 (**e**) GABA 2. Corpus Luteum (CL), Growing follicles (GF), Oocyte (O), Atertic follicle (AF), Cystic follicle (CF) (4X magnfication)

Table 1 Mean ± SEM of body weight, glucose level, body mass index, body mass gain, ovarian diameter, abdominal and thoracic circumference in control, PCOS, metformin, GAB 1 (100 mg/kg) and GABA 2 (500 mg/kg) treated groups before and after 36 days of experiment

Parameters	Control	PCOS	Metformin	GABA1	GABA2
Initial Body Weight (gm)	156 ± 01.37	156 ± 05.38	157 ± 07.57	150 ± 05.79	157 ± 04.22
Final Body Weight (gm)	181 ± 04.11	260 ± 02.81***	203 ± 03.29+	210 ± 04.57**++	222.2 ± 02.15**++
Initial Glucose (mg/dL)	117.20 ± 01.93	103.20 ± 02.81	122.41 ± 03.29	113.00 ± 04.57	120.40 ± 02.15
Final Glucose (mg/dL)	120.22 ± 03.21	166.46 ± 20.00***	135.21 ± 01.91++	129.00 ± 05.08+	138.40 ± 06.20+
Body mass Index (g/cm2)	0.49 ± 0.01	0.54 ± 0.02	0.47 ± 0.01	0.72 ± 0.03	0.69 ± 0.04
Body mass gain (g/kg)	4.34 ± 0.94	27.76 ± 8.61	16.21 ± 5.04	29.66 ± 6.47	15.17 ± 7.21
Right Ovary diameter (mm)	4.80 ± 00.37	5.10 ± 01.04	4.60 ± 00.25	6.10 ± 00.96	5.80 ± 00.12
Left Ovary diameter (mm)	5.00 ± 0.44	5.60 ± 0.24	5.20 ± 0.20	6.00 ± 0.15	5.70 ± 0.20
Abdominal Circumference (cm)	1.06 ± 0.09	1.05 ± 0.31	1.06 ± 0.51	1.04 ± 0.44	1.09 ± 0.34
Thoracic circumference (cm)	1.06 ± 0.23	1.05 ± 0.10	1.06 ± 0.18	1.16 ± 0.29	1.22 ± 0.24

Values are expressed as Mean ± SEM
*, **, *** indicate significance from the control group at *P* < 0.001, 0. 01 and 0.05 probability level
+, ++, +++ indicate significance from the PCOS group at P < 0.001, 0. 01 and 0.05 probability level

Table 2 Mean ± SEM of total protein, CAT, SOD, POD, GST, GSR, GSH, T-BARS, ROS, cholesterol, triglycerides, HDL, testosterone, progesterone and estradiol concentrations in control, PCOS, metformin, GAB 1 (100 mg/kg) and GABA 2 (500 mg/kg) treated female rats after 34 days of experiment

Parameters	Control	PCOS	Metformin	GABA1	GABA2
Total Protein (mg/g)	2.55 ± 0.23	3.09 ± 0.41	2.77 ± 0.26	2.04 ± 0.05	2.65 ± 0.26
CAT (u/mg)	29.44 ± 2.60	23.41 ± 4.06**	22.63 ± 2.35+	17.05 ± 2.28*	26.94 ± 2.28+
SOD (u/mg)	1.21 ± 0.24	0.99 ± 0.13**	1.90 ± 0.21+++	1.48 ± 0.11+	2.63 ± 0.37*+++
POD (nmole)	0.09 ± 0.16	0.04 ± 0.07*	0.47 ± 0.02+++	0.12 ± 0.09	0.18 ± 0.38++
GST (u/mol/mg)	61.14 ± 11.39	65.82 ± 03.13	55.48 ± 08.27	72.95 ± 17.41	59.31 ± 23.72
GSR (u/mol/mg)	174.36 ± 8.90	29.23 ± 13.30**	162.38 ± 16.60+++	97.66 ± 12.94++	161.09 ± 12.89+++
GSR-PX (u/mol/mg)	24.86 ± 02.97	10.71 ± 04.41	54.30 ± 05.55**+++	48.03 ± 08.81*+++	22.57 ± 03.04
GSH (u/mol/mg)	405.74 ± 36.39	558.79 ± 95.65	405.23 ± 27.63	359.62 ± 06.16	495.53 ± 50.12
T-BARS (nmol/mg)	206.46 ± 33.81	436.70 ± 63.74**	268.63 ± 56.98++	293.39 ± 24.38	245.63 ± 73.20+
ROS (u/min)	39.47 ± 13.63	79.19 ± 11.20*	38.14 ± 03.53+	18.78 ± 11.51+++	12.18 ± 08.60+++
Cholesterol (mg/dL)	215.60 ± 3.43	231.10 ± 4.27*	211.30 ± 6.81	222.21 ± 2.53+	210.10 ± 3.34++
Triglycerides (mg/dL)	185.11 ± 4.23	213.10 ± 5.16**	197.40 ± 5.82	204.20 ± 5.93	190.12 ± 6.32+
HDL (mg/dL)	160.70 ± 4.17	144.41 ± 3.63	153.21 ± 1.80	156.43 ± 5.52	165.34 ± 4.24+
Testosterone (ng/ml)	1.24 ± 0.14	2.07 ± 0.14**	1.24 ± 0.17++	1.50 ± 0.20	1.35 ± 0.10++
Progesterone (ng/ml)	6.96 ± 0.10	6.70 ± 0.15	6.82 ± 0.07	6.63 ± 0.11	6.70 ± 0.21
Estradiol (pg/ml)	4.89 ± 0.14	2.79 ± 0.18*	4.40 ± 0.17+	2.36 ± 0.24	4.46 ± 0.46++

Values are expressed as Mean ± SEM

*, **, *** indicate significance from the control group at P < 0.001, 0. 01 and 0.05 probability level

+, ++, +++ indicate significance from the PCOS group at $P < 0.001$, 0. 01 and 0.05 probability level

reduced (P < 0.05) as compared to the control group. GABA 2 group has significantly high levels of POD ($P < 0.001$) but GABA 1 did not increased POD activity as compared to PCOS group (Table 2).

GST, GSR and GSR-PX
There was no significant difference in the GST activity in all the treated groups as compared to the control group. GSR activity was significantly reduced (P < 0.001) in PCOS group as compared to control group but in metformin treated group, GSR activity was significantly high (P < 0.001) as compared to PCOS group. Similarly in GABA 1 and GABA 2 treated groups, GSR activity was significantly high ($P < 0.01$ and P < 0.001 respectively) when compared to the PCOS group (Table 2). There was significant difference observed in GSR-PX activity of PCOS and control group. In GABA 1 and Metformin treated groups, GSR-PX values were significantly high (P < 0.001) as compared to PCOS group but GABA 2 did not show any effect on GSR-PX activity as compared to the PCOS group (Table 2).

GSH, T-BARS and ROS
There was no significant change observed in the GSH levels in PCOS and in all the other groups (Table 2). The Mean ± SEM of T-BARS were significantly high (P < 0.01) in the ovarian tissues of PCOS group as compared to the control group, while Metformin treatment

significantly reduced ($P < 0.01$) in ovarian T-BARS levels as compared to the PCOS group. The ovarian T-BARS levels in the GABA 2 treated group were significantly reduced as compared to the PCOS group (Table 2). Reactive oxygen species (ROS) in the ovarian tissues were determined and was found significantly high ($P < 0.05$) in PCOS group as compared to the control group. Metformin and GABA treatment (1 and 2) resulted in significant reduction in the levels of ROS ($P < 0.05$ and $P < 0.001$) when comparison was made with PCOS group (Table 2).

Cholesterol, triglyceride and HDL
Cholesterol concentrations (mg/dL) in PCOS group was significantly high (P < 0.05) as compared to control group, while they were low in Metformin treated group. GABA 1 and GABA 2 treatment caused a significant decrease in cholesterol concertation as shown in Table 2.

The levels of Triglycerides in PCOS groups were significantly high ($P < 0.01$) as compared to the control group. While Metformin and GABA 1 treatment caused no reduction in triglycerides concentration however GABA 2 did cause a significant difference as compared to PCOS (Table 2).

HDL concentrations did not change in PCOS, metformin and GABA 1 treated groups; however, GABA 2 treatment caused significant increase in HDL concentration as compared to PCOS group (Table 2).

Hormonal analysis

Plasma testosterone concentration was measured because letrozole has been reported to cause hyperandrogenism that leads to PCOS. Testosterone concentration in the PCOS group was significantly high ($P < 0.01$) as compared to the control group. Testosterone concentrations in metformin and GABA 2 was significantly low ($P < 0.01$) as compared to the PCOS group. Plasma progesterone concentration was not affected in all the treated groups. However, Estradiol concentration was significantly reduced ($P < 0.05$) in PCOS animals as compared to the control group. However, GABA 2 group exhibited significantly high ($P < 0.01$) levels of Estradiol as compared to the PCOS group (Table 2).

Histological results

Number of different types of follicles were counted and presented in Table 3. Two methods were used for counting of different types of follicle. They were counted on the basis of diameter and type of follicle i.e. cystic, fibrotic and corpus leuteum [23].

Follicles with diameter 20–60, 60–100 μm

Mean ± SEM number of follicles with 20–60 and 60–100 μm diameters were not significantly different in different groups (Table 3).

Follicles with diameter 100–200, 600 and > 600 μm

The mean number of ovarian follicle with 100–200 μm diameter were significantly reduced ($P < 0.05$) in PCOS as compared to the control group. There was no significant increase noticed in GABA treated groups. Follicles with diameter ranging from 200 to 600 μm in all treated groups were found with no significant difference. The mean numbers of ovarian follicle was greater than 600 μm were non-significantly different in PCOS, Metformin and GABA treated groups (Table 3).

Cystic follicle

There was a significant decrease ($p < 0.001$) found in the number of cystic follicles of Metformin group as compared to PCOS. It was also observed that the number of cystic follicles in GABA 1 and 2 treated groups were significantly decreased ($p < 0.001$) as compared to PCOS group (Table 3).

Atretic follicle

PCOS group showed a highly significant ($p < 0.001$) increase in number of atretic follicles as compared to control group. There was Significant ($p < 0.05$) decrease observed in the number of atretic follicles in Metformin GABA 1 and GABA 2 treated groups as compared with PCOS group (Fig. 1).

Corpus luteum

The Number of Corpus Leuteum significantly reduced ($p < 0.001$) in PCOS group as compared to control group. There was also no significant ($p < 0.001$) difference found in in the number of Corpus Leuteum of Metformin and GABA 2 treated groups as compared to PCOS group (Table 3).

Discussion

The present study was designed to investigate the possible beneficial effects of GABA in mitigating PCOS by targeting insulin resistance in letrozole induced PCOS model of albino rats. There have been studies which show that outside of the brain, GAD and GABA receptors have been reported in the pancreatic islets, the gastrointestinal tract, ovaries and adrenal medulla. On the basis of previous studies, we targeted insulin resistance via oral administration of GABA to treat letrozole induced PCOS in rats. Results of present study showed normal glucose levels in GABA and metformin treated groups while glucose levels were elevated in the PCOS

Table 3 Mean ± SEM number of ovarian follicles in control, PCOS, metformin, GAB 1 (100 mg/kg) and GABA 2 (500 mg/kg) after 34 days of experiment

Developing follicles (μm)	CONTROL	PCOS	METFORMIN	GABA 1	GABA 2
D 20–60	8.66 ± 0.55	9.00 ± 0.73	7.16 ± 0.70	9.66 ± 0.55	8.50 ± 0.50
D 60–100	7.60 ± 0.50	7.60 ± 0.92	7.20 ± 0.66	5.20 ± 0.91	5.20 ± 0.58
D 100–200	7.00 ± 0.70	3.00 ± 0.54*	8.20 ± 1.06	3.80 ± 0.80	4.80 ± 0.37
D 200–400	8.00 ± 0.70	4.60 ± 0.74	6.60 ± 1.07	4.80 ± 0.73	4.20 ± 0.73
D 400–600	2.20 ± 0.37	0.80 ± 0.58	1.00 ± 0.44	0.80 ± 0.37	0.60 ± 0.24
>600	3.20 ± 0.37	0.80 ± 0.58	0.60 ± 0.24	0.40 ± 0.24	1.20 ± 0.37
Cystic Follicle	0.00 ± 0.00	9.17 ± 0.70 **	5.16 ± 0.30++	6.16 ± 0.47++	7.33 ± 0.42 +
Corpus Luteum	8.80 ± 0.37	2.40 ± 0.24 ***	4.20 ± 0.58 +	2.40 ± 0.50 ++	4.40 ± 0.24 ++
Atretic Follicle	4.00 ± 0.25	3.50 ± 0.34 **+++	2.83 ± 0.47	2.66 ± 0.33	2.83 ± 0.40 +

Values are expressed as Mean ± SEM
*, **, *** indicate significance from the control group at $P < 0.001$, 0.01 and 0.05 probability level
+, ++, +++ indicate significance from the PCOS group at $P < 0.05$, $P < 0.01$ and $P < 0.001$ probability level

group. These findings have provided base for the study of further complications related to PCOS and insulin resistance.

Antioxidant enzymes provide the first line defence mechanism which prevents biological molecules (lipids, proteins, DNA) from damage by inhibiting ROS formation. Hydrogen peroxide (H_2O_2), nitric oxide (NO), superoxide anion (O_2^-) and hydroxyl radical (OH) are central reactive oxygen and nitrogen species that are involved in tumorigenesis and mutagenesis. Superoxide dismutase (SOD) counteracts toxic effects of superoxide anion. Levels of antioxidant enzymes are important because dismutation of superoxide anion to form H_2O_2 is catalysed by SOD while H_2O_2 is converted to water molecules by the activity of catalase (CAT) and glutathione peroxidase (GSH-PX) while reduced glutathione (GSH) is used as an electron donor in such reactions [24]. Similarly, GSH levels are retained by thiol containing non-protein compound called glutathione reductase (GSR). GSR regenerates GSH (reduced form) from GSSG (oxidized form) for the constant activity of GSH-PX [25]. In PCOS group, SOD, POD, and CAT were significantly reduced as compared to the control group; similarly, POD activity was also low in PCOS as compared to the control group. However GABA and metformin treatment significantly recovered activity of CAT, SOD and POD in letrozole induced PCOS model. GSH levels were not different in PCOS group and were similar to control, however, GSR and GSR-PX levels were reduced in PCOS. Metformin treatment and GABA treatment significantly induced levels of GSR and GSR-PX levels suggesting the protective effect of GABA as described previously [15, 16].

NADPH oxidases are specialized enzymes that can generate superoxide anion which can be eliminated by CAT, POD and SOD, decreasing LPO in order to protect spermatozoa from oxidative stress [26]. In the PCOS, reduced levels of antioxidants have been reported previously and have been linked to the female infertility [27]. Similarly GABA has been reported as an inducer of macrophages infiltration and induces antioxidant enzymes activity [15, 16]. Similarly antioxidant potential and antioxidant enzymes inducer effect of GABA has been reported previously, by reducing ROS in the tissues and neurons. In present study, antioxidant enzymes levels were reduced in the PCOS group as compared to the control animals. Similarly, ROS was high in PCOS but less in control groups. Interesting results were observed when comparison was made between metformin treated groups, GABA treated groups and PCOS animals. Metformin and GABA treatment not only involved in reducing ROS level in the ovarian tissues but also induces antioxidant enzymes and glutathione levels in the ovarian tissues. This effect of GABA may be due to the effect of GABA on antioxidant recovery through overcoming

insulin resistance or effecting primary fatty acid amide (pFAA) disorder which is caused by insulin resistance. High levels of lipid peroxidation as observed in the PCOS group were also recovered by treatment with metformin and GABA. These results are in consistent with previous studies in which GABA treatment reduced ROS and induced antioxidant enzymes in sperm and Roman hens [1, 2]. Similarly, insulin resistance leads into disruption of antioxidant status of the body besides hyperglycemia and obesity, which are also major causing agents that disrupts body defense mechanism [28, 29]. It was reported that GABA treatment for 20 weeks restored glucose levels and muscular oxidation by treating hyperglycemia and pFAA disorder in mice. Cholesterol level was significantly high in the PCOS group as compared to the control; however GABA treatment significantly reduced Cholesterol level. These results are in accordance with the previous study [30], reported that treatment with GABA reduces cholesterol levels in chronic ethanol treated rats. However triglycerides were not significantly changed in all treated groups. Interestingly, HDL levels were significantly high by (500 mg/kg) dose of GABA. Elevated levels of triglyceride were found in men who consumed GABA enriched white rice while HDL levels were not affected. Similarly cholesterol levels were found low in men who consumed white rice [31].

High levels of testosterone in PCOS, as an indicator of the disorder, were significantly reduced by metformin and GABA 2 treatment, while low level of estradiol in PCOS group were induced by treatment with metformin and GABA however, progesterone levels were not affected. These results suggest the healing of the ovarian tissues and reduction in the number of cysts in the tissues. Similarly, increase in number of healthy follicles may be induced by GABA treatment. These results can be supported by the normal levels of glucose found in metformin and GABA treated groups because insulin resistance is the major contributory factor in altering hormonal levels among PCOS patients.

Finally, histological observations supported the protective and beneficial effect of GABA in letrozole induced PCOS model of rats. Number of cystic follicles was reduced in GABA treated groups as compared to PCOS group same as in metformin treated group. Number of atratic follicles was also reduced in metformin and GABA treated groups as compared to the PCOS group. Number of corpus luteum was increased in metformin and GABA treated groups as compared to the PCOS group.

Conclusion

In conclusion present findings demonstrate the antiandrogenic properties of GABA in treating PCOS. GABA also protected the ovarian tissue and prevented cyst development in this study. This effect of GABA may be because of inducing first line defence mechanism of the body and by reducing insulin resistance that improves the reproductive health by acting on the ovarian tissues. However, GABA also showed estrogenic and antiandrogenic effects by recovering the ovarian cysts which could be supportive in managing PCOS. GABA also showed to boost the antioxidant status by reducing the oxidative stress, lipid peroxidation and ROS..It displayed a significant role in subsiding the hyperlipidemic state and hyperglycemic state and it can be used as a possible ameliorative medication for curing clinical and biochemical characteristics of polycystic ovary syndrome. Further studies are required to investigate the exact mechanism of action of GABA in PCOS Rats model and also to investigate the possible role of GABA in curing PCOS management in women so that it can be used as an adjunct therapy for the treatment pf PCOS.

Abbreviations
17 – β –E$_2$: 17 - β -estradiol; AC: Abdominal circumference; BMI: Body mass index; DPX: Di –n-butyl phthalate in xylene; E$_2$: Estradiol; ELISA: Enzyme linked immunosorbent assay; ER: Estrogen receptor; FSH: Follicle Stimulating Hormone; GABA: Gamma-Aminobutyric acid; GnRH: Gonadotrophin releasing hormone; HRP: Horseradish peroxidase; LH: Luteinizing Hormone; Ml: Milli liter; PCOS: Poly Cystic Ovarian Syndrome; ROS: Reactive Oxygen Specie; T: Testosterone; TC: Thoracic circumference; TMB: Tetra methyl benzidine; Ml: Micro liter; Mm: Micro meter

Acknowledgements
This piece of work was funded by the Department of Animal Sciences Quaid-i-Azam University Islamabad, Pakistan. Furthermore we are grateful to the Deanship of Scientific Research at King Saud University for its funding of this research through Research Group Project number 193.

Funding
The project was partially funded by the Higher Education Commission (HEC) of Pakistan. We are grateful to the Deanship of Scientific Research at King Saud University for its funding of this research through Research Group Project number 193.

Authors' contributions
SJ designed the study, conceived the study and analyzed the results. AU and MP conceived an initial part of the study, performed the experiment, histology and helped in compiling the results. HW performed antioxidant enzymes estimation. AU performed tissue histology and helped in writing the results. HW and AU wrote the paper with input from all other authors SJ, SR, TA and AA made substantial contribution in interpretation of data and revising the manuscript for intellectual content. All authors read and approved the final manuscript.

Competing interests
The authors declare that they have no competing interests.

Author details
[1]Department of Animal Sciences, Quaid-i-Azam University, Islamabad, Pakistan. [2]Department of Community Health Sciences, College of Applied Medical Sciences, King Saud University, Riyadh, Saudi Arabia. [3]Department of biochemistry, Quaid-i-Azam University, Islamabad, Pakistan.

References
1. Abbott DH, Tarantal AF, Dumesic DA. Am J Primatol. 2009;71(9):776–84.
2. Zhang HY, Guo CX, Zhu FF, Qu PP, Lin WJ, Xiong J. Arch Gynecol Obstet. 2013;287(3):525–31.
3. Sam S, Dunaif A. Trends Endocrinol Metab. 2003;14(8):365–70.
4. Singh B, Panda S, Nanda R, Pati S, Mangaraj M, Sahu PK, Mohapatra PC. Indian J Clin Biochem. 2010;25(4):367–70.
5. Tsilchorozidou T, Conway GS. Clin Endocrin. 2004;61(5):567–72.
6. Dunaif A. Endocr Rev. 1997;18(6):774–800.
7. Moran C, Tena G, Moran S, Ruiz P, Reyna R, Duque X. Gynecol Obstet Investig. 2010;69(4):274–80.
8. Yen HC, Katz MH, Krop S. Toxicol Appl Pharm. 1970;17(3):597–604.
9. Franks S, Gilling-Smith C, Watson H, Willis D. Endocrinol Metab Clin N Am. 1999;28(2):361–78.
10. Nawrocka J, Starczewski A. Gynecol Endocrinol. 2007;23(4):231–7.
11. Cibula D, Fanta M, Vrbikova J, Stanicka S, Dvorakova K, Hill M, Skrha J, Zivny J, Skrenkova J. Hum Reprod. 2005;20(1):180–4.
12. Attia GR, Rainey WE, Carr BR. Fertil Steril. 2001;76(3):517–24.
13. Mansfield R, Galea R, Brincat M, Hole D, Mason H. Fertil Steril. 2003;79(4):956–62.
14. Tian J, Dang H, Kaufman DL. PLoS One. 2011;6(9):e25337.
15. Tian J, Chau C, Hales TG, Kaufman DL. J Neuroimmunol. 1999;96(1):21–8.
16. Reyes-García MG, Hernández-Hernández F, Hernández-Téllez B, García-Tamayo F. J Neuroimmunol. 2007;188(1):64–8.
17. Aebi H. Methods Enzymol. 1984;105:121–6.
18. Carlberg I, Mannervik B. J Biol Chem. 1975;250(14):5475–80.
19. Goldberg D, Spooner R. Methods Enzymatic Anal. 1983;3:258–65.
20. P. I. Tyan, A. H. Radwan, A. Eid, A. G. Haddad, D. Wehbe, A. T. Taher, BioMed research international 2014, 2014.
21. Burtis CA, Ashwood E, Tietz N. Philadelphia London L WB Saunders Company. 1994;32:610–2.
22. Iqbal M, Sharma S, Rezazadeh H, Hasan N, Abdulla M, Athar M. Redox Rep. 1996;2(6):385–91.
23. Maharjan R, Nagar PS, Nampoothiri L. Effect of Aloe barbadensis Mill. formulation on Letrozole induced polycystic ovarian syndrome rat model. Journal of Ayurveda and integrative medicine. 2010;1(4):273–279.
24. Usoh I, Akpan E, Etim E, Farombi E. Pak J Nutr. 2005;4(3):135–41.
25. Williams AC, Ford WCL. Fertil Steril. 2005;83(4):929–36.
26. Aitken RJ. Reprod Fertil Dev. 1995;7(4):659–68.
27. Mohan S, Priya V. Biol Med. 2009;1(3):44–9.
28. Li X, Wang X, Liu R, Ma Y, Guo H, Hao L, Yao P, Liu L, Sun X, He K. Mol Nutr Food Res. 2013;57(6):1067–79.
29. Felig P, Marliss E, Cahill GF Jr. N Engl J Med. 1969;281(15):811–6.
30. Soh J-R, Yamamoto TT, Cha Y-S. Nutraceuticals Food. 2003;8(2):119–23.
31. Nishimura M, Yoshida S-i, Haramoto M, Mizuno H, Fukuda T, Kagami-Katsuyama H, Tanaka A, Ohkawara T, Sato Y, Nishihira J. J Tradit Complement Med. 2016;6(1):66–71.

23

Expression and activity of Rac1 is negatively affected in the dehydroepiandrosterone induced polycystic ovary of mouse

Vineet Kumar Maurya[1], Chadchan Sangappa[1], Vijay Kumar[1], Sahil Mahfooz[1], Archana Singh[1], Singh Rajender[2] and Rajesh Kumar Jha[1*]

Abstract

Background: Polycystic ovarian syndrome (PCOS) is characterized by the presence of multiple follicular cysts, giving rise to infertility due to anovulation. This syndrome affects about 10% of women, worldwide. The exact molecular mechanism leading to PCOS remains obscure. RhoGTPase has been associated with oogenesis, but its role in PCOS remains unexplored. Therefore, we attempted to elucidate the Vav-Rac1 signaling in PCOS mice model.

Methods: We generated a PCOS mice model by injecting dehydroepiandrosterone (DHEA) for a period of 20 days. The expression levels of Rac1, pRac1, Vav, pVav and Caveolin1 were analyzed by employing immuno-blotting and densitometry. The association between Vav and Rac1 proteins were studied by immuno-precipitation. Furthermore, we analyzed the activity of Rac1 and levels of inhibin B and 17β-estradiol in ovary using biochemical assays.

Results: The presence of multiple follicular cysts in ovary were confirmed by histology. The activity of Rac1 (GTP bound state) was significantly reduced in the PCOS ovary. Similarly, the expression levels of Rac1 and its phosphorylated form (pRac1) were decreased in PCOS in comparison to the sham ovary. The expression level and activity (phosphorylated form) of guanine nucleotide exchanger of Rac1, Vav, was moderately down-regulated. We observed comparatively increased expressions of Caveolin1, 17β-estradiol, and inhibin B in the polycystic ovary.

Conclusion: We conclude that hyperandrogenization (PCOS) by DHEA diminishes ovarian Rac1 and Vav expression and activity along with an increase in expression of Caveolin1. This is accompanied by an increase in the intra-ovarian level of '17 β-estradiol and inhibin B.

Keywords: Polycystic ovary, Dehydroepiandrosterone, Rac1, Estradiol, Vav, Caveolin1

Introduction

The pool of primordial follicles in the ovary supply eggs for the entire reproductive life in mammals. To maintain fertility for the whole reproductive period, the primordial follicles are reserved in a quiescent state for regulated successive ovulation [1-3]. Primordial follicles are recruited from the reserve of dormant follicles into the pool of growing follicles through their activation process during which they undergo a series of developments [3].

Polycystic ovarian syndrome (PCOS) is characterized by anovulation and in the presence of multiple small cysts typically arranged in the periphery of one or both ovaries. PCOS can affect 5–10% of women during their reproductive age and contributes to this etiology in about 10% of the infertile women [4-6]. This disorder is considered to be a manifestation of the disturbance in the endocrine system, which causes secondary disorders contributing to female infertility [7]. The most commonly seen endocrine disturbance is hyperandrogenism accompanied by chronic oligo or anovulation [8]. The hypothalamic-pituitary synchrony is disrupted that increases pulsatile secretion of gonadotropin, disturbs oocyte-granulosa cell interaction, enhances

---
* Correspondence: rajesh_jha@cdri.res.in
[1]Division of Endocrinology, Life Science North 111B/101, CSIR-Central Drug Research Institute, B.S. 10/1, Sector-10, Jankipuram Extension, Sitapur Road, Lucknow 226031, India
Full list of author information is available at the end of the article

ovarian androgen production and causes excess insulin production and that leads to insulin resistance [9]. As a result, metabolic syndrome (MS) is seen in about 46% of the PCOS cases [10].

However, the intra-ovarian pathophysiology of PCOS is not yet explicit at cellular and molecular levels. The available data till date is insufficient to precisely delineate the intra-ovarian pathway that contributes to the development of this disorder. Therefore, we need further investigations to pinpoint the correct mechanism leading to the development of this disorder. The G-protein family member, Ras, has already been shown to participate in the pathophysiology of PCOS [11]. Another member of Rho family protein, Rac, is involved in gonad formation [12] and acts downstream to integrin signaling [13]. Its expression/activity is controlled by estrogen [14]. Rho guanine dissociation inhibitor (RhoGDI) antagonizes Rac1 and keeps it in the inactive state [15,16]. The Rho assists in actin dynamics through cofilin regulation by Luteinizing hormone signaling [17] in the granulosa cells [18]. Furthermore, Rac modulates cell cycle [19], which is activated by guanine exchange factor Vav [20,21]. Further, it is reported that Rac gets phosphorylated in the process of its activation [22]. Similarly, Vav also gets phosphorylated before it executes Rac activation [23,24]. Looking at the role of Rac/Vav signaling in ovarian physiology, we designed the present study to analyze expression and activity of Rac1 and Vav proteins in the ovary of a mice model of PCOS.

Materials and methods
Reagents
Dehydroisoandrosterone 3'-sulphate (cat no. D5297), hematoxylin (cat no. H3136), anti-beta-actin (cat no. A2668) and goat anti-Mouse IgG (γ-chain specific)-HRP (cat no. A3673) were purchased from Sigma Aldrich Inc., St Louis, MO, USA. Immobilon-P PVDF membrane (0.45 μm), ECL reagent kits (cat no. WBKLS0500), Protein-A-Agarose suspension (cat no. IP02) and goat anti-rabbit-HRP IgG (cat no.621140380011730) were procured from Merck-Millipore, Cedex, France. Other primary antibodies against phospho-Vav (Y174) (cat no. ab47282), phospho-Rac1/Cdc42 (S71) (cat no. ab5482) and Rac1 (cat no. ab33186) were purchased from Abcam, Cambridge, MA, USA. Anti-Vav (cat no. sc132) and anti-Caveolin1 (cat no. sc894) were purchased from Santa Cruz Biotechnology, CA, USA. Non-fat milk (cat no.170-6404) and precision plus protein standard marker (cat no. 161-0374) were obtained from Bio-Rad Lab., Inc., Hercules, CA., USA. Protein assay kit (cat no. 23225) was procured from Thermo-Scientific, Rockford, USA. The G-LISA Rac1 activation assay Biochem Kit (cat no. BK128) was purchased from Cytoskeleton, Denver, CO, USA. Inhibin B Enzyme Immunoassay kit (cat no. EIA-INB-1) was purchased from RayBiotech, Inc., Norcross, GA, USA. 17 β-estradiol assay

kit (cat no. ADI-900-008) was obtained from Enzo Life Science, Inc., Farmingdale New York, USA.

PCOS experimental animal model
The murine model of PCOS was developed by administering *Mus musculus* (strain C57/BL6) with dehydroisoandrosterone (DHEA). PCOS was induced in 22 days old mice (12 gm) by injecting DHEA (6 mg/100gm body weight; dissolved in 0.01 ml 95% ethanol, which was further diluted with corn oil) subcutaneously for 20 consecutive days as described previously [25-28]. The model is characterized by higher levels of serum testosterone, androstenedione and 5-alpha-dihydrotestosterone similar to that seen in PCOS patients. Previous studies have established that the DHEA-PCOS murine model represents some of the salient features of human PCOS, such as hyperandrogenism, abnormal maturation of ovarian follicles and anovulation [26,27,29-31]. We administered corn oil along with 95% ethanol in the control (sham) group. Animal usage and the protocols were duly approved by the Institutional Animal Ethics Committee of the CDRI, Lucknow, India. The animals were housed in a temperature-controlled facility (25 ± 1°C) with required illumination (12 h light and 12 h dark). Free access to food and water were provided to the animals. At the end of the experiments, animals were sacrificed by cervical dislocation followed by excision of ovaries, which were snap frozen at −80°C until further use. Each treatment/control group consisted of six animals.

Ovarian tissue histology and staining
To evaluate the histological alteration in the ovary, DHEA treated and sham/control ovaries were dissected and allowed to fix overnight at 4°C in 4% paraformaldehyde (PFA)-phosphate buffered saline (PBS). On subsequent day, tissue samples were kept in the tissue cassette and dehydrated using acetone (two times for 30 min each), acetone + benzene (1:1, 30 min) and cleared in benzene (two times for 30 min each). Subsequently, the tissues were removed and embedded in paraffin wax (Fisher Scientific, Rockford, USA) for 4 h at 65°C. This was followed by preparation of tissue paraffin moulds.

Embedded ovarian tissues were sectioned (5 μm) using microtome (Leica Biosystem, Germany) and mounted on poly-L-lysine (Sigma-Aldrich, MO, USA) coated glass slides. Sections were deparaffinized with two changes of xylene (10 min each) and rehydrated with subsequent changes of absolute alcohol (two times, five min each), 95% (two min) and 70% alcohol (two min). Sections were briefly washed (three times) and stained with hematoxylin solution for eight min. After staining, sections were again washed and kept for blue color development in 1.5% ammonium hydroxide (30% stock) for 30 sec. The tissue section mounted slides were washed in distilled water for five min, rinsed in 95% alcohol (10 repeats) and counterstained with 0.5% eosin for 30 sec. This was followed by dehydration through 95% and absolute alcohol two times for five min each. Finally, the slides were cleared in xylene two times for five min each and mounted with DPX mountant. The tissue sections were imaged through Inverted Phase Contrast Microscope (TS100-F, Nikon, Japan) using 5.2 megapixels digital camera (DS-Fi2-U3, Nikon, Japan).

Ovarian protein extract preparation

After excision, the ovaries were processed for total (cytosol + plasma membrane) protein extract preparation. The ovarian tissue was minced and homogenized in a buffer containing 100 mM KCl, 3 mM NaCl, 3.5 mM $MgCl_2$, 10 mM PIPES, 1.5 mM EGTA, 1 mM PMSF, 50 g/ml, phosphatase, and protease inhibitors (pH-7.4) [32]. The tissue homogenate was centrifuged at 200 × g for 10 min at 4°C to pellet-out unbroken cells and tissue debris. Later, the mitochondrial fraction was removed by centrifuging the preparation at 12,000 × g. The concentration of protein was estimated using Pierce BCA protein assay kit as per the manufacturer's instructions. Suitable concentration (20μg) of protein extract was prepared for down-stream purposes.

Rac1 activity assay

The activity of Rac1 (GTP bound form) was assayed in the ovarian protein extract using G-LISA Rac1 activation assay Biochem Kit, as per the manufacturer's instructions and that is already validated [33]. Briefly, a total of 50 μg protein extract was added to each corresponding well pre-coated with Rac-GTP-binding protein. This was incubated at 4°C for 30 min followed by successive incubation with 50 μl of anti-Rac1 for 45 min. Later, secondary antibody conjugated with HRP (50 μl) was incubated for 45 minutes. Subsequently, 50 μl of HRP detection reagent was added to each well, followed by incubation for another 20 min. The reaction was stopped by the addition of 50 μl of HRP stop solution and the absorbance was recorded at 490 nm.

Inhibin B assay

The level of inhibin B was determined in the ovarian protein extract using RayBio Inhibin B Enzyme Immunoassay kit as per the manufacturer's instructions. We added 100 μl of inhibin B antibody in each well of micro-plate, which was pre-coated with anti-rabbit antibody. The plate was incubated overnight at 4°C with gentle shaking. This was followed by the addition of 100 μl of protein sample to each well and incubation overnight at 4°C. HRP-Streptavidin was added followed by incubation at room temperature for 45 min. Subsequently, 100 μl of 5'-tetramethylbenzimide (TMB) was added as HRP

detection reagent and incubated at room temperature in dark for 30 min. The reaction was terminated by adding 50 μl stop solution and absorbance was recorded at 450 nm.

17 β-estradiol hormone estimation

The assay was performed as per instructions provided by the manufacturer. A total of 40 μg (100 μl) ovarian protein (n = 4; sample pooled from 10 animals to form 4 replicate in each group) was used for this assay. The standard of 17 β-estradiol was prepared by the addition of 100 μl standards (30,000 pg/ml, 7,500 pg/ml, 1,875 pg/ml, 468.8 pg/ml, 117.2 pg/ml and 29.3 pg/ml) and assay buffer3 (50 μl) into respective standard wells, whereas the standard diluent (100 μl) was added to well B_0 (maximum binding well). The NSB (negative control) received standard diluents (100 μl), assay buffer3 (50 μl) and conjugate (phosphatase conjugated with 17β-estradiol) (50 μl). Blank was prepared by adding only substrate (200 μl) and stop solution (50 μl). Next, we added 50 μl of conjugate in all the wells except blank. Antibody against 17β-estradiol (50 μl) was added in wells B_0, standard, and samples only followed by incubation of plate at room-temperature (RT) for 2 h. The unbound/excess content was decanted and micro-plate was washed thrice with 400 μl of wash buffer by gentle tapping on paper towel. Thereafter, a substrate (p-nitrophenyl phosphate; 200 μl) was added in each well followed by incubation at RT for 45 min. Finally, a stop solution (trisodium phosphate; 50 μl) was added to each well and micro-plate was read at 405 nm using micro-plate reader (SPECTRO star Nano, BMG LABTECH, GmbH, Germany). The graph was plotted with absorbance versus standards (17β-estradiol; pg/ml) after subtraction of NSB values. The concentration of 17β-estradiol was calculated based on the standard curve.

Co-immuno-precipitation assay

The ovarian protein lysate (100 μg, sham group) from each replicate was immuno-precipitated by incubation with anti-Vav overnight at 4°C. To collect the immune complexes, Protein-A-Agarose (20 μl) was added and the lysate-bead mixture was incubated at 4°C under rotary agitation for 4 h. It was followed by centrifugation at 10,000 × g for 10 min at 4°C and washing three times with PBS. Protein was eluted with Laemmli buffer and boiled for 5 min. The supernatant was subjected to 12% SDS-PAGE and immuno-blotted with anti-Rac1 according to a previously described method [32].

SDS-PAGE and Western blotting

Protein sample (20 μg) was denatured by boiling in Laemmli buffer [34] for 5 min at 95°C and applied on a 10-12% SDS-PAGE. The proteins resolved on the gel were transferred to PVDF membrane (0.45 μm) in transfer buffer (20% methanol, vol/vol; 0.19 M glycine; 0.025 M Tris-Base, pH = 8.3) [35]. The membrane was blocked with 5% non-fat milk/goat serum and incubated overnight at 4°C with antibodies against Rac1 (1:1000 dilution), pRac1 (1:1000 dilution), Vav (1:250 dilution), pVav (1:1000 dilution), Caveolin1 (1:1000 dilution) and beta-actin (1:6000 dilution). Thereafter, the membranes were incubated for one h with goat anti-rabbit IgG or goat anti-mouse IgG conjugated with Horseradish Peroxidase in a paraffin boat. Phosphate buffered saline (10 mM, pH 7.4 containing 0.1% Tween-20, PBS-T) was used throughout the procedure. Later, the membranes were exposed to ECL reagents to visualize the protein bands and imaged through Chemi-Imager (ImageQuant LAS4000, Buckinghamshire, UK). Immuno-positive bands were analyzed by densitometry using Total Lab Quant 1D software (Nonlinear Dynamics Ltd., UK). The beta-actin blot values were used to normalize the blots value of Rac1, pRac1, Caveolin1, Vav and pVav.

Statistical analysis

All the experiments were performed in three replicates using six animals in each group. Ovarian tissue samples were pooled from two animals to form one replicates to increase the yield of protein extract. Protein band intensities were averaged and the standard error of the mean (SE) was calculated. The data were subjected to one-way ANOVA using Microsoft Excel 2007. P values less than 0.05 were considered significant for statistical inference.

Results

Characterization of PCOS by histological analysis

To demonstrate the effect of DHEA, ovaries were sectioned and stained with hematoxylin/eosin. Ovarian sections of control (sham) group showed the presence of follicles at different stages of maturation (Figure 1). Atretic, graffian and healthy follicles were clearly visible along with corpora lutea (Figure 1A). The presence of healthy oocytes in the follicles was seen (Figure 1C). In contrast, DHEA treated ovary exhibited a bit distorted morphology (Figure 1B). The numbers of antral and pre-natal follicles were increased with arrangement typically that of the polycystic ovary; however, the granulosa cells appeared to be degenerated (Figure 1D). The size of the polycystic ovary was increased, perhaps due to an increase in the number of follicles. Oocytes and corpora-lutea were not seen in the polycystic ovary.

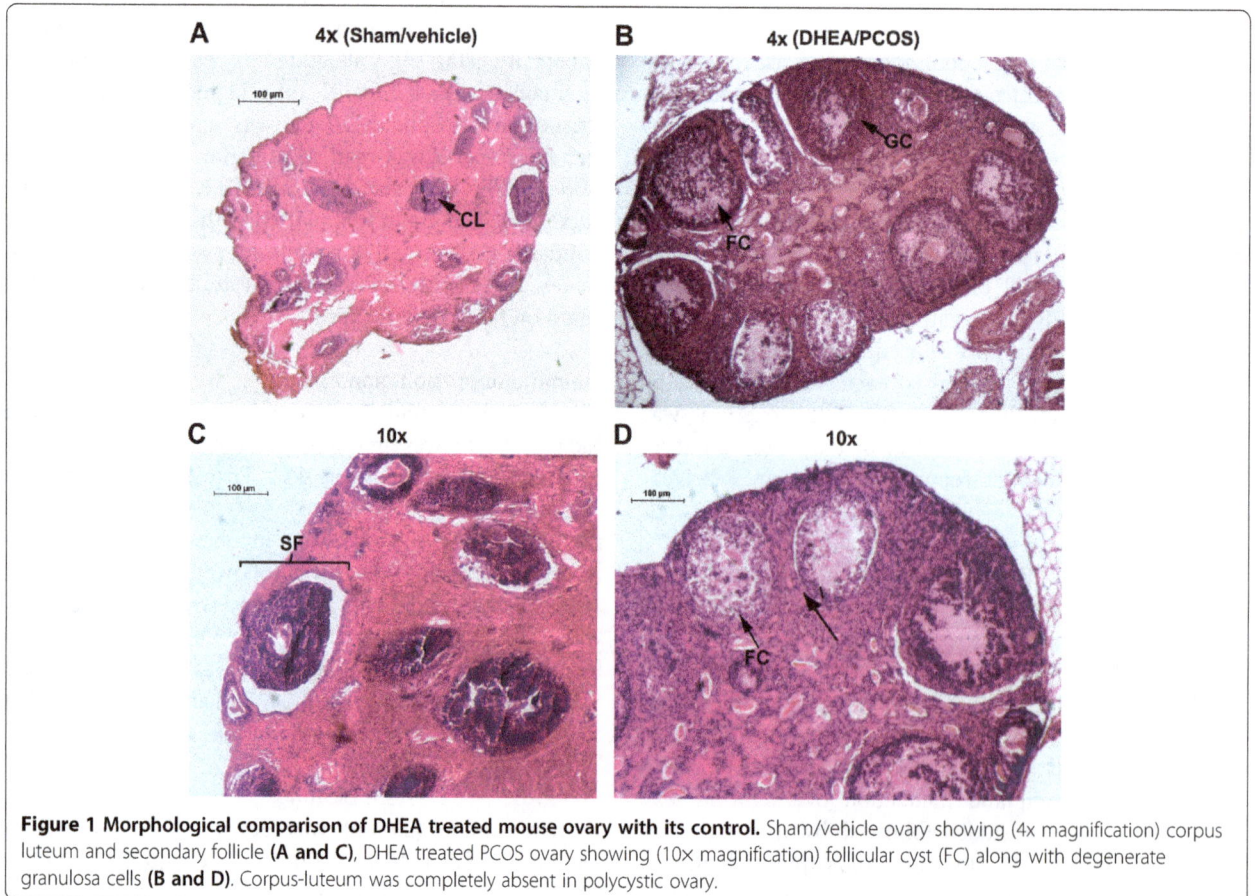

Figure 1 Morphological comparison of DHEA treated mouse ovary with its control. Sham/vehicle ovary showing (4x magnification) corpus luteum and secondary follicle **(A and C)**, DHEA treated PCOS ovary showing (10x magnification) follicular cyst (FC) along with degenerate granulosa cells **(B and D)**. Corpus-luteum was completely absent in polycystic ovary.

Increased expression level of inhibin B in polycystic ovary

The level of inhibin B correlates with the number of follicles recruited to undergo maturation [36]. Earlier studies have reported high concentrations of serum inhibin B in polycystic ovaries [37-39]. Herein, we performed assay of inhibin B in ovarian tissue protein extract to validate the pathophysiology of PCOS in our animal model. We observed a significant increase ($p < 0.015$) in level of inhibin B in the polycystic ovaries in comparison to sham (control) ovaries. Our result showed ~61% elevation in the level of inhibin B (Figure 2A).

Elevated level of 17 β-estradiol in the PCOS ovary

Serum level of 17β-estradiol (E_2) indicates the development of dominant follicles [36]. Therefore, we analyzed intra-ovarian level of 17β-estradiol in the PCOS and control groups. We observed about three folds elevation in the level of estradiol in PCOS ovary in comparison to the control ovary ($p < 0.03$) (Figure 2B).

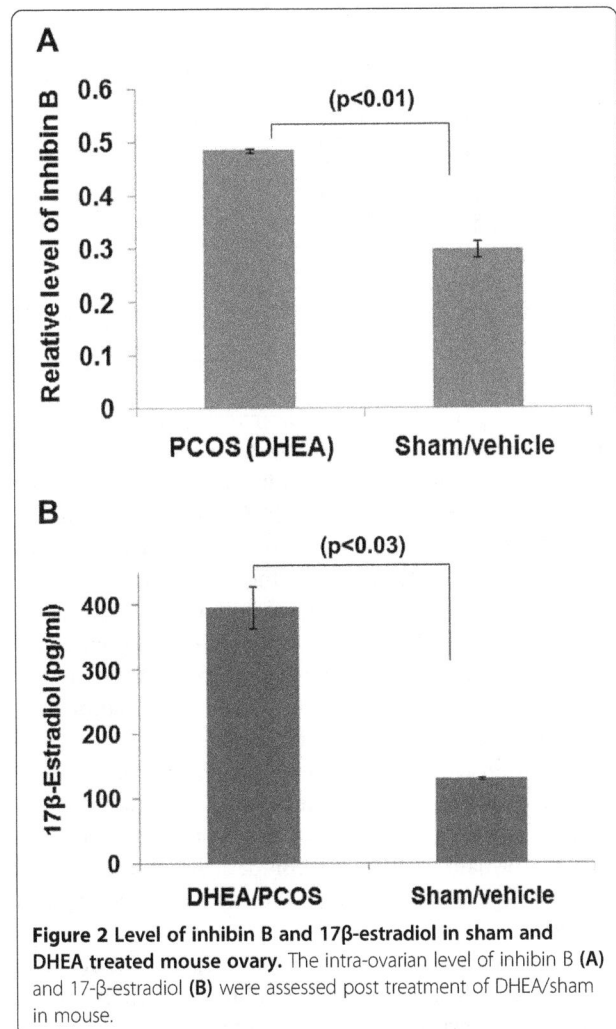

Figure 2 Level of inhibin B and 17β-estradiol in sham and DHEA treated mouse ovary. The intra-ovarian level of inhibin B (A) and 17-β-estradiol (B) were assessed post treatment of DHEA/sham in mouse.

Down regulation of activity and expression of Rac1 in PCOS ovary

In order to decipher the possible involvement of Rac1 signaling in PCOS, we detected the expression level of Rac1 and phosphorylated-Rac1 (S71) (pRac1) in the ovarian tissue protein extract prepared from the experimental model of PCOS. As shown in Figure 3A, compared with the sham/vehicle treated ovaries, the activity level of Rac1 was significantly decreased in the PCOS ovary. Similarly, the expression level of Rac1 protein was significantly down-regulated in DHEA treated/PCOS ovary (Figure 3B and C).

Further, to determine whether the activity of Rac1 in terms of its phosphorylation was affected in the DHEA treated (polycystic) ovary, the phosphorylation level of Rac1 was analyzed employing immuno-blotting. Treatment of ovary with DHEA resulted in down-regulation of pRac1 (Figure 3D and E). Thus, this domain of information suggests that DHEA/polycystic ovary may adversely affect the activity of Rac1.

Association of Vav activity in PCOS ovary

Rac1 is activated by Vav, which gets phosphorylated at tyrosine (Y) 174 [40]. To evaluate whether DHEA can also modulate of intra-ovarian activity of Rac1, we further evaluated the activity and expression level of Vav in the ovary after DHEA treatment (polycystic ovary). The activity of Vav in terms of its phosphorylation was analyzed through phosphorylation assay/Western blots (Figure 4). We found reduced expression level of total Vav in the hyper-androgenized ovary, but the difference in comparison to control was not statistically significant (Figure 4A and B). Similarly, the intensity of anti-pVav (Y174) positive band was found to be lower in PCOS in comparison to the control (sham) group ($p > 0.05$) (Figure 4C and D).

Vav can interact with Rac1 in ovary

It is well known that Vav displays guanidine exchange factor activity for Rho GTPases. We performed co-immuno-precipitation analysis to confirm the Rac1 association with Vav in the sham ovary. The Vav presence in the Vav antibody IP was confirmed by its immuno-blotting (Figure 5A). As shown in Figure 5B, the immuno-precipitated protein samples by Vav antibody from the ovary of sham administered displayed immuno-positive band of Rac1, which is an indication that Rac1 interacts with Vav in the ovary.

Caveolin1 is up-regulated in PCOS ovary

Caveolin1 is known to be an important scaffolding domain containing caveolae protein, which is involved in the regulation of several signaling cascades [41]. Since, Caveolin1 is linked to Rac1 degradation pathway, we

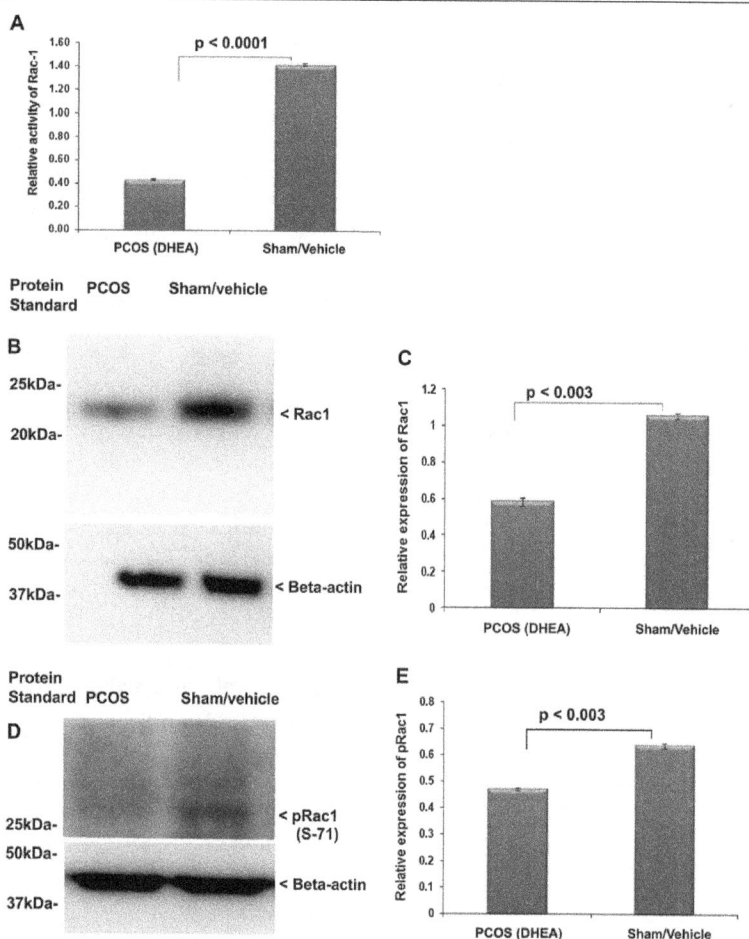

Figure 3 Determination of expression and activity of Rac1 in DHEA induced PCOS ovary. Relative activity of Rac1 was analyzed in the DHEA (PCOS) and sham treated ovary **(A)**. Expression level analysis of Rac1 was determined by immuno-blotting and densitometry in the ovary of PCOS and sham **(B and C)**. The activity Rac1was assayed by analysis of its phosphorylated form **(D and E)**.

investigated the expression level of Caveolin1 in the ovarian samples. We observed a significantly increased level of Caveolin1 in PCOS ovary in comparison to the control (sham) group (Figure 6A and B).

Discussion

Intra-ovarian signaling stimulates some of the primordial follicles to grow out of a cohort. The quiescent follicles remain in the inactive stage due to inhibitory mechanism operational either within the follicles or by the signals from the ovary [3]. During the post-natal development in mice, a large number of oocytes/follicles are depleted in comparison to the growing population of follicles [42,43]. This phenomenon is similar in the humans as well [3] and depletion of the pool of primodial follicles compromises female fertility. The condition of follicle insufficiency to ovulate is not understood precisely. Previous studies have demonstrated the association of Ras and Rho signaling in the process of ovarian follicle development [43-48]. Rac1 is a member of the Ras family,

making it a good candidate for investigation of its role in the regulation of follicular maturation.

The presence of multiple cysts in the ovaries are considered as a key diagnostic trait of PCOS [49-51], which was precisely mimicked in our PCOS mice model. This provided us with a platform for further biochemical and expression analysis. Our histological findings in PCOS ovary correlated well with the earlier reports showing increased ovarian size, absence of ovum and corpus-luteum in the ovaries of DHEA treated mice [52]. A relation between decrease in ovarian volume and the number of follicles with age of women with PCOS has been shown [53]. Increased level of inhibin B and 17β-estradiol in the PCOS group demonstrated elevation in the number of recruited dormant follicles in comparison to the control ovary [36]. Collectively, this confirmed a phenotype of polycystic ovary in our model system.

The estradiol negatively affects Rac1 activation [14], and in turn Rac1 regulates inhibin B [54]; however, this is not known in the ovarian tissue. Rac is a member

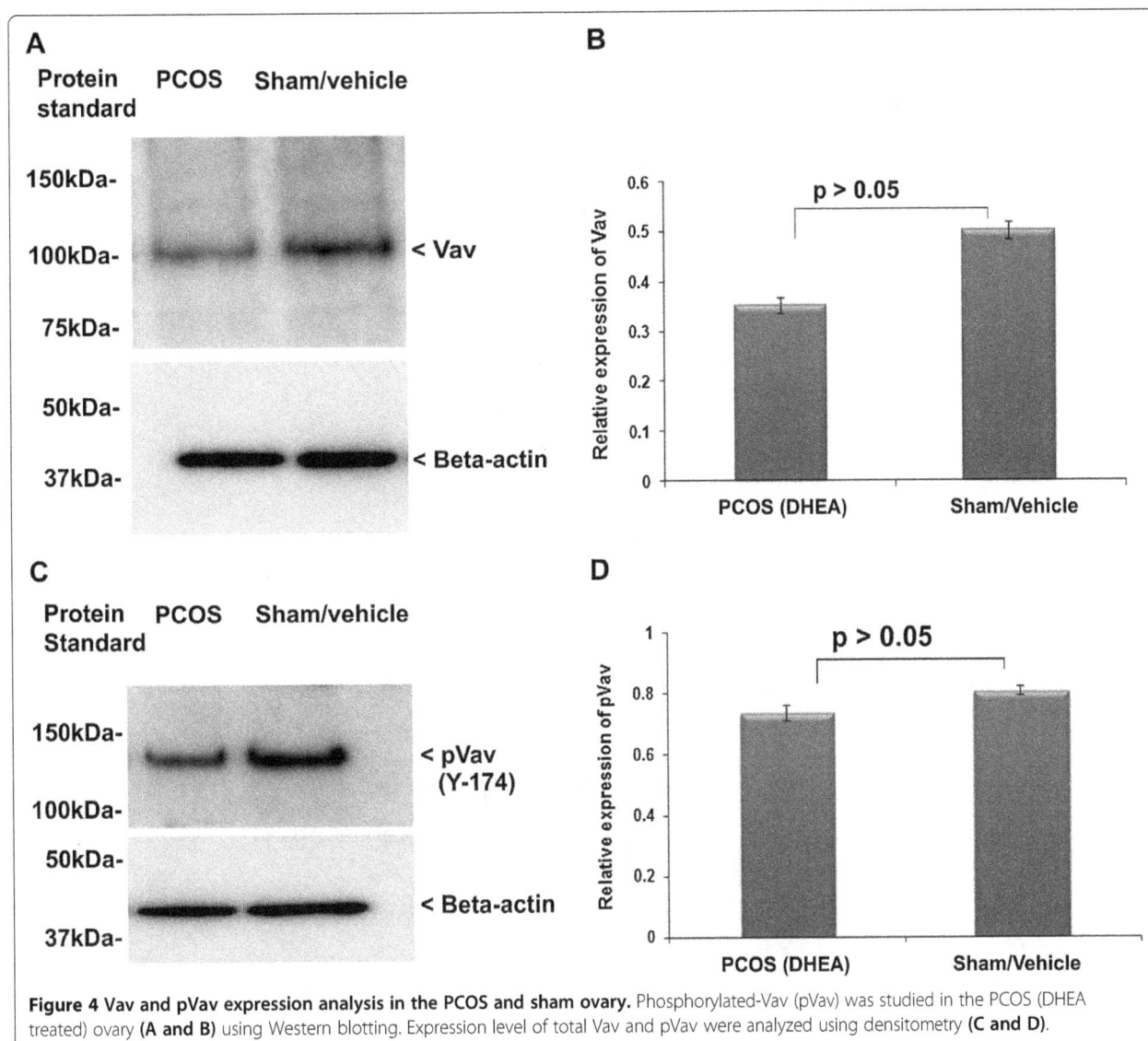

Figure 4 Vav and pVav expression analysis in the PCOS and sham ovary. Phosphorylated-Vav (pVav) was studied in the PCOS (DHEA) treated) ovary **(A and B)** using Western blotting. Expression level of total Vav and pVav were analyzed using densitometry **(C and D)**.

of small G-protein family (RhoGTPase) and other member of this G-protein family, Ras, has already been implicated in the pathophysiology of ovary [11]. A previous study has suggested involvement of Rac1in gonad formation [12], but its association with follicular maturation and function has not been shown. Our results suggested that expression of Rac1, pRac1 and its activity were significantly reduced in the hyperandrogenized ovary with DHEA (polycystic ovary). Activity of Rac1 was also lowered as compared to sham. It has been reported that higher production of estrogen in vascular smooth muscle cells causes down-regulation of Rac1 [14]. We observed a similar combination of elevated level of intra-ovarian 17β-estradiol and down-regulation of Rac1 on polycystic ovary. Further to confirm the involvement of Rac1, we studied the expression level of total Vav along with its phosphorylated form, which is a known activator

of Rac1 [24]. As expected, we observed a reduction in total Vav and its phosphorylated form. The association between Rac1-Vav was further confirmed by immuno-precipitation (IP), which showed Rac1 presence in the immuno-precipitates prepared using anti-Vav from sham treated group. Collectively, all the above results suggest that elevated 17β-estradiol levels might have down-regulated the activity/expression of Rac1 and Vav favoring the development of PCOS phenotype.

Several studies have also shown the interaction of Rac1 with caveolae protein, Caveolin1. Caveolin1 is known to control Rac1 protein levels by regulating ubiquitylation and degradation of activated Rac1 in an adhesion-dependent fashion [55]. The absence of Caveo-lin1 has been reported to increase the proliferation and anchorage-independent growth by a Rac-dependent, Erk-independent mechanism [56]. Since, there is no

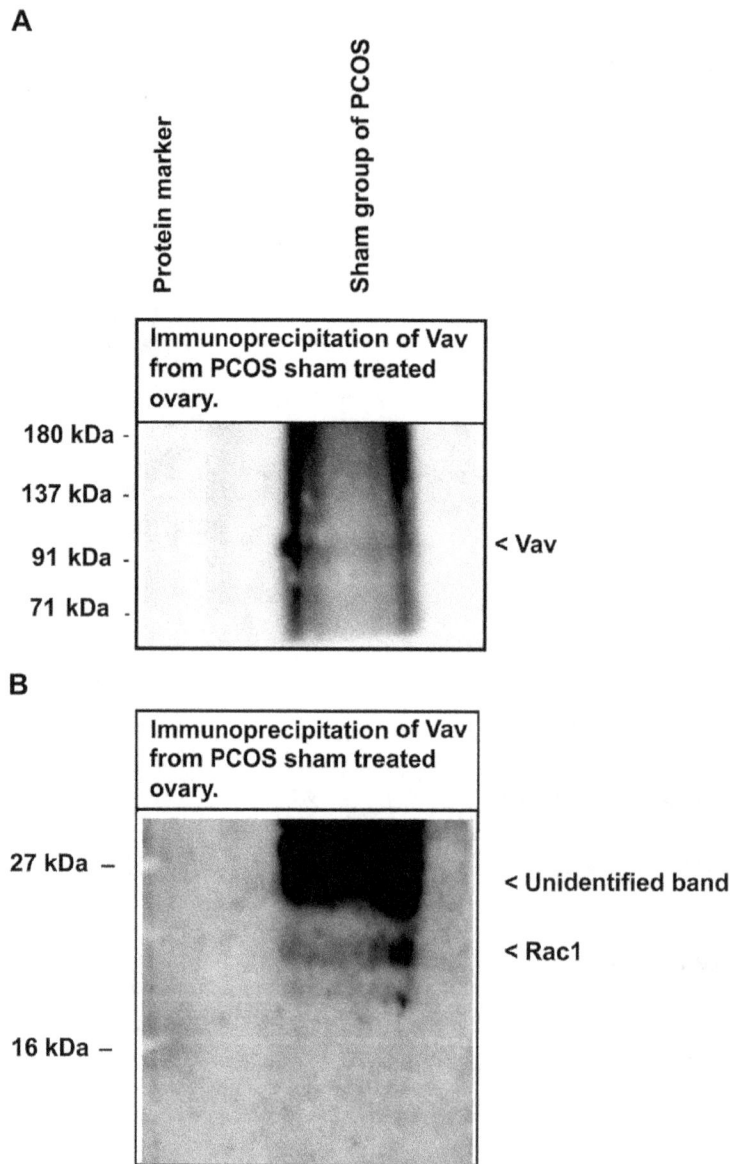

Figure 5 Analysis of Rac1 and Vav interaction in the ovary. Lysate from PCOS ovary was processed for Vav immuno-precipitation followed by immuno-blotting with Rac1 antibody **(A)**; presence of Rac1 in the Vav IP was confirmed by its immuno-blotting **(B)**.

evidence that Caveolin1 regulates Rac1 in the ovarian tissue, particularly in PCOS, we analyzed the expression of Caveolin1. A higher level of caveolin1 in PCOS ovary might have signaled a decrease in Rac1 and Vav levels that favors the development of PCOS phenotype. However, this is purely a speculation and further evidence is required to conclude the exact role of Caveolin1 in pathophysiology of PCOS. Rac1 and Caveolin1 are known to associate during cell proliferation signaling [56]; however, Caveolin1 antagonizing function for Rac1 activity in PCOS pathophysiology needs further validation. Herein, our study can infer that Caveolin1 is dysregulated in the PCOS ovary.

On the basis of our observations, we propose that increased androgens levels result in enhanced conversion of estradiol that initiates a series of events leading to the condition of PCOS. It is perhaps increased 17β-estradiol level that results in down regulation of Rac1 and Vav, ultimately, resulting in suspension of follicular development. This leads to arrest of follicular development, and promotes the to accumulation of immature follicles typical to PCOS ovaries. Elevated level of inhibin B is an indicator of repeated recruitment of follicles in the developmental process that is suspended before follicular maturation. How increased 17β-estradiol levels act on Rac/Vav needs to be studied further.

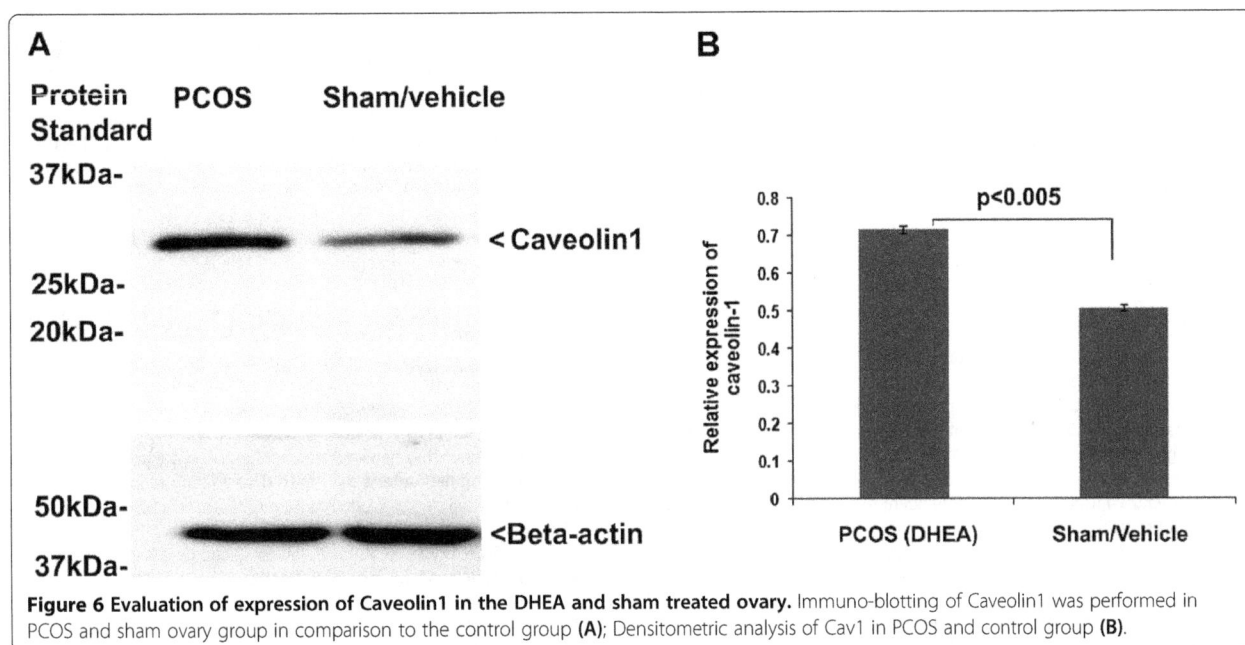

Figure 6 Evaluation of expression of Caveolin1 in the DHEA and sham treated ovary. Immuno-blotting of Caveolin1 was performed in PCOS and sham ovary group in comparison to the control group **(A)**; Densitometric analysis of Cav1 in PCOS and control group **(B)**.

Conclusion

The results of this study demonstrate for the first time diminished activity of Rac1 and Vav in hyperandrogenized mouse ovaries. Our findings might provide some explanation through small G-protein in the pathogenesis of follicular hyperplasia in PCOS. Altogether, these observations suggest a contribution of elevated estradiol and inhibin B levels due to the DHEA in pathophysiology of PCOS.

Abbreviations

PCOS: Polycystic ovarian syndrome; DHEA: Dehydroepiandrosterone; CL: Corpus luteum; FC: Follicle cyst; MS: Metabolic syndrome; PVDF: Polyvinylidene fluoride; ECL: Enhanced chemiluminescence; HRP: Horseradish peroxidase; Cat: Catalogue; h: Hour; PFA: Paraformaldehyde; PBS: Phosphate buffer saline; RhoA: Ras homolog gene family member A; Cdc42: Cell division control protein 42 homolog; Rac: Ras-related C3 botulinum toxin substrate; LH: Luteinizing hormone; IP: Immuno-precipitation.

Competing interests

The authors declare that they have no competing interests.

Authors' contributions

VKM carried out PCOS model preparation and development of Rac1, pRac1, Vav and pVav immuno-blot. SC performed Western blotting of Caveolin1, Rac1, pRac1, Vav and pVav along with the 17β-estradiol assay. VK performed the Rac1 activity assay, tissue paraffin embedding and microtomy. SM did the histological examination of ovarian tissue sections and helped in manuscript drafting. AS performed the immuno-precipitation of Vav, immuno-blotting with Rac1 and Vav along with the inhibin B assay. RS assisted in drafting the manuscript and experimental design. RKJ designed, analyzed the data and finalized the manuscript. All authors read and approved the final manuscript.

Authors' information

Rajesh Kumar Jha: http://www.cdriindia.org/Rajesh.htm.
Rajender Singh: http://www.cdriindia.org/Rajinder.htm.

Acknowledgments

Authors would like to acknowledge help of Mr. Geet Kumar Nagar in the histopathology and laboratory facilities of Dr. Anila Dwivedi. CSIR-CDRI manuscript number is 203/2012/RKJ.

Grant support

This research work received support from BSC0101Council of Scientific and Industrial Research (CSIR), New Delhi India.

Author details

[1]Division of Endocrinology, Life Science North 111B/101, CSIR-Central Drug Research Institute, B.S. 10/1, Sector-10, Jankipuram Extension, Sitapur Road, Lucknow 226031, India. [2]Division of Endocrinology, Life Science South, CSIR-Central Drug Research Institute, B.S. 10/1, Sector-10, Jankipuram Extension, Sitapur Road, Lucknow 226031, India.

References

1. Adhikari D, Liu K: Molecular mechanisms underlying the activation of mammalian primordial follicles. Endocr Rev 2009, 30:438–464.
2. Hirshfield AN: Development of follicles in the mammalian ovary. Int Rev Cytol 1991, 124:43–101. 43-101.
3. McGee EA, Hsueh AJ: Initial and cyclic recruitment of ovarian follicles. Endocr Rev 2000, 21:200–214.
4. Goodarzi MO, Dumesic DA, Chazenbalk G, Azziz R: Polycystic ovary syndrome: etiology, pathogenesis and diagnosis. Nat Rev Endocrinol 2011, 7:219–231.
5. Petrikova J, Lazurova I: Ovarian failure and polycystic ovary syndrome. Autoimmun Rev 2012, 11:A471–A478.
6. Wang S, Alvero R: Racial and ethnic differences in physiology and clinical symptoms of polycystic ovary syndrome. Semin Reprod Med 2013, 31:365–369.
7. Shayya R, Chang RJ: Reproductive endocrinology of adolescent polycystic ovary syndrome. BJOG 2010, 117:150–155.
8. Franks S, Gharani N, Waterworth D, Batty S, White D, Williamson R, McCarthy M: The genetic basis of polycystic ovary syndrome. Hum Reprod 1997, 12:2641–2648.
9. Kahsar-Miller M, Azziz R: The development of the polycystic ovary syndrome: family history as a risk factor. Trends Endocrinol Metab 1998, 9:55–58.

10. Bhattacharya SM: **Metabolic syndrome in females with polycystic ovary syndrome and International Diabetes Federation criteria.** *J Obstet Gynaecol Res* 2008, **34**:62–66.

11. Fan HY, Richards JS: **Minireview: physiological and pathological actions of RAS in the ovary.** *Mol Endocrinol* 2010, **24**:286–298.

12. Lee M, Shen B, Schwarzbauer JE, Ahn J, Kwon J: **Connections between integrins and Rac GTPase pathways control gonad formation and function in C. elegans.** *Biochim Biophys Acta* 2005, **1723**:248–255.

13. Cailleteau L, Estrach S, Thyss R, Boyer L, Doye A, Domange B, Johnsson N, Rubinstein E, Boucheix C, Ebrahimian T, Silvestre JS, Lemichez E, Meneguzzi G, Mettouchi A: **alpha2beta1 integrin controls association of Rac with the membrane and triggers quiescence of endothelial cells.** *J Cell Sci* 2010, **123**:2491–2501.

14. Laufs U, Adam O, Strehlow K, Wassmann S, Konkol C, Laufs K, Schmidt W, Bohm M, Nickenig G: **Down-regulation of Rac-1 GTPase by Estrogen.** *J Biol Chem* 2003, **278**:5956–5962.

15. Abramovici H, Mojtabaie P, Parks RJ, Zhong XP, Koretzky GA, Topham MK, Gee SH: **Diacylglycerol kinase zeta regulates actin cytoskeleton reorganization through dissociation of Rac1 from RhoGDI.** *Mol Biol Cell* 2009, **20**:2049–2059.

16. Sauzeau V, Sevilla MA, Montero MJ, Bustelo XR: **The Rho/Rac exchange factor Vav2 controls nitric oxide-dependent responses in mouse vascular smooth muscle cells.** *J Clin Invest* 2010, **120**:315–330.

17. Karlsson AB, Maizels ET, Flynn MP, Jones JC, Shelden EA, Bamburg JR, Hunzicker-Dunn M: **Luteinizing hormone receptor-stimulated progesterone production by preovulatory granulosa cells requires protein kinase A-dependent activation/dephosphorylation of the actin dynamizing protein cofilin.** *Mol Endocrinol* 2010, **24**:1765–1781.

18. Bristow JM, Sellers MH, Majumdar D, Anderson B, Hu L, Webb DJ: **The Rho-family GEF Asef2 activates Rac to modulate adhesion and actin dynamics and thereby regulate cell migration.** *J Cell Sci* 2009, **122**:4535–4546.

19. Mettouchi A, Klein S, Guo W, Lopez-Lago M, Lemichez E, Westwick JK, Giancotti FG: **Integrin-specific activation of Rac controls progression through the G(1) phase of the cell cycle.** *Mol Cell* 2001, **8**:115–127.

20. Garrett TA, Van Buul JD, Burridge K: **VEGF-induced Rac1 activation in endothelial cells is regulated by the guanine nucleotide exchange factor Vav2.** *Exp Cell Res* 2007, **313**:3285–3297.

21. Vedham V, Phee H, Coggeshall KM: **Vav activation and function as a rac guanine nucleotide exchange factor in macrophage colony-stimulating factor-induced macrophage chemotaxis.** *Mol Cell Biol* 2005, **25**:4211–4220.

22. Shyu KG, Chua SK, Wang BW, Kuan P: **Mechanism of inhibitory effect of atorvastatin on resistin expression induced by tumor necrosis factor-alpha in macrophages.** *J Biomed Sci* 2009, **16**:50. 50.

23. Aoukaty A, Tan R: **Role for glycogen synthase kinase-3 in NK cell cytotoxicity and X-linked lymphoproliferative disease.** *J Immunol* 2005, **174**:4551–4558.

24. Crespo P, Schuebel KE, Ostrom AA, Gutkind JS, Bustelo XR: **Phosphotyrosine-dependent activation of Rac-1 GDP/GTP exchange by the vav proto-oncogene product.** *Nature* 1997, **385**:169–172.

25. Elia E, Sander V, Luchetti CG, Solano ME, Di GG, Gonzalez C, Motta AB: **The mechanisms involved in the action of metformin in regulating ovarian function in hyperandrogenized mice.** *Mol Hum Reprod* 2006, **12**:475–481.

26. Luchetti CG, Solano ME, Sander V, Arcos ML, Gonzalez C, Di GG, Chiocchio S, Cremaschi G, Motta AB: **Effects of dehydroepiandrosterone on ovarian cystogenesis and immune function.** *J Reprod Immunol* 2004, **64**:59–74.

27. Sander V, Luchetti CG, Solano ME, Elia E, Di GG, Gonzalez C, Motta AB: **Role of the N, N'-dimethylbiguanide metformin in the treatment of female prepuberal BALB/c mice hyperandrogenized with dehydroepiandrosterone.** *Reproduction* 2006, **131**:591–602.

28. Zhu JQ, Zhu L, Liang XW, Xing FQ, Schatten H, Sun QY: **Demethylation of LHR in dehydroepiandrosterone-induced mouse model of polycystic ovary syndrome.** *Mol Hum Reprod* 2010, **16**:260–266.

29. Anderson E, Lee MT, Lee GY: **Cystogenesis of the ovarian antral follicle of the rat: ultrastructural changes and hormonal profile following the administration of dehydroepiandrosterone.** *Anat Rec* 1992, **234**:359–382.

30. Henmi H, Endo T, Nagasawa K, Hayashi T, Chida M, Akutagawa N, Iwasaki M, Kitajima Y, Kiya T, Nishikawa A, Manase K, Kudo R: **Lysyl oxidase and MMP-2 expression in dehydroepiandrosterone-induced polycystic ovary in rats.** *Biol Reprod* 2001, **64**:157–162.

31. Lee GY, Croop JM, Anderson E: **Multidrug resistance gene expression correlates with progesterone production in dehydroepiandrosterone-induced polycystic and equine chorionic gonadotropin-stimulated ovaries of prepubertal rats.** *Biol Reprod* 1998, **58**:330–337.

32. Maurya VK, Jha RK, Kumar V, Joshi A, Chadchan S, Mohan JJ, Laloraya M: **Transforming growth factor-beta 1 (TGF-B1) liberation from its latent complex during embryo implantation and its regulation by estradiol in mouse.** *Biol Reprod* 2013, **89**:84.

33. Hayashida T, Jones JC, Lee CK, Schnaper HW: **Loss of beta1-integrin enhances TGF-beta1-induced collagen expression in epithelial cells via increased alphavbeta3-integrin and Rac1 activity.** *J Biol Chem* 2010, **285**:30741–30751.

34. Laemmli UK: **Cleavage of structural proteins during the assembly of the head of bacteriophage T4.** *Nature* 1970, **227**:680–685.

35. Towbin H, Staehelin T, Gordon J: **Electrophoretic transfer of proteins from polyacrylamide gels to nitrocellulose sheets: procedure and some applications. 1979.** *Biotechnology* 1992, **24**:145–149. 145-9.

36. Eldar-Geva T, Robertson DM, Cahir N, Groome N, Gabbe MP, Maclachlan V, Healy DL: **Relationship between serum inhibin A and B and ovarian follicle development after a daily fixed dose administration of recombinant follicle-stimulating hormone.** *J Clin Endocrinol Metab* 2000, **85**:607–613.

37. Anderson RA, Groome NP, Baird DT: **Inhibin A and inhibin B in women with polycystic ovarian syndrome during treatment with FSH to induce mono-ovulation.** *Clin Endocrinol (Oxf)* 1998, **48**:577–584.

38. Dafopoulos K, Venetis C, Messini CI, Pournaras S, Anifandis G, Garas A, Messinis IE: **Inhibin secretion in women with the polycystic ovary syndrome before and after treatment with progesterone.** *Reprod Biol Endocrinol* 2011, **9**:59. doi: 10.1186/1477-7827-9-59.: 59.

39. Lockwood GM, Muttukrishna S, Groome NP, Matthews DR, Ledger WL: **Mid-follicular phase pulses of inhibin B are absent in polycystic ovarian syndrome and are initiated by successful laparoscopic ovarian diathermy: a possible mechanism regulating emergence of the dominant follicle.** *J Clin Endocrinol Metab* 1998, **83**:1730–1735.

40. Tong H, Zhao B, Shi H, Ba X, Wang X, Jiang Y, Zeng X: **c-Abl tyrosine kinase plays a critical role in beta2 integrin-dependent neutrophil migration by regulating Vav1 activity.** *J Leukoc Biol* 2013, **93**:611–622.

41. Minshall RD, Sessa WC, Stan RV, Anderson RG, Malik AB: **Caveolin regulation of endothelial function.** *Am J Physiol Lung Cell Mol Physiol* 2003, **285**:L1179–L1183.

42. Bristol-Gould SK, Kreeger PK, Selkirk CG, Kilen SM, Mayo KE, Shea LD, Woodruff TK: **Fate of the initial follicle pool: empirical and mathematical evidence supporting its sufficiency for adult fertility.** *Dev Biol* 2006, **298**:149–154.

43. Faddy MJ, Telfer E, Gosden RG: **The kinetics of pre-antral follicle development in ovaries of CBA/Ca mice during the first 14 weeks of life.** *Cell Tissue Kinet* 1987, **20**:551–560.

44. Fan HY, Liu Z, Mullany LK, Richards JS: **Consequences of RAS and MAPK activation in the ovary: the good, the bad and the ugly.** *Mol Cell Endocrinol* 2012, **356**:74–79.

45. Hackney JF, Pucci C, Naes E, Dobens L: **Ras signaling modulates activity of the ecdysone receptor EcR during cell migration in the Drosophila ovary.** *Dev Dyn* 2007, **236**:1213–1226.

46. Lee T, Montell DJ: **Multiple Ras signals pattern the Drosophila ovarian follicle cells.** *Dev Biol* 1997, **185**:25–33.

47. Yodoi R, Tamba S, Morimoto K, Segi-Nishida E, Nishihara M, Ichikawa A, Narumiya S, Sugimoto Y: **RhoA/Rho kinase signaling in the cumulus mediates extracellular matrix assembly.** *Endocrinology* 2009, **150**:3345–3352.

48. Vlachos S, Harden N: **Genetic evidence for antagonism between Pak protein kinase and Rho1 small GTPase signaling in regulation of the actin cytoskeleton during Drosophila oogenesis.** *Genetics* 2011, **187**:501–512.

49. Dunaif A, Thomas A: **Current concepts in the polycystic ovary syndrome.** *Annu Rev Med* 2001, **52**:401–419. 401-19.

50. Ehrmann DA: **Polycystic ovary syndrome.** *N Engl J Med* 2005, **352**:1223–1236.

51. Norman RJ, Dewailly D, Legro RS, Hickey TE: **Polycystic ovary syndrome.** *Lancet* 2007, **370**:685–697.

52. Aragno M, Brignardello E, Tamagno E, Gatto V, Danni O, Boccuzzi G: **Dehydroepiandrosterone administration prevents the oxidative damage induced by acute hyperglycemia in rats.** *J Endocrinol* 1997, **155**:233–240.

53. Alsamarai S, Adams JM, Murphy MK, Post MD, Hayden DL, Hall JE, Welt CK: **Criteria for polycystic ovarian morphology in polycystic ovary syndrome as a function of age.** *J Clin Endocrinol Metab* 2009, **94**:4961–4970.

54. Citterio C, Menacho-Marquez M, Garcia-Escudero R, Larive RM, Barreiro O, Sanchez-Madrid F, Paramio JM, Bustelo XR: **The rho exchange factors vav2 and vav3 control a lung metastasis-specific transcriptional program in breast cancer cells.** *Sci Signal* 2012, **5**:ra71.

55. Nethe M, Hordijk PL: **The role of ubiquitylation and degradation in RhoGTPase signalling.** *J Cell Sci* 2010, **123**:4011–4018.

56. Cerezo A, Guadamillas MC, Goetz JG, Sanchez-Perales S, Klein E, Assoian RK, del Pozo MA: **The absence of caveolin-1 increases proliferation and anchorage-independent growth by a Rac-dependent, Erk-independent mechanism.** *Mol Cell Biol* 2009, **29**:5046–5059.

24

Copeptin, a surrogate marker for arginine vasopressin, is associated with cardiovascular risk in patients with polycystic ovary syndrome

Basak Karbek[1*], Mustafa Ozbek[2], Melia Karakose[2], Oya Topaloglu[2], Nujen Colak Bozkurt[2], Evrim Cakır[3], Muyesser Sayki Aslan[2] and Tuncay Delibasi[2]

Abstract

Background: Women with polycystic ovary syndrome (PCOS) have higher risk for cardiovascular disease (CVD). Copeptin has been found to be predictive for myocardial ischemia. We tested whether copeptin is the predictor for CVD in PCOS patients, who have an increased risk of cardiovascular disease.

Methods: This was a cross sectional controlled study conducted in a training and research hospital. The study population consisted of 40 reproductive-age PCOS women and 43 control subjects. We evaluated anthropometric and metabolic parameters, carotid intima media thickness and copeptin levels in both PCOS patients and control group.

Results: Mean fasting insulin, homeostasis model assessment insulin resistance index (HOMA-IR), triglyceride, total cholesterol, low density lipoprotein cholesterol (LDL-C), free testosterone, 17-OH progesterone, Dehydroepiandrosterone sulfate (DHEAS), carotid intima media thickness (CIMT) levels were significantly higher in PCOS patients. Mean copeptin level was in 12.61 ± 3.05 pmol/L in PCOS patients while mean copeptin level was 9.60 ± 2.80 pmol/L in healthy control women ($p < 0.001$). After adjustment for age and BMI, copeptin level was positive correlated with fasting insulin, free testosterone levels, CIMT, and HOM A-IR.

Conclusions: Copeptin appeared to have an important role in metabolic response and subsequent development of atherosclerosis in insulin resistant, hyperandrogenemic PCOS patients.

Keywords: Polycystic ovary syndrome, Copeptin, Carotid intima media thickness, Insulin resistance, Cardiovascular disease risk

Introduction

Polycystic ovary syndrome is a common endocrine disorder affecting at least 5 to 10% of women of reproductive age [1]. Polycystic ovary syndrome is characterized by hyperandrogenism, menstrual disturbance, anovulation, infertility and obesity [2], and also associated with an increased number of cardiovascular risk factors [3], and early atherosclerosis [4,5]. Hyperinsulinism and insulin resistance are frequent findings in PCOS patients, and these traits have cause-consequence relationships with low-grade chronic inflammation [6], and increased cardiovascular disease risk [7].

Arginine vasopressin (AVP), which is also called antidiuretic hormone, is released from the neurohypophysis as a response to increased plasma osmolality and decreased blood volume. AVP exerts an antidiuretic effect in the kidney and a vasoconstrictive and blood platelet aggregating effect in the vessels. In addition, animal studies have shown effects of AVP on glucose metabolism. AVP influences gluconeogenesis and glycogenolysis in the liver [8,9], insulin and glucagon release by the Langerhans islets of the pancreas [10] and adrenocorticotrophic hormone release from the anterior hypophysis [11]. Vasopressin is a short-lived peptide and most assays have relatively limited sensitivity. An assay has been developed to measure plasma copeptin (copeptin), the

* Correspondence: b_karbek@yahoo.com
[1]Department of Endocrinology and Metabolic Diseases, Gaziantep Dr. Ersin Arslan Hospital, Milli Egemenlik bulvarı, Sanlılar Apt, no:51 daire:9 Şehitkamil/Gaziantep, Gaziantep, Turkey
Full list of author information is available at the end of the article

C-terminal portion of the precursor of AVP. Copeptin is considered to be a reliable and clinically useful surrogate marker for AVP [12]. In healthy populations and in patients with various cardiovascular diseases, there is a significant positive association between copeptin and AVP levels. However, the association between copeptin and patients with PCOS remains unknown. The present study was, therefore, undertaken to investigate the correlations between copeptin, and the progression of atherosclerosis in PCOS patients.

Subjects, materials and methods

We studied 40 patients with PCOS and age- body mass index (BMI) matched 43 healthy controls consisting of women with regular ovulatory cycles and normal androgen levels. All patients gave a written consent. All patients were female and nonsmokers. Participants recruited from Turkey, ethnicity of the participants' is Caucasian (Europe and Middle East). The diagnosis of PCOS was made according to the Rotterdam European Society for Human reproduction and Embryology/American Society for Reproductive Medicine–sponsored PCOS Consensus Workshop Group [13]. The revised diagnostic criteria of PCOS is as follows, with at least two of the following being required;

1. Oligo and/or anovulation that is menstrual disturbance
2. Clinical and/or biochemical signs of hyperandrogenism
3. Polycystic ovarian appearance on ultrasound

Participants who had smoking history, diabetes mellitus, hyperprolactinemia, congenital adrenal hyperplasia, androgen-secreting tumours, thyroid disorders, Cushing syndrome (1 mg dexamethasone suppression test), infection diseases, hypertension, hepatic or renal dysfunction were excluded from the study. Patients were also excluded if they had used within 3 months before enrollment confounding medications, including oral contraceptive agents, antilipidemic drugs, hypertensive medications, and insulin-sensitizing drugs.

Control group (n = 43) consisted of healthy patients who were admitted to check-up unit without any systemic disorder. All of the women in the control group had hirsutism score <8. All women in the control group had regular menses, every 21–35 days. None of the women in the control group had polycystic ovary in ultrasound.

Weight and height were measured in light clothing without shoes. BMI was calculated, dividing the weight divided by square of height (kg/m^2). Waist circumference was measured at the narrowest level between the costal margin and iliac crest, and the hip circumference was measured at the widest level over the buttocks while the subjects were standing and breathing normally. The waist-to-hip ratio (WHR) was calculated.

The degree of hirsutism was determined by Ferriman-Gallwey (FG) scoring [14]. The BMI, WHR and hirsutism scores were assessed by a single investigator for all of the subjects.

Measurement of carotid intima media thickness

Carotid intima media thickness (CIMT) was derived from noninvasive ultrasound of the common carotid arteries, using a high-resolution ultrasound machine (Sonoline G 40, Siemens) with 7.5 MHz mechanical sector transducer. The intima media thickness was defined as the distance between the blood-intima and media-adventitia boundaries on B-mode imaging. All scans and image measurements were carried out by the same investigator, who was blinded to the diagnosis of the participants.

Biochemical evaluation

Venous blood samples were obtained in the follicular phase of a spontaneous or progesterone induced menstrual cycle. Before the study, blood samples were drawn from each patient after 12 h overnight fasting for the determination of hormones, lipid profile, high-sensitive C- reactive protein (hs-CRP), insulin levels, glucose levels.

Plasma glucose was determined with glucose oxidase/peroxidase method (Gordion Diagnostic, Ankara, Turkey). Serum levels of follicle-stimulating hormone (FSH), luteinizing hormone (LH), prolactin, dehydroepiandrosterone sulfate (DHEAS), total testosterone (T), insulin and thyroid stimulating hormone (TSH) were measured with specific electrochemiluminescence immunoassays (Elecsys 2010 Cobas, Roche Diagnostics, Mannheim, Germany). Serum 17 hydroxyprogesterone was measured by radioimmunoassay. Levels of total-cholesterol, high density lipoprotein cholesterol (HDL-C), and triglyceride (TG) were determined with enzymatic colorimetric assays by spectrophotometry (BioSystems S.A., Barcelona, Spain). Low density lipoprotein cholesterol (LDL-C) was calculated using the Friedewald formula.

Serum hs-CRP was determined using high-sensitive CRP immunonephelometry (BN, Dade-Behring; Marburg, Germany). The cut off for hsCRP was taken 1.5 [15].

Insulin resistance was calculated by using the homeostasis model assessment insulin resistance index (HOMA-IR) [16], according to the formula, fasting plasma glucose (mmol/L) x fasting serum insulin (mU/mL) /22.5. The cut off value was taken 2.7 for HOMA-IR [17].

Copeptin

Blood samples collected into the tubes which contain EDTA. The blood centrifuged at 1.600 × g for 15 minutes, the plasma was separated and stored at –80°C until assessment of copeptin. Measurements of copeptin were performed in an EPOCH system (BioTek Instruments, Inc,

USA) using the commercially available enzyme-linked immunosorbent assay (ELISA) kit (Phoenix Pharmaceuticals, California, USA) in accordance with the manufactures' instructions. The assay range of the copeptin, ELISA kit was 0-100 pmol/L. Copeptin levels were expressed as ng/ml. The samples were carried out together in the same experiment.

Statistical analyses

Collected data was entered to SPSS version 17. Continuous data were shown as mean ± SD. Chi-squared tests were used to compare differences in rates. Normally distributed variables were compared by using Student T test. Data that were not normally distributed, as determined using Kolmogorov–Smirnov test, were logarithmically transformed before analysis. Data are expressed as mean ± SD or median with interquartile range as appropriate. Degree of association between continuous variables was calculated by Pearson correlation coefficient, nonnormally distributed variables was evaluated by spearman's rho correlation coefficient. The multiple linear regression enter method was used to determine the independent predictors. p value lower than 0.05 was accepted as statistically significant.

Results

Clinical and endocrinological parameters screened in patients with PCOS and in healthy control subjects were shown in Table 1. We studied 40 PCOS patients (22.97 ± 5.18 years; BMI; 24.40 ± 5.82 kg /m^2) and 43 age and BMI matched healthy control group (23.63 ± 4.60 years, BMI; 25.44 ± 4.82 kg/m^2).

Mean fasting insulin, HOMA-IR, triglyceride, total cholesterol, LDL-C, free testosterone, total testosterone, 17 OH progesterone, DHEAS, CIMT levels were significantly higher and estradiol were significantly lower in PCOS patients ($p < 0.05$) (Table 1).

Mean copeptin level was in 12.61 ± 3.05 pmol/L in PCOS patients while mean copeptin level was 9.60 ± 2.80 pmol/L in healthy control women ($p < 0.001$). After adjustment for age and BMI, copeptin level was positive correlated with fasting insulin, TG, free testosterone levels, CIMT, HOM A-IR, FG score and negative correlated with HDL- C and estradiol levels (Table 2). In multiple linear regression analyses copeptin was found to be significantly associated with CIMT (beta coefficient = 0.86, p = 0.002) (age, BMI were included in the model). The correlation between copeptin and CIMT was shown in Figure 1.

Mean CIMT level was 0.51 ± 0.052 millimeter in PCOS patients while mean CIMT level was 0.42 ± 0.043 millimeter in healthy control women ($p < 0.01$). A significant positive correlation was found between copeptin, fasting insulin, triglyceride, free testosterone , HOMA-IR and CIMT measurement (Table 3).

Table 1 The Clinical and biochemical/ hormonal data in women with polycistic ovary syndrome (PCOS) patients and healthy controls

Variable	Women with PCOS (n_40)	Healthy controls (n_43)	p
Age, years	22.97 ± 5.18	23.63 ± 4.60	>0.05
BMI, kg/m2	24.40 ± 5.82	25.44 ± 4.82	>0.05
Waist/hip ratio	0.84 ± 0.78	0.83 ± 0.73	>0.05
Fasting insulin, μ IU/ml	14.92 ± 9.96	9.25 ± 7.90	**<0.01***
HOMA-IR	3.98(1.4-7.9)	1.91(0.74-4.84)	**<0.01***
Total cholesterol, mg/dl	179.63 ± 26.62	151.46 ± 26.74	**<0.01***
Triglyceride, mg/dl	109.75 ± 54.92	78.82 ± 32.55	**<0.01***
LDL-C, mg/dl	99.45 ± 26.60	84.72 ± 23.51	**<0.01***
FSH, m IU/ml	5.39 ± 1.82	5.88 ± 1.76	>0.05
LH, m IU/ml	5.79 ± 1.94	5.76 ± 2.44	>0.05
Estradiol, pg/ml	43.44 ± 22.32	72.43 ± 38.00	**<0.01***
Free testosterone,pg/m	2.81 ± 1.02	1.44 ± 0.62	**<0.01***
17-OHprogesterone, ng/ml	1.41 ± 0.55	0.90 ± 0.64	**<0.01***
DHEAS, μq/dl	275.65 ± 115.45	195.67 ± 92.75	**<0.01***
CIMT, mm	0.51 ± 0.052	0.42 ± 0.043	**<0.01***
Copeptin, pmol/L	12.61 ± 3.05	9.60 ± 2.80	**<0.01***

*p <0.05 was accepted as statistically significant.
BMI body mass index, *HOMA-IR* homeostasis model assessment insulin resistance index, *HDL-C* high density lipoprotein cholesterol, *LDL-C* LOW density lipoprotein cholesterol, *hs-CRP* high-sensitive C- reactive protein, *TSH* thyroid stimulating hormone, *FSH* follicle-stimulating hormone, *LH* luteinizing hormone, *DHEAS* dehydroepiandrosterone sulfate, *CIMT* carotid intima media thickness.

The patient and control group examined separately and the correlations between copeptin and cardiometabolic parameters were not different for healthy and PCOS group.

Discussion

The present study confirms that serum levels of copeptin are increased in patients with PCOS, and, for the first time to our knowledge, demonstrates that elevated circulating serum levels of copeptin may provide important prognostic information in patients with PCOS. Copeptin showed significant correlations with cardiometabolic parameters in dependent of age and obesity.

PCOS women represent an intriguing biological model illustrating the relationship between hormonal pattern and cardiovascular risk profile, presenting a cluster of cardiovascular features, such as obesity, insulin resistance, hypertension, impaired cardiopulmonary functional capacity, autonomic dysfunction and low-grade chronic inflammation [18]. In recent substudy of the Women's Ischemia Evaluation Study (WISE) [15] shown that women with PCOS have a larger number of cardiovascular events. In this study, CVD was positively correlated with

Table 2 Correlation of age and body mass index adjusted copeptin levels with cardio-metabolic and endocrinologic parameters

Variable	r	P
Waist/hip ratio	0.11	0.253
Fasting glucose	0.10	0.533
Fasting insulin	0.41	**<0.001***
HOMA	0.47	**<0.01***
TC	-0.06	0.368
TG	0.01	0.470
HDL-C	-0.35	**<0.01***
LDL-C	0.10	0.290
hsCRP	0.04	0.422
CIMT	0.86	**<0.001***
Cortisol	-0.06	0.384
Estradiol	-0.24	**0.02***
17 OH-progesterone	0.15	0.181
ACTH	-0.02	0.457
Free testosterone	0.25	**0.02***
DHEA	0.06	0.359
FG score	0.38	**<0.001***

*p <0.05 was accepted as statistically significant.
ACTH: adrenocorticotropic hormone, CIMT: carotid intima-media thickness, CRP: C-reactive protein, DHEA: dehydroepiandrosterone, FG score: Ferriman–Gallwey score, HDL-C: high-density lipoprotein cholesterol, HOMA: homeostasis model assessment, LDL-C: low-density lipoprotein cholesterol, R: Pearson linear correlation coefficient.

Table 3 Correlation of carotid intima media thickness with cardiometabolic parameters

Variable	R	P
Waist/hip ratio	0.18	0.141
Fasting glucose	0.02	0.450
Fasting insulin	0.28	**0.02***
HOMA	0.29	**0.02***
TG	0.31	**0.01***
TC	0.11	0.254
HDL-C	-0.35	*0.013**
LDL-C	0.08	0.327
hsCRP	0.3	**<0.01***
Free testeron	0.28	**0.03***
Copeptin	0.39	**<0.001***
FG score	0.26	**0.04***

*p <0.05 was accepted as statistically significant.
CIMT: carotid intima-media thickness, hsCRP: high sensitivity C-reactive protein, FG score: Ferriman–Gallwey score, HDL-C: high-density lipoprotein cholesterol, HOMA: homeostasis model assessment, LDL-C: low-density lipoprotein cholesterol, R: Pearson linear correlation coefficient.

free testosterone. In addition, the event free survival (including fatal and non fatal events) was significantly lower in PCOS compared with non-PCOS women. In our study cardiometabolic parameters including HOMA-IR, TG, LDL-C, free testosterone, DHEAS, CIMT were significantly higher in PCOS patients and positively correlated with copeptin levels. Also, FG that reflects androgen effects was positively correlated with copeptin and CIMT.

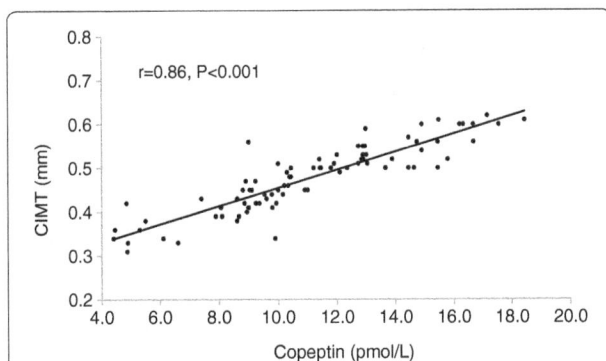

Figure 1 Linear correlation between copeptin and carotis intima media thickness (CIMT).

Orio F jr et al. [19] examined women with PCOS have significantly elevated PAI-1 activity independent of obesity. In Victor et al. [20] study an association was found between insulin resistance and an impaired endothelial and mitochondrial oxidative metabolism. They concluded that the inflammatory state related to insulin resistance in PCOS affects endothelial function. In presented study hsCRP and insulin resistance were found positive correlated with CIMT consistent with this hypothesis.

Copeptin, the C-terminal portion of provasopressin, is a glycosylated polypeptide comprising 39 amino acids and harboring a leucine-rich core segment [21]. It is a neurohormon (NH) of the AVP system [22] that is co-secreted with AVP from hypothalamus. It has also been termed AVP-associated glycopeptide, and was initially described by Holwerda in 1972 [21,23]. However, copeptin has recently come into clinical practice, and has been regarded as a novel NH. Recent studies showed that copeptin was elevated in acute myocardial infarction (AMI) and resulted in better diagnostic performance when assessed in combination with cardiac troponin, particularly during the first hour after onset of symptoms [24-26]. A negative test for both copeptin and troponin resulted in a remarkably high negative predictive value, that was helpful for a rapid rule out of AMI [24]. Furthermore, copeptin seems to have prognostic implications in patients with severe disorders such as severe congestive heart failure and patients with cardiac failure after AMI [27,28]. In patients with stable angina pectoris, copeptin showed a higher prognostic power regarding the endpoints death, stroke, or myocardial infarction than troponin [29]. Previous studies have shown that copeptin is not only a marker of cardiovascular diseases, but of other conditions as well. Potential links of copeptin with DM, metabolic syndrome (MetS) and microalbuminuria have drawn particular interest in the recent years. The AVP system has also been suggested to contribute to insulin resistance and DM potentially through a variety of mechanisms including stimulation of glucagon and ACTH secretion and glycogenolysis, etc. [30]. Therefore, copeptin, as a surrogate marker of this system, might also be associated with disrupted glucose homeostasis: a recent study demonstrated that increased copeptin levels were found to be associated with prevalent DM at baseline (p = 0.04) and insulin resistance (p < 0.001) in a large population of 4742 subjects (cross-sectionally) [30]. Consistent with this, copeptin was also reported to have a cross-sectional association with MetS in a large population of subjects [31]. In summary, based on the recent studies [30-32], copeptin may also be regarded as a promising marker of cardiometabolic risk (beyond established predictors of future cardiometabolic disease including fasting glucose, etc.) may serve as an additional guide in the early identification and management of subjects at risk for these conditions. However, in PCOS patients copeptin level has not been evaluated, yet. In our study we evaluated copeptin level in PCOS patients and we observed PCOS patients had higher copeptin levels. Additionally, we obtained positive correlation between copeptin and CIMT.

Copeptin may have a predictive role for detecting cardiometabolic risk in potential diseases. Therefore copeptin seems to be a marker that will enable the detection of cardiac injury in advancing age PCOS patients at an early stage. Copeptin appeared to have an important role in metabolic response and subsequent development of atherosclerosis in insulin resistant, hyperandrogenemic PCOS patients.

Competing interests
The authors declare that they have no competing interests.

Authors' contributions
BK: have made contributions to conception and design, acquisition of data, and analysis and interpretation of data. MO: have made contributions to conception and design, acquisition of data, and analysis and interpretation of data MK, OT: have made contributions to conception and design , acquisition of data, and analysis and interpretation of data. EC, NCB, MSA: have made contributions to acquisition of data. TD: have made contributions to conception, design and interpretation of data. All authors read and approved the final manuscript.

Author details
[1]Department of Endocrinology and Metabolic Diseases, Gaziantep Dr. Ersin Arslan Hospital, Milli Egemenlik bulvarı, Sanlılar Apt, no:51 daire:9 Şehitkamil/ Gaziantep, Gaziantep, Turkey. [2]Department of Endocrinology and Metabolic Diseases, Dışkapı Yıldırım Beyazıt Teaching and Research hospital, Ankara, Turkey. [3]Department of Endocrinology and Metabolic Diseases, Amasya Sabuncuoglu Serefettin Training and Research Hospital, Amasya, Turkey.

References
1. Norman RJ, Dewailly D, Legro RS, Hickey TE: Polycystic ovary syndrome. *Lancet* 2007, **370**:685–697.
2. Pasquali R, Gambineri A, Pagotto U: The impact of obesity on reproduction in women with polycystic ovary syndrome. *BJOG* 2006, **113**:1148–1159.
3. Orio F Jr, Palomba S, Spinelli L, Cascella T, Tauchmanova L, Zullo F, Lombardi G, Colao A: The cardiovascular risk of young women with polycystic ovary syndrome: an observational, analytical, prospective case –control study. *J Clin Endocrinol Metab* 2004, **89**:3696–3701.
4. Kelly CC, Lyall H, Petrie JR, Gould GW, Connell JM, Sattar N: Low grade chronic inflammation in women with polycystic ovarian syndrome. *J Clin Endocrinol Metab* 2001, **86**:2453–2455.
5. Kelly CJ, Speirs A, Gould GW, Petrie JR, Lyall H, Connell JM: Altered vascular function in young women with polycystic ovary syndrome. *J Clin Endocrinol Metab* 2002, **87**:742–746.
6. Escobar-Morreale HF, Luque-Ramirez M, San Millan JL: The molecular-genetic basis of functional hyperandrogenism and the polycystic ovary syndrome. *Endocr Rev* 2005, **26**:251–282.
7. Legro RS: Polycystic ovary syndrome and cardiovascular disease: a premature association? *Endocr Rev* 2003, **24**:302–312.
8. Whitton PD, Rodrigues LM, Hems DA: Stimulation by vasopressin, angiotensin and oxytocin of gluconeogenesis in hepatocyte suspensions. *Biochem J* 1978, **176**:893–898.
9. Keppens S, de Wulf H: The nature of the hepatic receptors involved in vaso-pressin-induced glycogenolysis. *Biochim Biophys Acta* 1979, **588**:63–69.
10. Abu-Basha EA, Yibchok-Anun S, Hsu WH: Glucose dependency of arginine vaso-pressin-induced insulin and glucagon release from the perfused rat pancreas. *Metabolism* 2002, **51**:1184–1190.
11. Holmes CL, Landry DW, Granton JT: Science review: vasopressin and the cardio-vascular system part 1—receptor physiology. *Crit care* 2003, **7**:427–434.
12. Morgenthaler NG, Struck J, Alonso C, Bergmann A: Assay for the measurement of copeptin, a stable peptide derived from the precursor of vasopressin. *Clin Chem* 2006, **52**:112–119.
13. Rotterdam ESHRE/ASRM-Sponsored PCOS Consensus Workshop Group: Revised 2003 consensus on diagnostic criteria and long-term health risks related to polycystic ovary syndrome. *Fertil Steril* 2004, **81**:19–25.
14. Ferriman D, Gallwey JD: Clinical assessment of body hair growth in women. *J Clin Endocrinol Metab* 1961, **21**:1440–1447.
15. Kilic T, Ural E, Oner G, Sahin T, Kilic M, Yavuz S, Kanko M, Kahraman G, Bildirici U, Berki KT, Ural D: [Which cut-off value of high sensitivity C-reactive protein is more valuable for determining long- term prognosis in patients with acute coronary syndrome?]. *Anadolu K Ardiyol Derg* 2009, **9**:280–289.
16. Matthews DR, Hosker JP, Rudenski AS, Naylor BA, Treacher DF, Turner RC: Homeostasis model assessment: insulin resistance and beta-cell function from fasting plasma glucose and insulin concentrations in man. *Diabetologia* 1985, **28**:412–419.
17. Gokcel A, Ozsahin AK, Sezgin N, Karakose H, Ertorer ME, Akbaba M, Baklaci N, Sengul A, Guvener N: High prevalence of diabetes in Adana, a southern province of Turkey. *Diabetes Care* 2003, **26**:3031–3034.
18. Giallauria F, Orio F, Palomba S, Lombardi G, Colao A, Vigorito C: Cardiovascular risk in women with polycystic ovary syndrome. *J Cardiovasc Med (Hagerstown)* 2008, **9**:987–992.
19. Orio F Jr, Palomba S, Cascella T, Tauchmanovà L, Nardo LG, Di Biase S, Labella D, Russo T, Savastano S, Tolino A, Zullo F, Colao A, Lombardi G: Is plasminogen activator inhibitor-1 a cardiovascular risk factor in young women with polycystic ovary syndrome? *Reprod Biomed Online* 2004, **9**:505–510.
20. Victor VM, Rocha M, Banuls C, Alvarez A, de Pablo C, Sanchez-Serrano M, Gomez M, Hernandez-Mijares A: Induction of oxidative stress and human leukocyte/endothelial cell interactions in polycystic ovary syndrome patients with insulin resistance. *J Clin Endocrinol Metab* 2011, **96**:3115–3122.
21. Morgenthaler NG, Struck J, Jochberger S, Dünser MW: Copeptin: clinical use of a new biomarker. *Trends Endocrinol Metab* 2008, **19**:43–49.
22. Voors AA, von Haehling S, Anker SD, Hillege HL, Struck J, Hartmann O, Bergmann A, Squire I, van Veldhuisen DJ, Dickstein K, OPTIMAAL Investigators: C-terminal provasopressin (copeptin) is a strong prognostic marker in

patients with heart failure after an acute myocardial infarction: results from the OPTIMAAL study. *Eur Heart J* 2009, **30**:1187–1194.

23. Holwerda DA: A glycope ptide from the posterior lobe of pig pituitaries. I. Isolation and characterization. *Eur J Biochem* 1972, **28**:334–339.

24. Reichlin T, Hochholzer W, Stelzig C, Laule K, Freidank H, Morgenthaler NG, Bergmann A, Potocki M, Noveanu M, Breidthardt T, Christ A, Boldanova T, Merki R, Schaub N, Bingisser R, Christ M, Mueller C: Incremental value of copeptin for rapid rule out of acute myocardial infarction. *J Am Coll Cardiol* 2009, **54**:60–68.

25. Keller T, Tzikas S, Zeller T, Czyz E, Lillpopp L, Ojeda FM, Roth A, Bickel C, Baldus S, Sinning CR, Wild PS, Lubos E, Peetz D, Kunde J, Hartmann O, Bergmann A, Post F, Lackner KJ, Genth-Zotz S, Nicaud V, Tiret L, Münzel TF, Blankenberg S: Copeptin improves early diagnosis of acute myocardial infarction. *J Am Coll Cardiol* 2010, **55**:2096–2106.

26. Gu YL, Voors AA, Zijlstra F, Hillege HL, Struck J, Masson S, Vago T, Anker SD, van den Heuvel AF, van Veldhuisen DJ, de Smet BJ: Comparison of temporal release pattern of copeptin with conventional biomarkers in acute myocardial infarction. *Clin Res Cardiol* 2011, **100**:1069–1076.

27. Stoiser B, Mörtl D, Hülsmann M, Berger R, Struck J, Morgenthaler NG, Bergmann A, Pacher R: Copeptin, a frag-ment of the vasopressin precursor, as a novel predictor of out-come in heart failure. *Eur J Clin Invest* 2006, **36**:771–778.

28. Khan SQ, Dhillon OS, O'Brien RJ, Struck J, Quinn PA, Morgenthaler NG, Squire IB, Davies JE, Bergmann A, Ng LL: C-terminal pro-vasopressin (copeptin) as a novel and prognostic marker in acute myocardial infarction: leicester acute myocardial infarction peptide (LAMP) study. *Circulation* 2007, **115**:2103–2110.

29. Von Haehling S, Papassotiriou J, Morgenthaler NG, Hartmann O, Doehner W, Stellos K, Wurster T, Schuster A, Nagel E, Gawaz M, Bigalke B: Copeptin as a prognostic factor for major adverse cardiovascular events in patients with coronary artery disease. *Int J Cardiol* 2012, **162**:27–32.

30. Enhörning S, Wang TJ, Nilsson PM, Almgren P, Hedblad B, Berglund G, Struck J, Morgenthaler NG, Bergmann A, Lindholm E, Groop L, Lyssenko V, Orho-Melander M, Newton-Cheh C, Melander O: Plasma copeptin and the risk of diabetes mellitus. *Circulation* 2010, **121**:2102–2108.

31. Enhörning S, Struck J, Wirfält E, Hedb lad B, Morgenthaler NG, Melander O: Plasma copeptin, a unifying factor behind the metabolic syndrome. *J Clin Endocrinol Metab* 2011, **96**:1065–1072.

32. Enhörning S, Bankir L, Bouby N, Struck J, Hedblad B, Persson M, Morgenthaler NG, Nilsson PM, Melander O: Copeptin, a marker of vasopre ssin, in abdominal obesity, diabetes and microalbuminuria: the prospective malmö diet and cancer study cardiovascular cohort. *Int J Obes (Lond)* 2013, **37**:598–603.

25

Epicardial adipose tissue thickness and NGAL levels in women with polycystic ovary syndrome

Serap Baydur Sahin[1,5*], Medine Cumhur Cure[2], Yavuz Ugurlu[3], Elif Ergul[3], Emine Uslu Gur[4], Nese Alyildiz[4] and Mehmet Bostan[3]

Abstract

Background: Polycystic ovary syndrome (PCOS) is associated with an increased cardiovascular disease (CVD) risk and early atherosclerosis. Epicardial adipose tissue thickness (EATT) is clinically related to subclinical atherosclerosis. In the present study, considering the major role of neutrophil gelatinase-associated lipocalin (NGAL) which is an acute phase protein rapidly releasing upon inflammation and tissue injury, we aimed to evaluate NGAL levels and EATT in PCOS patients and assess their relationship with cardiometabolic factors.

Methods: 64 patients with PCOS and 50 age- and body mass index-matched healthy controls were included in the study. We evaluated anthropometric, hormonal and metabolic parameters. EATT was measured by echocardiography above the free wall of the right ventricle. Serum NGAL and high-sensitive C- reactive protein (hsCRP) levels were measured by ELISA.

Results: Mean EATT was 0,38 +/-0,16 mm in the PCOS group and 0,34 +/-0,36 mm in the control group (p = 0,144). In the obese PCOS group (n = 44) EAT was thicker compared to the obese control group (n = 41) (p = 0.026). Mean NGAL levels of the patients with PCOS were 101,98 +/-21,53 pg/ml, while mean NGAL levels were 107,40 +/-26,44 pg/ml in the control group (p = 0,228). We found a significant positive correlation between EATT and age, BMI, waist circumference, fasting insulin, HOMA-IR, triglyceride and hsCRP levels in PCOS group.

Conclusions: Thickness of the epicardial adipose tissue can be used to follow the risk of CVD development in obese PCOS cases. However serum NGAL levels do not differ in patients with PCOS and control group.

Keywords: Polycystic ovary syndrome, Epicardial adipose tissue thickness, NGAL

Introduction

Polycystic ovary syndrome (PCOS) is a common endocrine disorder that affects about 5-10% of women of reproductive age and characterized by hyperandrogenism, menstrual disturbance, chronic anovulation and infertility [1]. PCOS is frequently associated with multiple risk factors for coronary heart disease (CHD), including insulin resistance (IR), dyslipidemia, visceral obesity and hypertension [2,3]. It is reported to be associated with elevation of various markers of endothelial inflammation and abnormal endothelial function which plays a critical role in cardiovascular disease and in particular in the development and progression of atherosclerosis [4].

Neutrophil gelatinase-associated lipocalin (NGAL), also known as lipocalin-2 is an acute phase protein, that is rapidly released from neutrophils upon inflammation and tissue injury [5]. Additionally, it has been found to be expressed in several types of cells, including kidney tubular cells, adipocytes, macrophages, brain endothelial cells and hepatocytes [6,7]. NGAL has been implicated in some pathophysiological processes, including apoptosis, iron transport, inflammation, cell survival, tumorigenesis, and atherosclerosis [6,7]. Evidence suggests that NGAL plays an important role in systemic insulin sensitivity and glucose homeostasis [8,9]. In a recent study, NGAL was determined to reflect the degree of inflammatory process in coronary artery disease [10].

* Correspondence: serapbaydur@gmail.com
[1]Department of Endocrinology and Metabolism Disease, Recep Tayyip Erdogan University Medical School, Rize, Turkey
[5]Department of Endocrinology and Metabolism Disease, Recep Tayyip Erdogan University Training and Research Hospital, 53020 Rize, Turkey
Full list of author information is available at the end of the article

Epicardial adipose tissue is true visceral fat deposited around the heart, between the myocardium and visceral epicard [11]. It mediates atherosclerosis via expression of several bioactive molecules [12] and has been reported to reflect the intraabdominal visceral fat [13]. Epicardial adipose tissue thickness (EATT) has been demonstrated to correlate with the severity of coronary artery disease (CAD) and the extent of coronary artery atherosclerosis [14-16].

In this study, our aim was to measure NGAL levels and EATT in women with PCOS and compare them with those of age and body mass index (BMI)-matched controls and to evaluate their relationship with cardio-metabolic factors.

Materials and methods
Study population
This study included 66 patients with PCOS and age- body mass index (BMI) matched 50 healthy controls. Women were all of the same ethnicity. All the patients gave a written consent. This study was approved by the Institutional Ethical Committee of the institution in which this study was conducted. All the patients were nonsmokers.

The diagnosis of PCOS was made according to the Rotterdam European Society for Human reproduction and Embryology/American Society for Reproductive Medicine– sponsored PCOS Consensus Workshop Group [17]. The revised diagnostic criteria of PCOS is as follows, with at least two of the following being required: i) Oligo and/or anovulation that is menstrual disturbance, ii) Clinical and/or biochemical signs of hyperandrogenism, iii) Polycystic ovarian appearance on ultrasound examination. Clinical hirsutism was defined by a modified Ferriman-Gallwey score of more than eight.

Patients and healthy subjects who had smoking history, diabetes mellitus, thyroid disorders, hyperprolactinemia, non-classical congenital adrenal hyperplasia (NCAH), androgen-secreting tumours, Cushing syndrome (1 mg dexamethasone suppression test), infection diseases, hypertension, hepatic or renal dysfunction were excluded from the study. The other exclusion criteria were; drug use within 3 months such as oral contraceptive agents, antilipidemic and hypertensive drugs, and insulin-sensitizing drugs. For the exclusion of NCAH, we measured 17OH-progesterone levels in the all patients. The patients who had basal 17OH-progesterone levels >4 ng/ml were diagnosed as NCAH. We performed ACTH stimulation test in patients who had >2 ng/ml 17-OHP levels. The diagnosis of NCAH was considered in patients with the poststimulation 17-OHP level exceed 10 ng/ml. These patients were not included in the study. We selected healthy volunteers from the subjects working at our hospital and students in our medical school and nursing school. Control group (n = 50) consisted of healthy patients who had hirsutism score <8, regular menses, every 21–35 days and normal androgen levels None of the women in the control group had polycystic ovary in ultrasound.

Clinical, biochemical and hormonal measurements
Weight, height, waist circumference and systolic and diastolic blood pressure (BP) were measured. The BMI was calculated by dividing the body weight in kilograms by the square of the height in meters (kg/m^2). Waist circumference was measured at the narrowest level between the costal margin and iliac crest. The BMI, waist circumference and hirsutism scores were assessed by a single investigator for all of the subjects.

Venous blood samples were obtained from all subjects following an 8–12 h overnight fast in the follicular phase of a spontaneous or progesterone induced menstrual cycle. The levels of fasting glucose, insulin, total cholesterol, triglyceride (TG), high-density lipoprotein cholesterol (HDL-cholesterol), low-density lipoprotein cholesterol (LDL-cholesterol) and high-sensitive C-reactive protein (hs-CRP) were measured. All the patients underwent a 75 gr oral glucose tolerance test (OGTT). An insulin resistance score Homeostasis Model Assessment-Insulin resistance (HOMA-IR) was computed by the following formula [18]: HOMA-IR = fasting plasma glucose (mmol/L) × fasting serum insulin (mU/mL)/22.5. The cut off value was taken 2.7 for HOMA-IR [19].

The hexokinase method was used to measure glucose levels, and photometric method (Abbott Architect c16000 otoanalyzer) was used to measure the total cholesterol, triglyceride (TG), high-density lipoprotein cholesterol (HDL-cholesterol), and low-density lipoprotein cholesterol (LDL-cholesterol) levels. Insulin was measured using CMIA (Chemiluminescent microparticle immunoassay) (Abbott, Architect system, USA). The concentration of high-sensitive C- reactive protein (hsCRP) was measured using immunotubidimetric method with Abbott Architect C16000 otoanalyzer (Abbott Diagnostic, USA). The cut off for hsCRP was taken <0.5 mg/dl.

Serum levels of insulin, follicle-stimulating hormone (FSH), luteinizing hormone (LH), prolactin, dehydroepiandrosterone sulfate (DHEAS), total testosterone, insulin and thyroid stimulating hormone (TSH) were measured using chemiluminescent microparticle enzyme immunoassay (CMIA) method with Abbott Architect i2000 (Abbott Diagnostic, USA). Serum 17 hydroxyprogesterone and free testosterone were measured by radioimmunoassay.

Measurement of NGAL
The serum levels of NGAL were measured using enzyme-linked immunosorbent assay (ELISA) method. We used commercially available human NGAL ELISA kit (MyBiosource, USA). The procedure for the ELISA method was according to the instructions provided by the manufacturer. Absorbance was measured at a wavelength of 450 ηm using

ELISA reader. The levels of NGAL are presented as ng/ml. The intra-assay and inter-assay coefficient of variation were 4.1% and 3.9%, respectively. The limit of detection (LOD) for the NGAL assay was <10 pg/ml.

Measurement of epicardial adipose tissue thickness

All patients underwent 2D Doppler echocardiography with a Philips IE-33 system and S5-1 transducer (1e5 mHz, Philips, Bothell, WA, USA). The epicardial fat thickness (EFT) was identified as the echo-free space between the outer wall of the myocardium and the visceral layer of the pericardium, and its thickness was measured perpendicularly on the free wall of the right ventricle at end-systole in three cardiac cycles. Parasternal long- and short-axis views were used. The average value of three cardiac cycles from each echocardiographic view was considered [20,21]. All the measurements were done by the same cardiologist.

Statistical analysis

Data were analyzed using SPSS Software (Version 17, SPSS, Inc., Chicago, IL, USA). Results were expressed as mean ± standard deviation. The Mann–Whitney U test was used to compare the continuous variables and the Chi-square test was used to compare categorical variables. Spearman's rank correlation test was used for calculation of associations between variables. A p value of less than 0.05 was considered to be statistically significant.

Results

We enrolled 66 patients with PCOS (mean age; 23,29 ±5,05 years, BMI; 32,09 ±9,80 kg/m^2) and 50 age and BMI matched healthy control group (mean age; 22,02 ±5,05 years, BMI; 29,80 ±5,5 kg/m^2) in the current study. The clinical and biochemical results of the study population are shown in Table 1.

Fasting plasma glucose, hsCRP, triglyceride, total and LDL cholesterol levels were significantly higher in women with PCOS (Table 1).

Mean EATT was 0,38 ±0,16 mm in the PCOS group and 0,34 ±0,36 mm in the control group (p = 0,144). Although EATT was higher in PCOS patients, the difference did not reach statistical significance. We found a significant correlation between EATT and age, BMI, waist circumference, fasting insulin, HOMA-IR, triglyceride and hsCRP in the patients with PCOS (Table 2). In the control group, EATT was also associated with.

Mean NGAL levels of the patients with PCOS were 101,98 ±21,53 pg/ml, while mean NGAL levels were 107,40 ±26,44 pg/ml in the control group (p = 0,228). Serum NGAL levels were not correlated with the metabolic parameters in both of the groups (Table 3).

The patients with PCOS were divided into 2 groups according to the HOMA-IR levels. The cut-off point was 2.7 [22]. 28 PCOS patients had an HOMA-IR greater

Table 1 The clinical, biochemical and hormonal results in women with polycystic ovary syndrome (PCOS) patients and healthy controls

Parameter	PCOS group (n = 66)	Control group (n = 50)	p
Age (years)	23.29 ±5.05	22.02 ±5.05	0.183
BMI (kg/m2)	32.09 ±9.80	29.80 ±5.5	0.148
Waist circumference (cm)	8.67 ±19.37	92.28 ±13.30	0.048
Systolic blood pressure (mmHg)	126.77 ±14.15	113.22 ±9.99	0.0001
Diastolic blood pressure (mmHg)	76.18 ±11.37	68.20 ±6.74	0.0001
Fasting insulin (μIU/ml)	11.16 ±6.58	9.47 ±6.06	0.160
Fasting glucose (mg/dl)	97.30 ±13.97	89.10 ±10.56	0.001
HOMA-IR	2.71 ±1.7	2.16 ± 1.5	0.072
Total cholesterol (mg/dl)	194.81 ±39.55	173.28 ±29.99	0,002
Triglyceride (mg/dl)	115.91 ±58.18	93.30 ±39.30	0.020
HDL-C (mg/dl)	49.61 ±11.09	47.08 ±10.30	0.213
LDL-C (mg/dl)	122.83 ±34.43	107.0 ±24.64	0.007
hsCRP (mg/dl)	0.54 ±0.95	0.19 ±0.31	0.015
TSH (μIU/ml)	2.11 ±1.47	2.58 ±3.24	0.295
Prolactin (ng/ml)	18.3 ± 15.4	17.4 ± 6.9	0.590
Total testosterone (ng/ml)	0.85 ± 0.3	0.56 ± 0.1	0.0001
FSH (mIU/ml)	4.5 ± 1.2	4.5 ± 0.7	0.950
LH (mIU/ml)	5.7 ± 2.7	3.5 ± 0.5	0.0001
Estradiol (pg/ml)	43.9 ± 33.3	41.02 ± 3.1	0.536
DHEAS (μg/dl)	266.3 ± 123	203.85 ± 40.3	0.0001
Free testosterone (pg/ml)	3,3 ± 2.3	2.3 ± 0.4	0.008
EATT (mm)	0.38 ±0.16	0.34 ±0.36	0.144
NGAL (pg/ml)	101.98 ±21.53	107.40 ±26.44	0.228

Values are expressed as means ± SD. BMI body mass index, HOMA-IR homeostasis model assessment insulin resistance index, HDL-C high density lipoprotein cholesterol, LDL-C low density lipoprotein cholesterol, hs-CRP high-sensitive C- reactive protein, TSH thyroid stimulating hormone, FSH follicle-stimulating hormone, LH luteinizing hormone, DHEAS dehydroepiandrosterone sulfat, EATT epicardial adipose tissue thickness, NGAL neutrophil gelatinase-associated lipocalin.

than 2.7, while 38 patients had an HOMA-IR lower than 2.7. EATT and hsCRP levels were higher in the insulin resistant group, however NGAL levels were similar in both of the groups (Table 4). The insulin resistant control group (n = 14) had also higher hsCRP levels, but EATT was similar.

When we evaluate the PCOS patients according to the hsCRP values, 16 patients had hsCRP values higher than 0.5 mg/L and EATT was found to be higher in this subgroup (p = 0.007). In the control group, 4 patients had hsCRP levels ≥ 0.5 mg/L and EATT was similar in the PCOS and control group. NGAL levels did not differ in both of the groups according to hsCRP levels.

When we divide the PCOS patients according to BMI, 21 patients had BMI < 25 kg/m^2. We compared the lean and obese patients with PCOS and found that NGAL and

Table 2 The correlation between epicardial adipose tissue thickness and metabolic parameters in patients with PCOS and control group

Parameter	PCOS group (n = 66)		Control group (n = 50)	
	r	p value	r	p value
Age	0,248	0,045[*]	0,231	0,106
BMI	0,641	0,0001[**]	0,314	0,027[*]
WC	0,563	0,0001[**]	0,258	0,070
FG score	0,061	0,626		
Fasting glucose	0,072	0,565	0,137	0,342
Fasting insulin	0,472	0,0001[**]	0,088	0,545
HOMA-IR	0,641	0,0001[**]	0,300	0,034[*]
Total cholesterol	0,216	0,081	0,299	0,035[*]
Triglyceride	0,363	0,003[**]	0,382	0,006[**]
LDL cholesterol	0,213	0,085	0,274	0,054
HDL cholesterol	−0,200	0,108	−0,243	0,093
hsCRP	0,324	0,008[**]	0,096	0,507
NGAL	0,086	0,494	−0,051	0,727
TSH	−0,110	0,377	0,010	0,946
Estradiol	0,026	0,834	0,029	0,846
LH/FSH	−0,367	0,068		
DHEAS	−0,133	0,286	−0,011	0,939
Total testosterone	0,185	0,137	0,078	0,596

r indicates Spearman's rho correlation coefficient; *Correlation is significant at the 0.05 level. **Correlation is significant at the 0.01 level. a log transformed. BMI body mass index, HOMA-IR homeostasis model assessment insulin resistance index, HDL-C high density lipoprotein cholesterol, LDL-C low density lipoprotein cholesterol, hs-CRP high-sensitive C- reactive protein, NGAL neutrophil gelatinase-associated lipocalin, TSH thyroid stimulating hormone, FSH follicle-stimulating hormone, LH luteinizing hormone, DHEAS dehydroepiandrosterone sulfat.

Table 3 The correlation between NGAL levels and metabolic parameters in patients with PCOS

Parameter	r	p value
Age	0,042	0,738
BMI	0,149	0,235
WC	0,148	0,239
FG score	0,051	0,684
Fasting glucose	0,088	0,487
Fasting insulin	−0,109	0,880
HOMA-IR	0,031	0,808
Total cholesterol	0,013	0,917
Triglyceride	0,037	0,772
LDL cholesterol	0,019	0,882
HDL cholesterol	−0,081	0,523
hsCRP	0,064	0,612
EATT	0,086	0,494
TSH	0,176	0,162
Estradiol	−0,001	0,993
LH/FSH	−0,089	0,702
DHEAS	0,216	0,085
Total testosteron	−0,043	0,733

r indicates Spearman's rho correlation coefficient. BMI body mass index, HOMA-IR homeostasis model assessment insulin resistance index, HDL-C high density lipoprotein cholesterol, LDL-C low density lipoprotein cholesterol, hs-CRP high-sensitive C- reactive protein, EATT epicardial adipose tissue thickness, TSH thyroid stimulating hormone, FSH follicle-stimulating hormone, LH luteinizing hormone, DHEAS dehydroepiandrosterone sulfat.

hsCRP levels were similar in both of the groups. However HOMA-IR and EATT was higher in the obese patients (p = 0.001, p = 0.007). In the control group, 41 patients had BMI > 25 kg/m^2 and EATT, serum NGAL and hsCRP levels did not differ in the obese and healthy subjects (p = 0.902, p = 0.057, p = 0.342). When we compared the obese PCOS (n = 44) and obese control group (n = 41), EAT was thicker in the PCOS group (p = 0.026), however NGAL levels did not differ (Table 5).

Discussion

Our study shows that epicardial adipose tissue thickness is higher in obese PCOS patients compared with obese control subjects, however NGAL levels are similar in both of the groups. We demonstrated that EATT was positively correlated with age, BMI, waist circumference, fasting insulin, HOMA-IR, triglyceride and hsCRP levels. Therefore, EATT can be used to follow the risk of CVD development in obese PCOS cases.

Women with PCOS have multiple risk factors for cardiovascular disease (CVD) and is considered as a major long-term health risk. The risk factors for premature atherosclerosis and CVD, such as increased central adiposity, elevated blood pressure, higher total and LDL cholesterol levels, higher triglyceride levels, and higher plasma glucose levels were more prevalent in our PCOS population, compared with matched-for-age and BMI control women, as have been shown in previous studies [23,24]. These metabolic risk factors may predict the development of atherosclerosis in women with PCOS.

Although an increase in mortality due to coronary artery disease in patients with PCOS was not shown in the long term follow up [2], there is strong evidence that women with PCOS are at increased risk of metabolic cardiovascular syndrome [25]. In a study, coronary artery calcification was evaluated in younger women with PCOS 30–45 years as a measure of subclinical atherosclerotic disease burden, and it was found to be more prevalent in PCOS women [3]. In the other study, postmenopausal women noted 2.5 higher odds of obstructive coronary artery disease for those with clinical features of PCOS, even when controlling for metabolic and common cardiac risk factors [26].

Highly sensitive C-reactive protein (hsCRP) levels are good predictors of subclinical atherosclerosis and vascular

Table 4 The comparison of PCOS and control group according to HOMA-IR levels

Variable	HOMA-IR ≥ 2.7 PCOS group (n = 28)	HOMA-IR < 2.7 PCOS group (n = 38)	p	HOMA-IR ≥ 2.7 Control group (n = 14)	HOMA-IR < 2.7 Control group (n = 36)	p
EATT (mm)	0.44 ± 1.1	0.34 ± 1.4	0.019	0.35 ± 0.16	0.33 ± 0.12	0.592
NGAL (pg/ml)	100.4 ± 23.2	103.1 ± 20.3	0.610	113.5 ± 21.4	105 ± 28.1	0.310
hsCRP (mg/dl)	0.89 ± 1.1	0.27 ± 0.6	0.009	0.38 ± 0.5	0.11 ± 0.14	0.004
BMI (kg/m2)	37.5 ± 10.3	28.1 ± 7.3	0.0001	34.06 ± 5.5	28.1 ± 4.6	0.0001

Values are expressed as means ± SD.

events [22]. Many studies have also shown high hsCRP levels in women with PCOS [22,27] in contrast to others that say it is related only to obesity [28]. In our study, serum hsCRP levels were significantly higher in women with PCOS than the controls and it was correlated with BMI, EATT and decreased insulin sensitivity. Kim et al. have reported higher hsCRP levels even in lean PCOS women [22]. In our study, hsCRP levels did not differ in lean PCOS and lean control subjects.

NGAL is highly expressed in adipocytes, that its expression is regulated by obesity, and that it induces insulin resistance [8]. Studies investigating the relationship between NGAL levels and PCOS found confusing results. Cakal E et al. demonstrated that NGAL levels were higher in PCOS patients and was related with insulin resistance [29]. However, in the other study, NGAL levels were found to be lower in PCOS patients [30]. In our study, NGAL levels were similar in PCOS patients and healthy subjects. NGAL measurements also did not differ in groups based on the HOMA-IR and hsCRP levels and BMI.

In the recent studies it was found that serum levels of NGAL were significantly elevated in patients with angiographically confirmed CAD compared to those with normal arteries or controls [10,31,32]. The authors explain that these diffrences can result because of the expression of NGAL from vascular cells during atherogenesis. In our study, NGAL levels did not correlate with the cardiometabolic risk factors.

Epicardial adipose tissue thickness is clinically related to abdominal visceral adiposity which has significant impact on cardiovascular diasease risk [13]. In recent

studies, EATT was found to be associated with coronary heart diseases [14-16].

There are only few studies evaluating the EATT in PCOS patients and in both of the studies EAT was thicker in the PCOS patients [33,34]. In our study, EAT was thicker in the PCOS group, but the difference was not significant. EATT was associated with the cardiometabolic risk factors, such as HOMA-IR and triglyceride in PCOS and control group. EATT was also associated with hsCRP in the PCOS patients, while it was not in the control group. When we compared the PCOS and control group according to HOMA-IR, hsCRP levels and BMI, we showed that EAT was thicker in the PCOS group who were obese and had higher HOMA-IR and hsCRP levels. However we did not demonstrate such a relationship in the control group. Additionally, in obese PCOS patients EATT was higher compared to obese healthy subjects. All obese subjects, whether PCOS or controls had similar EATT compared to the lean subjects. Therefore, we suggest that obesity does not solely influence EATT.

In conclusion, measurement of epicardial adipose tissue thickness is a non-invasive tool and easy to perform and appears to be a good method to follow the risk of cardiovascular disease development in obese and insulin resistant PCOS patients.

Competing interests
The authors declare that they have no competing interests.

Authors' contributions
SBS, MCC and MB conceived the study and participated in its design. YU and EE performed the ultrasound examinations. SBS, EUG, NA and MB participated in the analysis and interpretation of data. SBS, NA and EUG collected the data. SBS, MCC, YU, EE, EUG, NA and MB wrote the paper. All authors read and approved the final manuscript.

Author details
[1]Department of Endocrinology and Metabolism Disease, Recep Tayyip Erdogan University Medical School, Rize, Turkey. [2]Department of Biochemistry, Recep Tayyip Erdogan University Medical School, Rize, Turkey. [3]Department of Cardiology, Recep Tayyip Erdogan University Medical School, Rize, Turkey. [4]Department of Internal Medicine, Recep Tayyip Erdogan University Medical School, Rize, Turkey. [5]Department of Endocrinology and Metabolism Disease, Recep Tayyip Erdogan University Training and Research Hospital, 53020 Rize, Turkey.

Table 5 The comparison of obese PCOS and control subjects

	Obese PCOS group (n = 44)	Obese control group (n = 41)	p
EATT (mm)	0.42 ± 0.1	0.34 ± 0.1	0.026
NGAL (pg/ml)	104.2 ± 22.9	110.7 ± 27.1	0.235
HOMA-IR	3.1 ± 1.7	2.4 ± 1.5	0.045
hsCRP (mg/dl)	0.62 ± 0.9	0.21 ± 0.33	0.012

Values are expressed as means ± SD.

References

1. Azziz R, Woods KS, Reyna R, Key TJ, Knochenhauer ES, Yildiz BO: **The prevalence and features of the polycystic ovary syndrome in an unselected population.** *J Clin Endocrinol Metab* 2004, **89**(6):2745–2749.
2. Wild S, Pierpoint T, McKeigue P, Jacobs H: **Cardiovascular disease in women with polycystic ovary syndrome at long-term follow-up: a retrospective cohort study.** *Clin Endocrinol (Oxf)* 2000, **52**(5):595–600.
3. Christian RC, Dumesic DA, Behrenbeck T, Oberg AL, Sheedy PF 2nd, Fitzpatrick LA: **Prevalence and predictors of coronary artery calcification in women with polycystic ovary syndrome.** *J Clin Endocrinol Metab* 2003, **88**(6):2562–2568.
4. Ross R: **Atherosclerosis–an inflammatory disease.** *N Engl J Med* 1999, **340**(2):115–126.
5. Schmidt-Ott KM, Mori K, Li JY, Kalandadze A, Cohen DJ, Devarajan P, et al: **Dual action of neutrophil gelatinase-associated lipocalin.** *J Am Soc Nephrol* 2007, **18**(2):407–413.
6. Chen X, Jia X, Qiao J, Guan Y, Kang J: **Adipokines in reproductive function: a link between obesity and polycystic ovary syndrome.** *Mol Endocrinol* 2013, **50**(2):R21–R37.
7. Zhang J, Wu Y, Zhang Y, Leroith D, Bernlohr DA, Chen X: **The role of lipocalin 2 in the regulation of inflammation in adipocytes and macrophages.** *Mol Endocrinol* 2008, **22**(6):1416–1426.
8. Yan QW, Yang Q, Mody N, Graham TE, Hsu CH, Xu Z, et al: **The adipokine lipocalin 2 is regulated by obesity and promotes insulin resistance.** *Diabetes* 2007, **56**(10):2533–2540.
9. Wang Y, Lam KS, Kraegen EW, Sweeney G, Zhang J, Tso AW, et al: **Lipocalin-2 is an inflammatory marker closely associated with obesity, insulin resistance, and hyperglycemia in humans.** *Clin Chem* 2007, **53**(1):34–41.
10. Kafkas N, Demponeras C, Zoubouloglou F, Spanou L, Babalis D, Makris K: **Serum levels of gelatinase associated lipocalin as indicator of the inflammatory status in coronary artery disease.** *Int J Inflam* 2012, **2012**:189797.
11. Iacobellis G, Corradi D, Sharma AM: **Epicardial adipose tissue: anatomic, biomolecular and clinical relationships with the heart.** *Nat Clin Pract Cardiovasc Med* 2005, **2**(10):536–543.
12. Baker AR, Silva NF, Quinn DW, Harte AL, Pagano D, Bonser RS, et al: **Human epicardial adipose tissue expresses a pathogenic profile of adipocytokines in patients with cardiovascular disease.** *Cardiovasc Diabetol* 2006, **5**:1.
13. Iacobellis G, Assael F, Ribaudo MC, Zappaterreno A, Alessi G, Di Mario U, et al: **Epicardial fat from echocardiography: a new method for visceral adipose tissue prediction.** *Obes Res* 2003, **11**(2):304–310.
14. Ahn SG, Lim HS, Joe DY, Kang SJ, Choi BJ, Choi SY, et al: **Relationship of epicardial adipose tissue by echocardiography to coronary artery disease.** *Heart* 2008, **94**(3):e7.
15. Eroglu S, Sade LE, Yildirir A, Bal U, Ozbicer S, Ozgul AS, et al: **Epicardial adipose tissue thickness by echocardiography is a marker for the presence and severity of coronary artery disease.** *Nutr Metab Cardiovasc Dis* 2009, **19**(3):211–217.
16. Djaberi R, Schuijf JD, van Werkhoven JM, Nucifora G, Jukema JW, Bax JJ: **Relation of epicardial adipose tissue to coronary atherosclerosis.** *Am J Cardiol* 2008, **102**(12):1602–1607.
17. Rotterdam ESHRE/ASRM-Sponsored PCOS Consensus Workshop Group: **Revised 2003 consensus on diagnostic criteria and long-term health risks related to polycystic ovary syndrome.** *Fertil Steril* 2004, **81**:19–25.
18. Matthews DR, Hosker JP, Rudenski AS, Naylor BA, Treacher DF, Turner RC: **Homeostasis model assessment: insulin resistance and beta-cell function from fasting plasma glucose and insulin concentrations in man.** *Diabetologia* 1985, **28**:412–419.
19. Gokcel A, Ozsahin AK, Sezgin N, et al: **High prevalence of diabetes in Adana, a southern province of Turkey.** *Diabetes Care* 2003, **26**:3031–3034.
20. Iacobellis G, Willens HJ, Barbaro G, Sharma AM: **Threshold values of high-risk echocardiographic epicardial Fat thickness.** *Obesity (Silver Spring)* 2008, **16**(4):887–892.
21. Mariani S, Fiore D, Barbaro G, Basciani S, Saponara M, D'Arcangelo E, et al: **Association of epicardial fat thickness with the severity of obstructive sleep apnea in obese patients.** *Int J Cardiol* 2013, **167**(5):2244–2249.
22. Kim JW, Han JE, Kim YS, Won HJ, Yoon TK, Lee WS: **High sensitivity C-reactive protein and its relationship with impaired glucose regulation in lean patients with polycystic ovary syndrome.** *Gynecol Endocrinol* 2012, **28**(4):259–263.
23. Talbott E, Guzick D, Clerici A, Berga S, Detre K, Weimer K, et al: **Coronary heart disease risk factors in women with polycystic ovary syndrome.** *Arterioscler Thromb Vasc Biol* 1995, **15**(7):821–826.
24. Graf M, Richards C, Brown V, Meissner L, Dunaif A: **The independent effects of hyperandrogenaemia, hyperinsulinaemia and obesity on lipid and lipoprotein profiles in women.** *Clin Endocrinol (Oxf)* 1990, **33**(1):119–131.
25. Talbott EO, Zborowski JV, Rager JR, Boudreaux MY, Edmundowicz DA, Guzick DS: **Evidence for an association between metabolic cardiovascular syndrome and coronary and aortic calcification among women with polycystic ovary syndrome.** *J Clin Endocrinol Metab* 2004, **89**:5454–5461.
26. Shaw LJ, Bairey Merz CN, Azziz R, Stanczyk FZ, Sopko G, Braunstein GD, et al: **Postmenopausal women with a history of irregular menses and elevated androgen measurements at high risk for worsening cardiovascular event-free survival: results from the national institutes of health–national heart, lung, and blood institute sponsored Women's ischemia syndrome evaluatio.** *J Clin Endocrinol Metab* 2008, **93**(4):1276–1284.
27. Talbott EO, Zborowski JV, Boudreaux MY, McHugh-Pemu KP, Sutton-Tyrrell K, Guzick DS: **The relationship between C-reactive protein and carotid intima-media wall thickness in middle-aged women with polycystic ovary syndrome.** *J Clin Endocrinol Metab* 2004, **89**(12):6061–6067.
28. Ketel IJ, Stehouwer CD, Henry RM, Serné EH, Hompes P, Homburg R, et al: **Greater arterial stiffness in polycystic ovary syndrome (PCOS) is an obesity–but not a PCOS-associated phenomenon.** *J Clin Endocrinol Metab* 2010, **95**(10):4566–4575.
29. Cakal E, Ozkaya M, Engin-Ustun Y, Ustun Y: **Serum lipocalin-2 as an insulin resistance marker in patients with polycystic ovary syndrome.** *J Endocrinol Invest* 2011, **34**(2):97–100.
30. Diamanti-Kandarakis E, Livadas S, Kandarakis SA, Margeli A, Papassotiriou I: **Serum concentrations of atherogenic proteins neutrophil gelatinase-associated lipocalin and its complex with matrix metalloproteinase-9 are significantly lower in women with polycystic ovary syndrome: hint of a protective mechanism?** *Eur J Endocrinol* 2008, **158**(4):525–531.
31. Choi KM, Lee JS, Kim EJ, Baik SH, Seo HS, Choi DS, et al: **Implication of lipocalin-2 and visfatin levels in patients with coronary heart disease.** *Eur J Endocrinol* 2008, **158**(2):203–207.
32. Zografos T, Haliassos A, Korovesis S, Giazitzoglou E, Voridis E, Katritsis D: **Association of neutrophil gelatinase-associated lipocalin with the severity of coronary artery disease.** *Am J Cardiol* 2009, **104**(7):917–920.
33. Aydogdu A, Uckaya G, Tasci I, Baysan O, Tapan S, Bugan B, et al: **The relationship of epicardial adipose tissue thickness to clinical and biochemical features in women with polycystic ovary syndrome.** *Endocr J* 2012, **59**(6):509–516.
34. Cakir E, Doğan M, Topaloglu O, Ozbek M, Cakal E, Vural MG, et al: **Subclinical atherosclerosis and hyperandrogenemia are independent risk factors for increased epicardial fat thickness in patients with PCOS and idiopathic hirsutism.** *Atherosclerosis* 2013, **226**(1):291–295.

Permissions

List of Contributors

Saira Saeed Mirza
Department of Epidemiology, University of Rotterdam, Rotterdam, The Netherlands

Kashif Shafique
Institute of Health and Wellbeing, University of Glasgow, 1-Lilybank Gardens, G12 8RZ Glasgow, UK
School of Public Health, Dow University of Health Sciences, Karachi, Pakistan

Abdul Rauf Shaikh
Department of Community Medicine, Dow University of Health Sciences, Karachi, Pakistan

Naveed Ali Khan
Department of Surgery, Dow University of Health Sciences, Karachi, Pakistan

Masood Anwar Qureshi
Institute of Basic Medical Sciences, Dow University of Health Sciences, Karachi, Pakistan

Maryamosadat Miri
Exercise Physiology, Jahrom University of Medical Sciences, Jahrom, Fars, Iran

Hojatolah Karimi Jashni
Department of Anatomy, Jahrom University of Medical Sciences, Jahrom, Iran

Farzaneh Alipour
Student Research Committee, Jahrom University of Medical Sciences, Jahrom, Fars, Iran

Toshifumi Takahashi, Hideki Igarashi, Shuichiro Hara, Mitsuyoshi Amita, Koki Matsuo, Ayumi Hasegawa and Hirohisa Kurachi
Department of Obstetrics and Gynecology, Yamagata University Faculty of Medicine, Yamagata 990-9585, Japan

Ming-Wei Lin
Institute of Public Health, National Yang-Ming University, Taipei, Taiwan

Mei-Feng Huang and Meng-Hsing Wu
Departments of Physiology, National Cheng Kung University College of Medicine, Tainan, Taiwan
Departments of Obstetrics and Gynecology, National Cheng Kung University College of Medicine and Hospital, 138 Sheng-Li Road, 70428 Tainan, Taiwan

Marie Louise Wissing, Thomas Høst and Anne Lis Mikkelsen
Department of Gynecology-Obstetrics, Holbaek Fertility Clinic, Holbaek Hospital, Smedelundsgade 60, 4300 Holbaek, Denmark

Si Brask Sonne
Institute of Biology, University of Copenhagen, 2100 Copenhagen, Denmark

David Westergaard and Kirstine Belling
Department of Systems Biology, Center for Biological Sequence Analysis, Technical University of Denmark, Kemitorvet building 208, 2800 Lyngby, Denmark

Kho do Nguyen
DTU Multi Assay Core, Technical University of Denmark DTU, 2800 Lyngby, Denmark

Jie Chen and Yong Tan
First Clinical Medicine College, Nanjing University of Chinese Medicine, Nanjing 210046, China

Jie Chen, Dong Xia, Yanjie Xia, Hongwei Wang, Long Yi, Qian Gao and Yong Wang
State Key Laboratory of Chemistry for Life Science and Jiangsu Key Laboratory of Molecular Medicine, Medical School of Nanjing University, Nanjing 210093, China

Shanmei Shen
Divisions of Endocrinology, the Affiliated Drum Tower Hospital, Medical School, Nanjing University, Nanjing 210093, China

Yunxia Cao
Department of Obstetrics and Gynecology, Anhui Medical University, Hefei 230022, China

Wenjun Wang
Centre of Reproduction, Department of Obstetric and Gynaecology, Memorial Hospital of Sun Yat-Sen University, Guangzhou 510120, China

Xiaoke Wu
Department of Obstetrics and Gynecology, the First Affiliated Hospital, Heilongjiang University of Chinese Medicine, Harbin 150040, China

Dessie Salilew-Wondim, Dawit Tesfaye, Karl Schellander and Michael Hoelker
Institute of Animal Science, Animal Breeding and Husbandry Group, University of Bonn, Endenicher Allee 15, Bonn 53115, Germany

Qi Wang and Benjamin K Tsang
Reproductive Biology Unit and Division of Reproductive Medicine, Department of Obstetrics & Gynecology and Cellular & Molecular Medicine, Interdisciplinary School of Health Sciences, University of Ottawa, Ottawa K1H 8L6, ON, Canada

Qi Wang and Benjamin K Tsang
Chronic Disease Program, Ottawa Hospital Research Institute, The Ottawa Hospital (General Campus), Critical Care Wing, 3rd Floor, Room W3107, 501 Smyth Road, Ottawa K1H 8L6, ON, Canada

Md Munir Hossain
Department of Animal Breeding and Genetics, Bangladesh Agricultural University, Mymensingh 2202, Bangladesh

Benjamin K Tsang
Department of Agricultural Biotechnology, World Class University Major in Biomodulation, College of Agriculture and Life Sciences, Seoul National University, Seoul 151-921, South Korea

Shigang Zhao, Ye Tian and Zi-Jiang Chen
Shanghai Key Laboratory for Assisted Reproduction and Reproductive Genetics, Center for Reproductive Medicine, Renji Hospital, School of Medicine, Shanghai Jiaotong University, Shanghai 200135, China

Shigang Zhao, Xiuye Xing, Tao Li, Hongbin Liu, Tao Huang, Yunna Ning, Han Zhao and Zi-Jiang Chen
Center for Reproductive Medicine, Provincial Hospital Affiliated to Shandong University, Jinan, China

National Research Center for Assisted Reproductive Technology and Reproductive Genetics, Jinan, China
The Key laboratory for Reproductive Endocrinology of Ministry of Education, Jinan, China
Shandong Provincial Key Laboratory of Reproductive Medicine, Jinan 250021, China

Wei Zhang
Department of joint and bone oncology, Provincial Hospital Affiliated to Shandong University, Jinan 250021, China

Mojca Jensterle, Tomaz Kocjan and Andrej Janez
Department of Endocrinology, Diabetes and Metabolic Diseases, University Medical Centre Ljubljana, Zaloska 7, SI-1000 Ljubljana, Slovenia

Vesna Salamun and Eda Vrtacnik Bokal
Department of Obstetrics and Gynecology, Reproductive Unit, University Medical Centre Ljubljana, Zaloska 7, 1525 Ljubljana, Slovenia

Vitaly A. Kushnir, David F. Albertini and Norbert Gleicher
Center for Human Reproduction, 21 East 69th Street, New York, NY 10021, USA

Vitaly A. Kushnir
Wake Forest School of Medicine, Winston-Salem, NC, USA

Noy Halevy
Sackler School of Medicine, Tel Aviv University, Tel Aviv, Israel

David H. Barad and Norbert Gleicher
Foundation for Reproductive Medicine, New York, NY, USA

David F. Albertini
University of Kansas, Lawrence, KS, USA

Norbert Gleicher
Rockefeller University, New York, NY, USA

Irene Tessaro, Silvia C. Modina, Federica Franciosi, Giulia Sivelli, Laura Terzaghi, Valentina Lodde and Alberto M. Luciano
Reproductive and Developmental Biology Laboratory, Department of Health, Animal Science and Food Safety, Università degli Studi di Milano, Via Celoria 10, Milan 20133, Italy

Silvia C. Modina and Alberto M. Luciano
Interdepartmental Research Centre for the Study of Biological Effects of Nano-concentrations (CREBION), Università degli Studi di Milano, Via Celoria 10, Milan 20133, Italy

Dilek Arpaci
Division of Endocrinology and Metabolism, Department of Internal Medicine, Faculty of Medicine, Bulent Ecevit University, Zonguldak, Turkey

Aysel Gurkan Tocoglu, Hasan Ergenc and Ali Tamer
Department of Internal Medicine, Faculty of Medicine, Sakarya University Training and Research Hospital, Sakarya, Turkey

Sabiye Yilmaz, Nurgul Keser and Huseyin Gunduz
Department of Cardiology, Sakarya University Training and Research Hospital, Sakarya, Turkey

Fakhroddin Mesbah, Mohsen Moslem, Zahra Vojdani and Hossein Mirkhani
Department of Anatomical Sciences, Shiraz University of Medical Sciences, Shiraz 71348-53185, Iran

Fakhroddin Mesbah and Zahra Vojdani
Embryonic Stem Cell Lab, Shiraz University of Medical Sciences, Shiraz, Iran

Hossein Mirkhani
Department of Pharmacology, School of Medicine, Shiraz University of Medical Sciences, Shiraz, Iran
Medicinal and Natural Products Chemistry Research Center, Shiraz University of Medical Sciences, Shiraz, Iran

Wenyan Xi, Hui Mao, Xiuhua Zhao, Ming Liu and Shengyu Fu
Department of Obstetrics and Gynaecology, The Second Affiliated Hospital of Xi'an Jiaotong University, No. 157, Xiwu Road, Xi'an City 710004 Shaanxi Prov., China

Yongkang Yang
Department of Obstetrics and Gynaecology, The Second Affiliated Hospital of Shaanxi University of Chinese Medicine, Xianyang City 712000 Shaanxi Prov., China

A Veiga-Lopez, J Moeller and V Padmanabhan
Department of Pediatrics, University of Michigan, 7641A Med Sci II, Ann Arbor, MI 48109-5622, USA

A Veiga-Lopez
Department of Animal Science, Michigan State University, East Lansing, MI 48824, USA

D. H. Abbott
Department of Obstetrics and Gynecology and Wisconsin National Primate Research Center, University of Wisconsin, Madison, WI 53715, USA

Pan Dou, Qing Xue and Yang Xu
Department of Clinical Nutrition, Peking University First Hospital, Beijing, China

Huiyan Ju, Jing Shang, Qing Xue and Yang Xu
Center of Reproduction and Genetics, Peking University First Hospital, Beijing, China

Xueying Li
Department of Biostatistics, Peking University First Hospital, Beijing, China

Xiaohui Guo
Department of Endocrinology, Peking University First Hospital, Beijing, China
No.7, Xishiku Road, Xicheng District, Beijing 100034, People's Republic of China

Minghui Chen, Yanwen Xu, Benyu Miao, Lu Luo and Canquan Zhou
Reproductive Medicine Center, The First Affiliated Hospital of Sun Yat-sen University, 58 2nd Zhongshan Road, Guangzhou GD510080, People's Republic of China

Minghui Chen, Yanwen Xu, Benyu Miao, Lu Luo and Canquan Zhou
Guangdong Provincial Key Laboratory of Reproductive Medicine, The First Affiliated Hospital of Sun Yat-sen University, 58 2nd Zhongshan Road, Guangzhou GD510080, People's Republic of China

Huijuan Shi
Department of Pathology, The First Affiliated Hospital of Sun Yat-sen University, 58 2nd Zhongshan Road, Guangzhou GD510080, People's Republic of China

Hui Zhao
Department of Hepatic Surgery, The Third Affiliated Hospital of Sun Yat-sen University, 600 Tianhe Road, Guangzhou GD510630, People's Republic of China

Sarwat Jahan, Faryal Munir, Suhail Razak, Anam Mehboob, Qurat Ul Ain and Hizb Ullah
Reproductive Physiology Laboratory, Department Of Animal Sciences, Quaid-i-Azam University, Islamabad, Pakistan

Suhail Razak and Ali Almajwal
Department of Community Health Sciences, College of Applied Medical Sciences, King Saud University, Riyadh, Saudi Arabia

Tayyaba Afsar
Department of Biochemistry, Quaid-i-Azam University, Islamabad, Pakistan

Weixi Xiong, Ying Lin, Lili Xu, Amin Tamadon and Yi Feng
Department of Integrative Medicine and Neurobiology, State Key Lab of Medical Neurobiology, School of Basic Medical Sciences, Shanghai Medical College; Institute of Acupuncture Research (WHO collaborating center for traditional medicine) and Institute of Brain Science, Brain Science Collaborative Innovation Center, Fudan University, Shanghai 200032, China

Weixi Xiong, Ying Lin and Lili Xu
Grade 2008 Clinical Medicine, Shanghai Medicine School, Fudan University, Shanghai 200032, China

Weixi Xiong
Department of Neurology, West China Hospital of Sichuan University, Chengdu, Sichuan 610041, China

Ying Lin
Department of Medical Oncology, Fudan University Shanghai Cancer Center, Shanghai 200032, China

Lili Xu
Department of Cardiology, Zhongshan Hospital, Fudan University, Shanghai 200032, China

Shien Zou, Fubo Tian and Xin Li
Department of Gynecology, Obstetrics and Gynecology Hospital, Fudan University, Shanghai 200011, China

Ruijin Shao
Institute of Neuroscience and Physiology, Department of Physiology, Sahlgrenska Academy, University of Gothenburg, Gothenburg 40530, Sweden

Eser Sefik Ozyurek and Gokhan Artar
Bagcilar Research and Training Hospital Obgyn Department, Merkez Mh., Mimar Sinan Caddesi, 6 Sokak, 34100 Bagcilar, Istanbul, Turkey

Tevfik Yoldemir
Marmara University Teaching and Research Hospital Obgyn Department, Fevzicakmak District Muhsin Yazicioglu Street 10 Ustkaynarca Pendik, Istanbul, Turkey

Ricardo Santos Simões, José Maria Soares-Jr, Manuel J. Simões, Maria Cândida P. Baracat, Gustavo Arantes R. Maciel, Paulo C. Serafini and Edmund C. Baracat
Disciplina de Ginecologia, Departamento de Obstetrícia e Ginecologia, Hospital das Clínicas, Faculdade de Medicina da Universidade de São Paulo, São Paulo, Brazil

Helena B. Nader
Department of Molecular Biology, Federal University of São Paulo, São Paulo, Brazil

Ricardo Azziz
Departments of Obstetrics and Gynecology and of Medicine, Medical College of Georgia, Augusta University, Augusta, GA, USA

José Maria Soares-Jr
Av. Dr. Enéas de Carvalho Aguiar, 255 - 10o.andar - Sala 10.167 - 05403-900,São Paulo, SP, Brazil

Asad Ullah, Sarwat Jahan, Suhail Razak, Madeeha Pirzada, Hizb Ullah and Naveed Rauf
Department of Animal Sciences, Quaid-i-Azam University, Islamabad, Pakistan

Suhail Razak and Ali Almajwal
Department of Community Health Sciences, College of Applied Medical Sciences, King Saud University, Riyadh, Saudi Arabia

Tayyaba Afsar
Department of biochemistry, Quaid-i-Azam University, Islamabad, Pakistan

Vineet Kumar Maurya, Chadchan Sangappa, Vijay Kumar, Sahil Mahfooz, Archana Singh and Rajesh Kumar Jha
Division of Endocrinology, Life Science North 111B/101, CSIR-Central Drug Research Institute, B.S. 10/1, Sector-10, Jankipuram Extension, Sitapur Road, Lucknow 226031, India

Singh Rajender
Division of Endocrinology, Life Science South, CSIR-Central Drug Research Institute, B.S. 10/1, Sector-10, Jankipuram Extension, Sitapur Road, Lucknow 226031, India

Basak Karbek
Department of Endocrinology and Metabolic Diseases, Gaziantep Dr. Ersin Arslan Hospital, Milli Egemenlik bulvarı, Sanlılar Apt, no:51 daire:9 Şehitkamil/ Gaziantep, Gaziantep, Turkey

Mustafa Ozbek, Melia Karakose, Oya Topaloglu, Nujen Colak Bozkurt, Muyesser Sayki Aslan and Tuncay Delibasi
Department of Endocrinology and Metabolic Diseases, Dışkapı Yıldırım Beyazıt Teaching and Research hospital, Ankara,Turkey

Evrim Cakır
Department of Endocrinology and Metabolic Diseases, Amasya Sabuncuoglu Serefettin Training and Research Hospital, Amasya, Turkey

Serap Baydur Sahin
Department of Endocrinology and Metabolism Disease, Recep Tayyip Erdogan University Medical School, Rize, Turkey

Medine Cumhur Cure
Department of Biochemistry, Recep Tayyip Erdogan University Medical School, Rize, Turkey

Yavuz Ugurlu, Elif Ergul and Mehmet Bostan
Department of Cardiology, Recep Tayyip Erdogan University Medical School, Rize, Turkey

Emine Uslu Gur and Nese Alyildiz
Department of Internal Medicine, Recep Tayyip Erdogan University Medical School, Rize, Turkey

Serap Baydur Sahin
Department of Endocrinology and Metabolism Disease, Recep Tayyip Erdogan University Training and Research Hospital, 53020 Rize, Turkey

Index